Diabetes Mellitus in Children and Adolescents

Luther B. Travis, M.D., F.A.A.P.

Professor of Pediatrics
Director of Divisions of Nephrology and Diabetes
Director, Children's Diabetes Management Center
University of Texas Medical Branch
Galveston, Texas

Ben H. Brouhard, M.D., F.A.A.P.

Professor of Pediatrics
Associate Director, Divisions of Nephrology and Diabetes
Associate Director, Children's Diabetes Management Center
University of Texas Medical Branch
Galveston, Texas

Barbara-Jo Schreiner, R.N., M.N.

Diabetes Nurse Specialist
Assistant Director, Children's Diabetes Management Center
University of Texas Medical Branch
Galveston, Texas

Volume 29 in the Series
MAJOR PROBLEMS IN CLINICAL PEDIATRICS

Milton Markowitz, *Consulting Editor*

1987   **W.B. SAUNDERS COMPANY**
Philadelphia   London   Toronto   Mexico City   Rio de Janeiro   Sydney   T

*This book is dedicated to
our children—
may God bless you all!*

Contributors

William R. Allen, M.D.
Associate Professor of Pediatrics, Texas A & M School of Medicine and Scott and White Clinic, Temple, Texas
(Chapter 20)

Michael J. Bourgeois, M.D.
Assistant Professor of Pediatrics, Division of Endocrinology, Texas Tech University School of Medicine, Lubbock, Texas
(Chapter 18)

Ben H. Brouhard, M.D.
Professor of Pediatrics; Associate Director, Divisions of Nephrology and Diabetes; Associate Director, Children's Diabetes Management Center, University of Texas Medical Branch, Galveston, Texas
(Chapters 1, 2, 5, 13, 22, 24)

Mary C. Cerreto, Ph.D.
Formerly Associate Professor of Pediatrics; Chief, Division of Child Psychology, University of Texas Medical Branch, Galveston, Texas
(Chapter 9)

Eileen N. Ellis, M.D.
Assistant Professor of Pediatrics, Division of Nephrology, University of Arkansas Medical School, Little Rock, Arkansas
(Chapter 17)

Jordan W. Finkelstein, M.D.
Professor of Pediatrics; Associate Professor of Psychiatry and Behavioral Sciences; Director, Division of Adolescent Medicine, University of Texas Medical Branch, Galveston, Texas
(Chapter 16)

Shaye Guidos Henderson, R.N., M.Ed.
Pediatric Diabetes Health Educator, Children's Diabetes Management Center, University of Texas Medical Branch, Galveston, Texas
(Appendix)

Terry A. Johnson, R.N., M.N.
Diabetes Nurse Specialist, Children's Diabetes Management Center, University of Texas Medical Branch, Galveston, Texas
(Chapter 6)

Alok Kalia, M.D.
Assistant Professor of Pediatrics, Division of Nephrology, University of Texas Medical Branch, Galveston, Texas
(Chapter 12)

Paula McMahon, R.D.
Dietitian and Nutrition Consultant, Children's Diabetes Management Center, University of Texas Medical Branch, Galveston, Texas
(Chapter 7)

Arlan L. Rosenbloom, M.D.
Professor of Pediatrics; Director, Diabetes Research, Education, and Treatment Center, University of Florida School of Medicine, Gainesville, Florida
(Chapter 25)

Barbara-Jo Schreiner, R.N., M.N.
Diabetes Nurse Specialist; Assistant Director, Children's Diabetes Management Center, University of Texas Medical Branch, Galveston, Texas
(Chapters 10, 15, 19, 21, Appendix)

Luther B. Travis, M.D.
Professor of Pediatrics; Director, Divisions of Nephrology and Diabetes; Director, Children's Diabetes Management Center, University of Texas Medical Branch, Galveston, Texas
(Chapters 3, 4, 6–8, 11, 12, 14, 15, 18–20, 23)

Foreword

The changes in how children with diabetes are managed since the time I completed my pediatric training in 1949 have been quite remarkable. At that time, and through all of the 1960s and much of the 1970s, discussions about childhood diabetes care were still dominated by the perennial arguments between advocates of permissive and rigid treatments. Many of us favored the former and, all too often, control of hyperglycemia was on a trial and error basis and far from satisfactory. This hit or miss approach is no longer acceptable now that it is generally agreed that there is an association between hyperglycemia and vascular disease. The trend toward tighter control led to the development of a number of a new techniques that have made it possible to monitor blood glucose more closely and to provide other information on how well the patient is being controlled.

The senior author of this monograph, Dr. Luther B. Travis, has treated children with diabetes throughout this period of change. He graduated from the Medical College of Georgia in 1955, completed his pediatric training at Baylor, and did a fellowship in metabolic and renal disease at the University of Texas Medical Branch in Galveston. He joined the faculty of that medical school in 1962, has been the Director of the Division of Pediatric Nephrology and Diabetes since 1972, and in 1973 was appointed Professor of Pediatrics. He is the author of nearly 100 articles and is known nationally for his work in nephrology as well as diabetes. He has contributed a great deal of time to the American Diabetes Association, and, in 1980, Dr. Travis received the Outstanding Service to Youth Award from that organization.

Dr. Ben H. Brouhard graduated from Indiana University School of Medicine in 1972 and received his pediatric training at Duke University. He began his association with Dr. Travis in 1974; starting as a Fellow, he moved up the academic ladder to full Professor in 1983. He is the author of 60 scientific publications. Barbara-Jo Schreiner is a Pediatric Clinical Nurse Specialist in Juvenile Diabetes. She received her Bachelor of Science degree from the College of Nursing, University of South Florida, Tampa, in 1975 and her Master of Nursing from the College of Nursing, University of Florida, Gainesville, in 1979. She joined Drs. Travis and Brouhard in 1982 and is a vital member of the diabetes team. She belongs to a number of professional societies and has been honored as one of the Outstanding Young Women of America. She holds the appointment of Clinical Instructor, School of Nursing, University of Texas Medical Branch, Galveston.

This is a book by clinicians who have personally treated hundreds of children with diabetes. While their orientation is clinical, it is based on sound scientific facts. The book contains practical advice and very specific details regarding management. Although the authors aim for tight control, their approach is not rigid and takes into consideration the individual needs of the child and the family. Considerable emphasis is placed on the developmental and behavioral aspects. The philosophy of the authors is that of trying to balance the medical needs and the lifestyles of the patients. Theirs is a very reasonable approach presented in a well written, easy to read text.

MILTON MARKOWITZ, M.D.

Preface

What is this? Another new book on diabetes? How many of these do we really need? Is this one any different from the others? For what purpose and to whom is this one directed?

We agree! The last few years have seen a large number of new and updated texts, and we've wondered about the desirability of yet another. This is the reason why one of us resisted the temptation for so long to write or edit another book on diabetes. But after a while, as the ego seems to override other considerations, we began to think about the prospect in more depth and to talk with various publishers. We (LBT, BHB) came to the conclusion that there might well be a need for another book on diabetes, and our perceptions were generally matched by most publishers, but our concepts as to the type of need differed. Most of the publishing companies either wanted a very traditional textbook or a cookbook of "how to," without even a hint of a biochemical-physiologic base. We felt that there was a middle ground (that is, a clinically oriented text with a scientific base). The people with whom we talked at W. B. Saunders agreed and have been supportive of this concept throughout. We hope that we've been able to find this middle ground and present it in this text.

The conceptual philosophy of this book might be summarized by the statement, "Diabetics are people first." Thus, we have tried to present our beliefs that diabetes care should be incorporated into the lifestyle of the individual and family, rather than the reverse. The authors realize that, at times, some degree of "tightness" of glucose control is probably lost, but in general, our experience of the last 25 years with well over a thousand families has reinforced this philosophic approach. And when one compares the mean, or range, of glycosylated hemoglobins from our clinic with those reported from clinics said to be more rigid in approach, they are identical.

To whom is this book directed? Certainly it is not directed to the academic diabetologist, for our omissions of certain basic information and our liberal use of other data will, undoubtedly, prove frustrating. It's directed to the clinician, whether physician, nurse, dietitian, health educator, physician assistant, or patient. It is hoped that all may benefit from our collective experience.

One of the worst fears one has about such a volume as this is that it will be out of date even before it's published. In an area such as diabetes, in which knowledge and application are changing so rapidly, this is always a concern, but the basic tenets around which this book is written will remain. Thus, we do not apologize for certain new items not mentioned. The reader will need to fill in the blanks wherever they exist.

It is difficult to comprehend, and even more to explain, the enormous changes that have occurred over the past 25 years in our understanding of insulin-dependent diabetes mellitus and in the translation of this understanding into day-to-day management. Only slightly more than a decade ago, almost 50 percent of insulin-dependent diabetics were treated with a single injection of insulin per day. Virtually everyone relied on semiquantitative urine glucose determinations and occasional blood sugar values to direct "the best" care possible. Complications were considered by most to be almost inevitable events, and there was little real hope that there was a "cure" in the immediate future. Additionally, care was directed almost solely by the physician with occasional assistance from a dietitian, and patient involvement in day-to-day decisions was popular in only a few centers.

How different today! Blood glucose monitoring at home, at work, or at play is now the rule for almost all insulin-requiring diabetics. We now have cumulative markers for precisely and objectively monitoring glucose control. Normalization of blood glucose, once a fantasy, is now a more realistic objective. Multiple-dose and continuous subcutaneous insulin therapies are now commonly used, even in the young. Diabetes care is delivered by multidisciplinary teams that incorporate the patient and family into the program. Complications are no longer considered inevitable. And there's more—with even more to come.

Newly diagnosed persons with insulin-dependent diabetes mellitus and their siblings are being screened for HLA-DR markers and islet-cell antibodies. Those with positive results are being considered for inclusion in research protocols dealing with immunosuppressive intervention. Over a half dozen centers have performed, in humans, either pancreas or islet-cell transplantation in highly selected persons. Several second-generation glucose monitors have memory banks for storing and accumulating results. New glucose sensors, not dependent on incorporation into the vascular system, are under development and, once available, will open the door to implantable closed-loop artificial beta cells. Meanwhile, we go along using purified insulins developed by the most sophisticated of synthetic or biosynthetic methodology that was unheard of a decade ago. Already there are plans for introducing nasal insulin, patch insulin, and oral insulins. And thoughts of the potential eradication of and cure for diabetes are in the minds of many.

All of these things are exciting for the future, and it is quite likely that standard therapy a decade from now will make our management of the 1980s archaic. This is our hope, but for now, we do the best we can with the tools we have available. It is to this end that this book is directed.

The authors would like to thank the copy editors at W. B. Saunders for their patience, as the date for publication got pushed further and further back by the tardiness of some of the manuscripts. Additional thanks go to Ms. Vi Quiroga, administrative assistant of the Children's Diabetes Management Center, who did most of the typing and who suffered with us through two "crashes" of the word processor. Thanks also go to the other members of our Team, who often worked so that we could write. But most of all, the three of us would like to thank our patients and their families for teaching us virtually all we know and for having patience with us when we were too dense to hear or learn.

LUTHER B. TRAVIS
BEN H. BROUHARD
BARBARA-JO SCHREINER

Contents

Classification

In an effort to bring some uniformity to diagnostic criteria for diabetes, an international group (National Diabetes Data Group, or NDDG) assembled in 1978 to gain consensus on classification criteria for the heterogenous group of metabolic disorders known as diabetes mellitus and to create a common nomenclature for the scientific community. The specific aims of the classification criteria were (1) to serve as a basis for planning and conducting research; (2) to serve as a framework for collecting epidemiologic data on etiology, natural history, and complications in various populations; and (3) to aid the clinician in categorizing patients with various degrees of glucose intolerance or ones with characteristics that placed them at increased risk for diabetes. The classification criteria that were developed were intended to have the following characteristics: (1) diagnostic classes defined as precisely as possible; (2) diagnostic classes that were mutually exclusive, even if a patient changed categories with time; (3) class assignment that required only clinical measurements; (4) terminology that described the phenotypic expression of the disease as much as possible; and (5) a classification that allowed incorporation of new research findings. The classification criteria, as currently published, identify five groups: diabetes mellitus, impaired glucose tolerance, gestational diabetes, previous glucose intolerance, and potential glucose intolerance.

PRIMARY DIABETES MELLITUS

Diabetes Mellitus

Under the heading of diabetes there are several subgroups (Table 1–1). The first of these is Type I diabetes, or insulin-dependent diabetes mellitus (IDDM). Affected dividuals are generally younger (hence the previous terminology of "juvenile-onset"), are insulinopenic, require injected insulin, and are prone to ketosis. This type is also associated with certain HLA types and immune responses and is the major form of the disease, which will be discussed throughout this book.

Patients with Type II diabetes, or noninsulin-dependent diabetes mellitus (NIDDM), are usually past 40 years of age, are not necessarily dependent on injected insulin, and are not prone to ketosis. These patients may have normal to low levels of plasma insulin or high plasma insulin concentrations with insulin resistance. Patients with this form of diabetes may be asymptomatic and show only slow progression of the disease. Inheritance patterns are important in both subgroups; however, obesity also seems to be a major epidemiologic factor in NIDDM. Other types of diabetes (Table 1–2) include those associated with pancreatic disease, hormonal abnormalities, certain drugs or chemicals (Table 1–3), insulin-re-

Table 1–1. CLASSIFICATION OF PRIMARY CARBOHYDRATE INTOLERANCE*

Diagnostic Class	Former Terminology
I. Diabetes Mellitus	
A. Insulin-dependent, Type I	Juvenile diabetes, juvenile-onset diabetes, JODM, brittle, childhood
B. Non–insulin-dependent, Type II	Adult-onset, AODM, stable, maturity-onset
1. Nonobese	
2. Obese	
C. Other types (Type III)	Secondary diabetes
II. Impaired Glucose Tolerance	
A. Nonobese	Asymptomatic diabetes, chemical diabetes, subclinical diabetes, borderline diabetes, latent diabetes
B. Obese	
C. Other types	
III. Gestational Diabetes	Gestational diabetes
IV. Previous Abnormalities of Glucose Tolerance	Latent diabetes, prediabetes
V. Potential Abnormality of Glucose Tolerance	Prediabetes, potential diabetes

*Modified from National Diabetes Data Group: Classification and diagnosis of diabetes and other categories of glucose intolerance. Diabetes 28:1039, 1979.

Table 1–2. CONDITIONS ASSOCIATED WITH DIABETES MELLITUS*

I. Pancreatic Disease
- Hereditary relapsing pancreatitis
- Cystic fibrosis
- Hemochromatosis
- Thalassemia
- α_1-Antitrypsin deficiency
- Trauma
- Infections
- Toxics
- Neoplasms

II. Hormonal Disorders
- Growth hormone deficiency
  - Type I
  - Type II
- Panhypopituitary dwarfism
- Laron dwarfism
- Pheochromocytoma
- Multiple endocrine adenomatosis
- Eosinophilic adenomas of the pituitary
- Cushing's disease
- Glucagon-secreting tumors

III. Inborn Errors of Metabolism
- Glycogen storage disease, Type I
- Acute intermittent porphyria
- Hyperlipidemias (Types III, IV, V)

IV. Genetic Disorders with Insulin Resistance
- Ataxia telangiectasia
- Myotonic dystrophy
- Lipoatrophic syndromes
- Leprechaunism
- Acanthosis nigricans
  - Type A
  - Type B
- Mendenhall's syndrome

V. Hereditary Neuromuscular Diseases
- Muscular dystrophy
- Late-onset proximal myopathy
- Huntington's chorea
- Machedo's disease
- Herrmann's syndrome
- Optic atrophy, diabetes mellitus, diabetes insipidus, neurosensory deafness syndrome
- Freidreich's ataxia
- Alstrom's syndrome
- Laurence-Moon-Biedl syndrome

VI. Progeroid Syndromes
- Cockayne's syndrome
- Werner's syndrome

VII. Obesity
- Prader-Willi syndrome
- Achondroplastic dwarfism

VIII. Cytogenetic Syndromes
- Trisomy 21 syndrome
- Klinefelter's syndrome
- Turner's syndrome

IX. Miscellaneous
- Steroid-induced ocular hypertension
- Epiphyseal dysplasia and infantile-onset diabetes mellitus
- Progressive cone dystrophy

*Modified from Rotter JI, Rimoin DL: Etiology. In Brownlee M (ed): *Handbook of Diabetes Mellitus*, Vol. 1. Garland STPM Press, New York, pp 3–93, 1981.

Table 1–3. DRUGS ASSOCIATED WITH ALTERED GLUCOSE TOLERANCE*

I. Diuretics Antihypertensives Chlorthalidone Clonidine Diazoxide Furosemide Metolazone	**IV. Catecholamines** Diphenylhydantoin Epinephrine Isoproterenol Levodopa Norepinephrine
II. Hormonally Active Agents Adrenocorticotropin Glucagon Glucocorticoids Oral contraceptives Somatotropin Thyroid hormones	**V. Analgesics** Indomethacin
III. Psychoactive Agents Chlorprothixene Haloperidol Lithium carbonate Phenothiazines Tricyclic antidepressants	**VI. Antineoplastic Agents** Alloxan L-Asparaginase Streptozocin **VII. Miscellaneous** Isoniazid Nicotinic acid

*Modified from National Diabetes Data Group: Classification and diagnosis of diabetes and other categories of glucose intolerance. Diabetes 28:1039, 1979.

This list is not all inclusive; certain drugs have not been listed because it is not clear if the hyperglycemic response reported represents solely a pharmacologic action or an interaction among several agents given simultaneously. Also, drugs were not listed for which the association is not clearly established.

ceptor abnormalities, and genetic syndromes (discussed further on).

Although an attempt has been made to avoid confusion, occasional misclassification may occur; for example, the distinction between a person with IDDM and a thin person with NIDDM who is receiving insulin may prove difficult. Furthermore, the early natural history of one type may mimic another (for example, the remissive phase of IDDM or the stress-related ketosis of NIDDM). Thus, if the stages are not viewed in the context of the whole but are examined as isolated events, an inappropriate assignment may result. Diagnostic criteria for children suspected of having diabetes differ only slightly from those of the adult and are covered in Chapter 3.

Impaired Glucose Tolerance (IGT)

This classification describes a group of patients who have either normal or mildly elevated fasting plasma glucose concentration (less than is required for a diagnosis of diabetes, or less than 140 mg/dl) and who during an oral glucose tolerance test have plasma glucose values that are between normal and diabetic values. Although these patients are clearly not diabetic, they are probably at higher risk than the general population for developing diabetes. It is estimated that up to 10 percent of such patients annually will proceed to overt diabetes. However, many with an initial abnormality will return to normal glucose tolerance spontaneously, and others will remain in this class. Thus, to avoid the potential stigma that the term "diabetes" might bring, modifiers such as "chemical," "borderline," "subclinical," "asymptomatic," and "latent" diabetes should be avoided in deference to "IGT." Since few children with the diagnosis of IGT appear to progress to symptomatic diabetes, repeated glucose tolerance testing seems neither necessary nor warranted, and the child may be monitored at home with blood or urine sugars. Rosenbloom and Hunt (1982) have shown that, in children with asymptomatic glucosuria, a two-hour glucose tolerance test may be all that is necessary to demonstrate carbohydrate intolerance. The greater the deviation from normal, the greater the risk of developing overt diabetes mellitus.

Gestational Diabetes (GD)

Gestational diabetes defines a group of women in whom the onset or recognition of diabetes or glucose intolerance occurs during pregnancy. Thus, diabetic women who become pregnant are not included in this class. Clinical recognition of this group is important, since appropriate management can prevent much of the perinatal morbidity and mortality often associated with it. These women are at higher risk for developing diabetes 5 to 10 years after the pregnancy than are women with neither overt diabetes nor an abnormal glucose tolerance test. Indications for investigating glucose tolerance during pregnancy include glycosuria, history of diabetes in a first-degree relative, history of stillbirth or spontaneous abortion, history of fetal malformation, previous large-for-gestational-date infant, maternal obesity, increased maternal age, and parity of five or more.

Previous Abnormality of Glucose Tolerance (PAGT)

This class defines persons who have normal glucose tolerance but had documented hyperglycemia or impaired glucose tolerance in the past. Women with gestational diabetes whose glucose tolerance returned to normal after delivery are a subset of this group. Another subset is formerly obese diabetic patients whose glucose tolerance has returned to normal after weight loss. Others in this group include patients who have had transient hyperglycemia or impaired tolerance secondary to stress such as burns, injuries, surgery, or infections. Such terms as "latent diabetes" and "prediabetes" have been previously used to describe such conditions, but the NDDG recommends that these terms be discontinued.

Potential Abnormality of Glucose Tolerance

This class includes individuals who have never exhibited glucose intolerance but who are at higher risk than the general population for developing diabetes. This is a category that has its greatest value either in epidemiologic studies or in the counseling of nondiabetic individuals. Such individuals might include twins or siblings of known diabetics, or offspring when one or both parents have diabetes. Previous terminology for this class has been "prediabetes" or "potential diabetes," but such terms imply that diabetes is

already present, which is inappropriate and unjustified.

In addition to the aforementioned classifications, there are many hereditary syndromes that have glucose intolerance or overt diabetes mellitus as a component. Certainly these syndromes represent a small part of the total diabetic population; however, they do demonstrate the heterogeneity of the symptom-complex of diabetes.

SECONDARY DIABETES MELLITUS (TYPE III)

Diabetes Associated with Pancreatic Disease

Hereditary relapsing pancreatitis is an autosomal dominant disorder that is characterized by recurrent episodes of severe abdominal pain. This disease, starting in childhood, eventually leads to fibrosis and inflammation of the pancreas with endocrine insufficiency resulting from the destruction of the entire gland.

Cystic fibrosis is associated with diabetes in almost 75 percent of such patients. The longer the patient survival, the greater the chance of developing beta-cell insufficiency. Even so, diabetes has been documented early in the course of the disease. Although ketosis and microvascular complications have not been demonstrated, this may be explained by the fact that the patients usually die from their primary disease before such complications are manifested. Anatomically, there is marked disorganization of the pancreas, with fibrosis and disruption of the islets.

Hemochromatosis has an associated glucose intolerance in over 50 percent of patients. Clinical characteristics are those of non–insulin-dependent diabetes, and secondary vascular complications, including retinopathy, have been reported. Although iron deposition with anatomic destruction of the islets was originally thought to play a role in the pathogenesis of the carbohydrate abnormality, evidence now suggests otherwise. The degree of iron overload is not different in these patients regardless of whether or not they have diabetes. Furthermore, the plasma insulin response to an oral glucose load is often increased, whereas a decrease would be expected if islet destruction were an on-going process. The prevalence of diabetes among parents of patients with hemochromatosis is similar to that of parents of patients with idiopathic diabetes, and some investigators have proposed that the diabetes is genetically determined and that the additional pancreatic damage uncovers this tendency.

Glucose intolerance has also been described in patients with *thalassemia major* and *alpha₁-antitrypsin deficiencies*. The diabetes in both cases may be secondary to pancreatic destruction.

Hormonal Disorders

A number of hereditary syndromes that are secondary to an abnormality of function in one of the nonpancreatic endocrine glands may also be associated with glucose intolerance. Thus, in these syndromes, diabetes is a secondary phenomenon. Two forms of *isolated growth hormone deficiency* have been described, both associated with glucose intolerance. Type I, characterized by insulinopenia following a glucose challenge, has an autosomal recessive inheritance pattern. Type II, inherited as an autosomal dominant, is characterized by a hyperinsulinemic response to glucose. Although glucose intolerance characterizes these syndromes, hypoglycemia may occur in children with subsequent pronounced intolerance in adulthood.

Patients with *hereditary panhypopituitary dwarfism* of the autosomal or x-linked recessive type exhibit glucose intolerance with insulinopenia, both of which are corrected with growth hormone replacement. *Laron dwarfism* is associated with elevated levels of growth hormone but low to undetectable levels of somatomedin. The abnormalities in carbohydrate metabolism are similar to those seen in Type I growth hormone deficiency with insulinopenia.

Hereditary pheochromocytoma may occur as an isolated disorder or in association with medullar thyroid carcinoma, neurofibromatosis, or von Hippel-Lindau disease, all inherited as autosomal dominants. Insulinopenia characterizes the glucose intolerance; this is corrected by ablation of the tumor or by the administration of catecholamine blockers, phenoxybenzamine, or phentolamine. Decreased circulating insulin in these patients is due to inhibition of insulin release via stimulation of alpha-adrenergic receptors. Thus, the diabetes of pheochromocytoma is secondary to the abnormal catecholamine output.

The dominantly inherited syndrome of *multiple endocrine adenomatosis* is characterized by hyperplasia or neoplasia of one or more endocrine glands. The parathyroid, pancreatic islets, and pituitary are most commonly involved. Usually severe hypoglycemia is encountered, but if the patient has eosinophilic adenomas of the pituitary, Cushing's disease, or glucagon-secreting tumors of the pancreas, without islet hyperplasia, glucose intolerance may occur.

Inborn Errors of Metabolism

Several inborn errors of metabolism have an associated glucose intolerance, but the exact relationship of the abnormality to carbohydrate metabolism is often not clear. *Glycogen storage disease, Type I* (von Gierke's disease), is a recessive disorder caused by a deficiency of glucose-6-phosphatase, which hydrolyzes glucose-6-phosphate to glucose. Fasting hypoglycemia is a prominent feature in these patients, which improves with age; although glucose intolerance grows increasingly severe with age. Insulinopenia in the basal state and in response to glucose challenge has been documented. *Acute intermittent porphyria* is an autosomal dominant disorder characterized by an error of porphyrin metabolism and has been associated with a variety of endocrine disturbances including inappropriate antidiuretic hormone (ADH) release, paradoxic increases in plasma growth hormone in response to glucose loading, and isolated adrenocorticotropic hormone (ACTH) deficiency. A high percentage of these patients have glucose intolerance but with elevated plasma insulin levels. The relationship between the porphyrin defect and the glucose intolerance is not known. Although Type IV hyperlipidemia is associated with IDDM, *Type III, IV,* and *V hyperlipidemias* have been associated with NIDDM. In these forms, the lipid abnormality is not affected by insulin therapy.

Genetic Disorders with Insulin Resistance

Several genetic disorders are associated with nonketotic insulin-resistant diabetes. *Ataxia telangiectasia*, characterized by cerebellar ataxia, conjunctival and cutaneous telangiectasia, IgA deficiency, thymic hypoplasia, and respiratory infections, has associated glucose intolerance in 50 percent of patients studied, but there is rarely glycosuria and never ketosis. Early studies suggested a peripheral insensitivity to insulin. Receptor studies, using insulin binding to monocytes, indicate an 80 to 85 percent decrease in receptor affinity. Further data suggest that this defect in insulin receptor affinity is caused by circulating inhibitors of insulin binding.

Patients with *myotonic dystrophy,* an autosomal dominant disorder characterized by myotonia, progressive muscular atrophy, frontal baldness, cataracts, and testicular atrophy, show impaired glucose tolerance with normal fasting sugars but marked hyperinsulinemia. Excessive insulin secretion occurs in response to various stimuli, but both epinephrine infusion and fasting result in normal suppression of insulin release. The response to the excessive rise in insulin is also blunted, since it is not accompanied by an exaggerated fall in blood glucose. The abnormal glucose tolerance does not appear to be associated with microangiopathy. The finding of insulin hyper-responsiveness with mild glucose intolerance suggests a defect in tissue sensitivity. Decreased binding of insulin to monocytes has been demonstrated without a decrease in receptor numbers. However, sera from myotonic patients did not inhibit insulin binding to normal cells. Thus, myotonic dystrophy appears to be associated with a decrease in affinity of insulin receptors, resulting in insulin resistance with a compensatory elevation of plasma insulin levels.

Several syndromes are characterized by absence of subcutaneous, intra-abdominal, and perinephric fat; hyperlipidemia; and insulin-resistant, nonketotic diabetes. The autosomal recessive form has its onset in infancy or early childhood (*Seip's syndrome*). The face is affected in this syndrome, and cirrhosis and hepatomegaly are frequent. Glucose tolerance is normal in childhood, but insulin-resistant, nonketotic diabetes occurs after puberty; hyperinsulinism has been documented. When this syndrome occurs after puberty, it is known as *Lawrence's syndrome.* The studies on insulin binding are conflicting, but different tissues have been used and no data concerning a circulating inhibitor are available.

Leprechaunism is a recessive syndrome characterized by unusual facies, hirsutism, clitoromegaly in females, decreased subcutaneous fat stores, mental and motor retardation, growth retardation, and early death. Abnormalities of glucose metabolism that have been documented include hypoglycemia with fasting, hyperplasia of the islets, and insulin hypersensitivity and resistance with increased plasma insulin levels. It has been proposed that because normal levels of insulin receptors were found in two patients with hyperinsulinism and resistance, a defect distal to the receptor is the origin of the diabetes.

Two varieties of insulin resistance with *acanthosis nigricans* have been described. Type A occurs predominantly in females and is associated with ovarian dysfunction, virilization, primary amenorrhea, and polycystic ovaries; Type B, an autoimmune disorder, is characterized by autoantibodies, hypocomplementemia, and systemic lupus erythematosus (SLE). The defect in Type A appears to be due to decreased insulin receptors on cell surfaces, Type B to a decrease in insulin receptor affinity rather than number.

Mendenhall's syndrome consists of severe insulin-resistant diabetes; old-appearing facies; hyperpigmentation; protuberant abdomen; thickened, hard nails; early dentition; and enlarged genitalia. The diabetes has its onset at age 3 to 7 years and is associated with severe insulin resistance. Of the three children described so far, all died from infection; at autopsy they showed severe fibrosis of the pancreas.

Three cytogenetic syndromes may be associated with diabetes: trisomy 21 syndrome, Klinefelter's syndrome, and Turner's syndrome. *Trisomy 21 syndrome* has been associated with carbohydrate intolerance; however, reports are conflicting. *Klinefelter's syndrome* (XXY) has a reported frequency of 8 to 10 percent for clinical diabetes and 24 to 40 percent for abnormal glucose tolerance. The carbohydrate intolerance is mild and may be related to obesity. Diabetes occurs in about 50 percent of patients with *Turner's syndrome* (XO), and of those under 16 years of age, 78 percent have abnormal glucose tolerance tests.

Neuromuscular Disorders

A number of neuromuscular diseases are associated with glucose intolerance. Both *facioscapulohumeral dystrophy* and *Duchenne type muscular dystrophy* have been associated with glucose intolerance. The etiology may be related to delay in disposal of glucose because of decreased metabolism of glucose with diminished muscle mass. One sibship of *late-onset proximal myopathy* with NIDDM has been reported. Hyperinsulinism has been described in *Huntington's chorea* with glucose intolerance. *Machedo's disease* is a slowly progressive neuromuscular disease characterized by nystagmus, mild dysarthria, and distal muscle atrophy. Again, decreased muscle mass has been proposed as the cause of the elevated blood sugars. *Herrmann's syndrome* is characterized by photomyoclonus, nerve deafness, nephropathy, dementia, and ketosis-resistant diabetes. The inheritance pattern is autosomal dominant. The combination of *optic atrophy, diabetes mellitus, diabetes insipidus, and neurosensory deafness* composes an autosomal recessive syndrome, in which the diabetes is of the ketosis-prone, insulin-dependent type. *Friedreich's ataxia* is characterized by ataxia, dysarthria, nystagmus, diminished to absent deep tendon reflexes, impaired position sensation, scoliosis, and pes cavas; the disease is inherited as an autosomal recessive. Insulin-dependent diabetes has been reported in 8 to 40 percent of patients. *Alstrom's syndrome* is characterized by obesity, nerve deafness in childhood, with the development of carbohydrate intolerance, and progressive renal disease in later life. Patients with *Laurence-Moon-Biedl syndrome* demonstrate retinitis pigmentosa, polydactyly, obesity, hypogonadism, and mental retardation. Glucose intolerance occurs in less than half these patients; furthermore, it may be secondary to the obesity.

Just as many of the neuromuscular disorders show carbohydrate intolerance possibly on the basis of decreased muscle mass, so also may some of the progeroid syndromes. *Cockayne's syndrome* is characterized by a cachectic appearance with premature aging, mental retardation, microcephaly, deafness, and intracranial calcifications. Increased plasma insulin secretion with a blunted glucose response suggests peripheral unresponsiveness. Patients with *Werner's syndrome*, an autosomal recessive disease, show premature aging, graying of the hair, atrophy, and hyperkeratosis of the skin cataracts, ulceration

of the feet, soft tissue and vascular calcifications, severe arteriosclerosis, and atherosclerosis. Glucose intolerance is present in about 50 percent of patients. No symptoms are related to the hyperglycemia; ketosis and microangiopathy are rare.

As with the Laurence-Moon-Biedl syndrome, glucose intolerance in patients with the Prader-Willi syndrome or achondroplastic dwarfism may be secondary to obesity. *Prader-Willi syndrome* is characterized by obesity, short stature, mental retardation, and hypogonadism. NIDDM with insulin resistance and absence of ketosis may develop in later childhood. The diabetes of *achondroplastic dwarfism* is most certainly due to obesity; plasma insulin concentrations following oral glucose in patients with abnormal glucose tolerance show a delayed peak with delayed return to normal, similar to other patients with obesity.

Miscellaneous Syndromes

There are also several miscellaneous syndromes that have been associated with diabetes. The *increase in ocular pressure following topical dexamethasone* is a genetically determined phenomenon that may be related to the inheritance of diabetes. The increase in pressure is greatest with the $P^H P^H$ genotype (> 15 mmHg), intermediate with $P^L P^H$ (6 to 15 mmHg), and least with $P^L P^L$ (<6 mmHg). In studying glucose tolerance in these patients, the frequency is greatest in the $P^H P^H$ group and least in the $P^L P^L$ group. *Epiphyseal dysplasia* and infantile-onset diabetes mellitus was described in three siblings with discolored teeth, scoliosis, and pigmentary abnormalities of the skin. It is presumed that this is a rare but distinct autosomal recessive syndrome. *Progressive cone dystrophy*, characterized by total color blindness, degenerative liver disease, neurosensory hearing loss, gonadotropic defects, and IDDM, has been described in a large kindred from Norway. The inheritance pattern is presumed to be autosomal recessive.

2

Current Concepts of Etiology and Pathogenesis

GENETICS

Diabetes mellitus comprises a genetically heterogeneous group of diseases; that is, different genetic or environmental etiologic factors, or both, can result in similar phenotypes. As such, "diabetes" is not a diagnostic term but is used to describe a symptom-complex or laboratory abnormality. As noted in Chapter 1, diabetes can be subdivided into several groups, including those associated with genetic syndromes; but there is strong evidence that even the well-recognized classifications of Type I (IDDM) and Type II (NIDDM) diabetes need to be further subdivided. Attempts at subclassification are important today but will become more and more important with time, as only by defining subgroups can appropriate etiologic studies be performed.

Although the familial nature of diabetes has been recognized for decades, specific inheritance patterns have not been delineated; all modes of inheritance have been proposed. Indeed, all proposals may be correct, depending on the specific subtype of the diabetic syndrome being considered. In part, confusion has arisen from various definitions of what constitutes diabetes, environmental modifications of the expression of the diabetic genotype, and variability in age of onset. Studies using only clinical techniques have limitations, as apparently healthy individuals with the diabetic genotype will not be recognized. Subclinical markers have been used in an attempt to detect these individuals and to define the population more precisely. Such markers include genetic (for example, ABO or HLA antigens), biochemical (for example, serum glucose insulin or C-peptide levels), physiologic (for example, insulin response to a glucose load), and immunologic (for example, insulin and pancreatic islet antibodies).

FAMILY STUDIES

Many investigators have shown that diabetics have an increased family history of diabetes. Most studies indicate that persons who have diabetes report a positive family history from 25 to 50 percent of the time, whereas nondiabetics report such a history less than 15 percent of the time. Although suggestive, these data are of little value for either epidemiologic studies or clinical use. A more sensitive technique is the comparison of the prevalence of diabetes among relatives of affected individuals to the prevalence

Table 2–1. **ETHNIC VARIABILITY IN DIABETES MELLITUS***

Ethnic Group	Diet			Vascular Complications
	Fat	*Carbohydrate*	*Ketosis*	
European	High	High	Common	Common
Ashkenazi Jew	High	High	Common	Common
Rhodesian Sephardic Jew	High	High	Uncommon	Common
Pima Amerind	High	High	Rare	Common
Albama-Coushatta Amerind	High	High	Rare	Common
Seneca Amerind	High	High	Rare	Common
Navajo Amerind	High	High	Rare	Uncommon
Lebanese	High	—	Uncommon	Common
Eskimo	High	Low	Rare	Rare
Japanese	Low	High	Rare	Uncommon
Ceylonese	Low	High	Rare	Uncommon
Indian	Low	High	Rare	Common
South African Indian	Low	High	Rare	Very common
South African Zulu	Low	High	Common	Rare
Rhodesian African	Low	High	Common	Rare

*Modified from Rotter JI, Rimoin DL: Etiology. In Brownlee M (ed): *Handbook of Diabetes Mellitus.* Garland STPM Press, New York, 1981.

among similar relatives of a control group (that is, unaffected individuals). Using biochemical markers such as the glucose tolerance test, the prevalence of affected individuals may be as high as 10 to 30 percent of parents, siblings, or close relatives of patients with diabetes, as compared with 6 to 15 percent of such relatives of nondiabetic individuals.

Since increased family prevalence may be the result of genetic or environmental factors, studies of twins represent one method of separating these variables. Using clinical diabetes as a marker, the concordance rate for monozygotic twins has been found to vary from 45 to 96 percent, whereas that for dizygotic twins ranges from 3 to 37 percent. Again, when more sensitive markers are used, the concordance rate for monozygotic twins is usually above 70 percent. Although these studies suggest that genetic factors are involved in the diabetic state, exact mechanisms of genetic transmission are unknown.

MODES OF INHERITANCE

Almost every conceivable mode of transmission has been proposed. Autosomal recessive inheritance was originally postulated by Pincus and White in 1933. Others have also presented data to support this hypothesis, but difficulties are encountered when offspring of two diabetic parents are studied. If diabetes were indeed a simple recessive trait, all children would be expected to have the diabetic genotype. However, at most, only 50 percent of such offspring have been found to have diabetes, and this fact led to the suggestion that there is incomplete penetrance. Other investigators have suggested that diabetes may be inherited as an autosomal dominant trait with incomplete penetrance. Since one mode of genetic transmission is not a satisfactory explanation for all cases, several authors have proposed a multifactorial or polygenic inheritance. Other proposals are that diabetes is inherited by a single gene that is influenced by a number of modifying genes and that there is a polyallelic recessive inheritance.

Reviewing these data, Rimoin in 1967 proposed that diabetes mellitus was a group of heterogeneous diseases, each with a different mode of inheritance. Strongly supporting this view are studies that have examined differences among various ethnic populations. Table 2–1 lists some of the various groups studied. Variability in the prevalence and pattern of disease among these ethnic groups may be secondary to both genetic and environmental factors but may also indicate heterogeneity. One environmental factor of note is the general correlation between "overnutrition" and prevalence of diabetes. When groups of individuals, such as the Kurdish and Yemenite Jews of Israel, migrated into different population environments, the prevalence of diabetes markedly increased with subsequent dietary changes. Nevertheless, differences exist among ethnic groups, which may not be secondary to environmental differences. Different ethnic groups with similar diets may still have markedly different prevalence of diabetic vascular complications (for example, Ceylonese versus Indian).

Probably the most commonly cited evidence for heterogeneity comes from comparisons of ketosis-resistant (NIDDM) and ketosis-prone diabetes (IDDM). Studies by Pyke and associates (1976) strongly suggest a distinct separation of these two entities. These investigators studied monozygotic twins by examining differences between concordant and discordant pairs. Evaluation of their studies and careful analysis of similar studies from others showed that when the pairs were divided into those who did and those who did not develop diabetes after the age of 40 years, 100 percent of the pairs were concordant. Comparison of pairs who manifested clinical diabetes before 40 years of age revealed that only 50 percent were concordant. These data suggest that the predisposition to diabetes (Type I) is modified or influenced by nongenetic factors.

GENETIC MARKERS

As previously mentioned, subclinical and genetic markers have been used to distinguish the two major subgroups of the diabetic phenotype. Subclinical markers are measures used to detect an abnormal genotype in the absence of the phenotype. Physiologic studies can occasionally serve as genetic markers; for example, the insulin response to glucose loading provided early evidence of heterogeneity. The relative hyperinsulinemic response of NIDDM may be contrasted against the insulinopenic response of IDDM.

Other markers such as blood group antigens and human leukocyte antigens (HLA) have been used in population groups to separate Type I and Type II diabetes. Early studies, which evaluated the association of red cell antigens and diabetes, found blood group A to be more commonly associated, but the association was weak and a pathogenetic relationship could not be found. This finding has been largely ignored, but it is notable that the blood group A association occurs only with Type II diabetes. Renewed interest in such associations emerged with studies of HLA, the loci for which are located on the sixth autosomal chromosome. The HLA region has at least four defined loci, three of which are serologically defined (known as the A, B, and C loci) and one of which is defined by the mixed lymphocyte

reaction (D locus). Other genes have also been localized to this region of the human genome (for example, those regulating several components of the complement sequence). Many investigators have reported increases in HLA-B8 and HLA-B15 in persons with insulin-dependent diabetes mellitus, and studies from England and France have demonstrated an increased frequency of HLA-B18. Combined data from several centers have suggested that HLA-B7 is decreased in frequency in the patient with ketosis-prone diabetes, and initial family studies seem to confirm the "protective" effect of this allele. Two alleles at the D locus, Dw3 and Dw4, have been associated with an increased risk for insulin-dependent diabetes. Although it is not clear which of these loci carry the greatest risk for the patient, the relative risk associated with Dw3 has been reported to be 4.5, whereas that for B8 is 2.5.

There also appear to be ethnic differences for HLA antigens. Reports from Japan indicate that B5, B12, B54, Dw3 and Dw4, B54, and B12 have increased frequency in IDDM. HLA typing in blacks and in Latin American populations suggest similar associations to the Caucasian population, but the frequency of the diabetes-associated genes is less. HLA typing for various ethnic groups may help to determine if such antigens are directly responsible for the phenotype or are linked to the antigens that are responsible. If, for example, the alleles with increased frequency are the genes that predispose an individual to IDDM, then they should be constant from population to population, as seems to be the case for HLA-B27 and ankylosing spondylitis. However, if they are only linked to these predisposing genes, then the specific alleles may differ among ethnic groups.

It has also been suggested that heterogeneity exists for patients within IDDM. Reports have indicated an increased relative risk with both B8 and B15 alleles versus those with only one such allele (for example, B8B15 versus B8X or B15X) or those with two identical alleles (for example, B8B8). Furthermore, Ludvigsson and associates (1977) have noted that diabetic patients with B8B15 are younger at onset and have a decreased frequency of detectable C-peptide than do individuals with only one of these antigens. Other evidence for heterogeneity comes from the antibody response to exogenous insulin therapy. Diabetic patients who later develop insulin antibodies have an increased frequency of HLA-B8 and a normal frequency of HLA-B15; whereas those individuals who immediately formed high titers of insulin antibodies have a normal frequency of HLA-B8 and an increased frequency of HLA-B15. IDDM patients with the HLA-B8 allele have a higher frequency of persistent islet-cell antibodies than do those with Dw3. The presence of the HLA-B8 antigen is more often associated with autoimmune diseases, such as thyroiditis, Graves' disease, Addison's disease, and myasthenia gravis. These and other differences are summarized in Table 2–2.

Heterogeneity may also exist for NIDDM. The best form delineated is the maturity-onset diabetes of youth (MODY). Affected patients, although less than 40 years of age at onset, behave physiologically the same as patients with NIDDM. Genetic studies provide evidence that suggests a separate entity from the usual patient with NIDDM. Eighty-five percent of MODY patients have a diabetic parent and 45 percent demonstrate three generations of direct vertical transmission, thus suggesting autosomal dominance. Fajans and coworkers (1978) identify two subgroups within this category: those who respond to a glucose load with hyperinsulinemia and those who do not. Only the latter progress to require insulin therapy. Another method of subdividing this group of diabetics has been chlorpropamide-primed, alcohol-induced flushing, reported as a preclinical marker of MODY. Studies have shown that most persons with diabetes flush in response to alcohol after prior administration of chlorpropamide; a response rarely observed in nondiabetics. The positive flush response is a dominantly inherited trait and antedates the diabetic phenotype.

COUNSELING

An obvious outcome of comprehensive genetic analysis is the prediction of risk to family members of patients with diabetes. In order for genetic counseling to be most effective, an accurate and precise diagnosis must be made. By merely identifying a person as having IDDM, NIDDM, or MODY, the counselor has information that is useful in predicting risk. From published studies of epidemiologic investigations, the relative risks of developing diabetes for first-degree relatives is low, particularly for IDDM. The sibling of a child with IDDM has about a 5 to 10 percent risk of developing the same disease, whereas the risk to the offspring of a single diabetic parent is thought to be 1 to 2 percent. Data collected from HLA typing may also contribute additionally to knowledge about relative risk (for example, if a sibling is known to have both HLA-B8 and HLA-B15). Gorsuch and co-workers (1982) examined the risk of Type I diabetes in 288 siblings of 160 affected children by identifying the number of HLA haplotypes they had in common. HLA-identical siblings were found to be at higher risk than siblings with only one common haplotype, and to have a 100-fold greater risk than the general population. Conversely, the risk to nonidentical siblings was not increased when compared with the general population. The risks to first-degree relatives of patients with IDDM is somewhat greater, being 5 to 10 percent for overt diabetes and 15 to 25 percent for an abnormal glucose tolerance test. For patients with MODY, the risk to siblings and offspring is 50 percent. As additional subgroups are better defined with improved techniques, risks will be better approximated.

Table 2–2. **HETEROGENEITY WITHIN IDDM**

Evidence	B8	B15	B(Dw3)/B15(Dw4)
Relative risk for diabetes	Additive		Increased relative risk
Linkage disequilibrium	Dw3, Drw3A1	Cw3, Drw4, Dw4	Increased occurrence in monozygotic twins
Insulin antibodies	Nonresponder (no antibodies)	High responder (high antibodies)	Increased risk
Islet-cell antibodies	Persistent	Transient	
Antipancreatic cell mediated immunity	Increased	Not increased	
Associated with other autoimmune endocrine disease	Yes	No	
Age of onset	Any age	Younger age	

Table 2–3. **VIRUSES IMPLICATED IN THE PATHOGENESIS OF DIABETES MELLITUS**

Type	Virus	Species Known (affected)
RNA	Mumps	Humans
		Humans (in vivo)
		Monkeys (in vitro)
	Coxsackie B4, 5	Humans
		Mice
	Encephalomyocarditis, M variant	Mice
	Foot and mouth disease	Guinea pigs
		Cattle
		Mice
	Venezuelan equine encephalomyelitis	Hamsters
		Monkeys
		Mice
	Rubella	Humans
		Rabbits
	Reovirus (Type 3)	Mice
DNA	Cytomegalovirus	Humans
	Epstein-Barr virus	Humans
	Varicella	Humans

VIRUSES

A number of studies have also addressed the temporal relationship of viral illness to onset of the disease process, particularly of IDDM. The concept of a viral etiology for IDDM comes from several sources: anatomic study of diabetic islets, genetic studies, epidemiologic studies correlating specific viral antibody titers with the incidence of newly diagnosed diabetics, and experimental models of virus-induced diabetes. Table 2–3 summarizes some of the data that have been reported concerning such pathogenetic mechanisms.

Epidemiologic observations from the United States and England have noted the highest frequency of onset for IDDM to be in the fall and winter, with the lowest in summer. Of significance is that when a city in the southern hemisphere is surveyed, the times of highest frequency were almost precisely six months removed, from May through August. These data are compatible with those of the highest incidence of viral respiratory disease and suggest viruses to be a significant factor in the etiology of IDDM.

Animal Models

Introduction of viral agents into some animal models is associated with the development of a syndrome similar to IDDM. The responsible factors and the relative strengths of their influence are noted in Table 2–4. Early studies described necrosis of exocrine pancreatic tissue and islet degeneration after suckling mice were infected with the Coxsackie B4 virus. This virus is one that has been associated with the disease in humans. Later studies found that this virus, after 14 passages in tissue culture, produced a diabetes-like syndrome in 80 percent of SJL/J mice. These mice demonstrated insulitis, beta-cell necrosis, Coxsackie B4 virus in beta cells, hypoinsulinemia, and hyperglycemia. It was further noted that, even though SWR/J and NIH Swiss mice were susceptible, other strains (C57, BL/6J, DBA/2) were resistant.

Another animal model of viral diabetes comes from data on the encephalomyocarditis (EMC) virus, M variant. Animals infected with this virus develop beta-cell degranulation, coagulation necrosis, and shrinkage of affected islets but maintain normal alpha cells. After only one to two days of inoculation, the virus replicates within the beta cells and is associated with unregulated release of insulin and resultant hypoglycemia. Subsequently, hypoinsulinemia and hyperglycemia develop in about 75 percent of animals. However, the hyperglycemia is permanent in only 10 to 15 percent and transient in the remainder; the degree of hyperglycemia correlating with the extent of beta-cell damage. The male animal is more susceptible to EMC than is the female, and administration of testosterone enhances susceptibility in castrated males and females. This emphasizes the importance of hormonal factors in susceptibility of mice to virus-induced diabetes.

Because mouse strains vary in their susceptibility to virus-induced diabetes, studies have been undertaken to examine more closely the genetics of this susceptibility. An encephalomyocarditis–susceptible strain and an EMC-resistant strain were bred, and the F_1 generation was infected with EMC as well as back-crossed against the parental strains. Data from these studies indicate a polygenic mode of inheritance, whereas other studies have suggested an autosomal recessive mode. Other studies have attempted to elucidate mechanisms for how genetic factors confer resistance or susceptibility. One such mechanism may be the genetic control of the degree of viral replication in the beta cells. Studies have demonstrated that EMC virus inoculated into susceptible mouse strains showed higher pancreatic viral titers than did those of resistant strains. The higher titers are the

Table 2–4. **FACTORS THAT INFLUENCE VIRUS-INDUCED DIABETES MELLITUS IN ANIMAL MODELS**

Factor	Degree of Influence	Comments
Characteristics of Virus		
Type	+	Mostly RNA-type, few DNA
Strain	+ +	B4, Coxsackie, M variant EMC
Dose	+	Must be large enough to cause moderate infection but not kill
Virulence	+ +	Should be attenuated in its primary illness in host to allow expression of diabetic state
Passage	+ +	Passage in vivo or in vitro through host is usually necessary for diabetogenic effect
Characteristics of Host		
Species	+ + +	Depends on presence of specific surface virus receptor on beta cell
Age	+	Young adults most susceptible (EMC virus)
Sex	+	M > F (EMC virus)
Hormonal factors	+	Estrogen, testosterone, adrenal corticosteroids (EMC virus)
Genetic background of host		M variant EMC and Coxsackie B4; C57 G 1/6 strain resistant

result of increased numbers of beta cells being infected rather than of greater numbers of virus in the individual beta cells. Even among resistant strains, variations occur in the percentage of beta cells that are infected, raising the possibility that only certain subpopulations of beta cells contain EMC virus receptors that allow viral penetration. Additionally, it has been found that at least twice as many EMC viruses attach to the beta cell from susceptible strains as from resistant strains. These data are also compatible with the concept that receptors for the virus on the cell surface, under genetic control, confer the relative susceptibility or resistance to the development of diabetes.

Other viruses that have been studied include rubella, reovirus, and the Trinidad strain of Venezuelan encephalitis virus in Golden Syrian hamsters and rhesus monkeys. These studies all demonstrate the ability of these agents to cause a diabetes-like syndrome. The details of genetic susceptibility such as outlined for the EMC virus have not yet been completely defined.

Viral Infection in Humans

Reports as early as 1894 noted an association between mumps infection and the development of diabetes mellitus. The variability in time of onset of diabetic symptoms from the mumps infection made the association vague. Large epidemiologic studies have not demonstrated a strong association of mumps and diabetes, even though studies in Erie County, New York, did show consistent and repetitive peaks in the onset of IDDM compared with those of mumps orchitis. In vitro studies have shown that the ABC strain of mumps virus is capable of infecting cultured human pancreatic beta cells.

Coxsackievirus has also been implicated as a pathogenic agent for diabetes in humans, as mentioned previously. One of the most convincing studies concerns a case report by Yoon and co-workers (1979). These investigators isolated a Coxsackie B4 virus from the pancreas of a 10-year-old boy who died one week after diabetes was diagnosed. At autopsy, infiltration of the islets of Langerhans with lymphocytes was noted along with beta-cell necrosis. Serologic studies confirmed a rising titer of neutralizing antibody titer to this virus (1:4 on the second day, increasing to 1:32 on the seventh day). The virus was isolated from the child's pancreas and inoculated in beta-cell tissue cultures. Subsequent inoculation of the SJL strain of mice produced insulitis, beta-cell necrosis, and hyperglycemia.

Champsour and associates (1982) presented a 16-month-old girl who had fever, acute thrombocytopenia, and insulin-dependent diabetes. Coxsackie B5 virus was isolated from the stool, and seroconversion was documented. This Coxsackie B5 virus was injected into four groups of mice, all of whom subsequently demonstrated an abnormal glucose tolerance. The child's HLA type was B18, BfF1; and islet cell antibodies were positive in a titer of 1/160 on days 8 and 18 after onset, 1/40 on day 112, and negative at 1 year. It was postulated that the association of genetic predisposition and viral stimulus produced the syndrome of IDDM.

Rubella virus has also been implicated; in studies of patients with the congenital rubella syndrome, overt diabetes has been reported in about 20 per cent of cases. Of these patients, about one half had HLA-B8. Long-term follow-up studies, HLA typing, and glucose tolerance testing of nonaffected siblings are required before any firm conclusions can be reached about the coexistence of diabetes and rubella.

Other viruses have also been implicated in some cases, particularly with EMC, in which neutralizing antibody titers have been found in 12 percent of patients with IDDM compared with about 6 percent of control subjects. Although temporal associations have also been made between diabetes and cytomegalovirus, measles, polio, influenza, and tick-borne encephalitis, conclusions cannot yet be drawn.

AUTOIMMUNITY

Another factor that may affect the emergence of the diabetic phenotype is development of antibodies directed against the islets or islet-cell cytoplasm (ICA). Such antibodies have been found in up to 67 percent of newly diagnosed cases of IDDM. They are of the IgG class, are at their highest level early in the disease process, and decrease with time. About 20 percent of IDDM patients have a persistently positive antibody titer, and most of these tend to have HLA-B8. A complement-fixing immunofluorescence assay for ICA appears more closely related to the acute phase of the disease than does the non–complement-fixing ICA IgG. Antibodies to islet-cell surface antigen (ICSA) have also been demonstrated and are also most closely associated with the acute phase of the disease. It has been demonstrated that serum from ICSA-positive patients causes release of chromium from islets of newborn rats when complement is added. This effect is not demonstrable when the serum is positive for ICA only. Thus, ICSA may be directly cytotoxic to islet cells. Antibodies to other cells have also been demonstrated in certain families; antibodies to thyroid, adrenal, and parietal cells have been isolated.

Cell-mediated immunity has been implicated in the pathogenesis of diabetes by some investigators. Lymphocytes from patients with diabetes have been found to be toxic to cultured insulinoma cells. Furthermore, these lymphocytes have been shown to inhibit insulin release from rat islet cells in vitro. Other evidence of an autoimmune etiology for diabetes includes circulating immune complexes in patients with recent onset of their disease, immunofluorescence of muscle membrane, altered levels of interferon, and lymphocytotoxic antibodies. Animal data also support an autoimmune mechanism as one factor in the etiology of diabetes. The BB/W rat spontaneously develops diabetes at 60 to 120 days of age. At this time there is round-cell invasion of the endocrine pancreas with subsequent development of glucose intolerance and often, lethal ketoacidosis. Antilymphocyte serum produces a much lower incidence of diabetes and indeed returns the blood glucose levels to normal in 30 percent of affected rats. If a clear role of cytotoxic antibodies or cell-mediated immunity could be established, then intervention would be strongly considered.

HORMONES

Several hormones—glucocorticoids, catecholamines, growth hormone, glucagon, and somatostatin—have been thought to play a possible etiologic role in development of diabetes. These hormones have been associated with and/or are known to influence insulin action or secretion.

Glucocorticoids

In physiologic amounts, glucocorticoids enhance gluconeogenesis in vivo and in vitro, enhance lipolysis, and inhibit glucose utilization. In pharmacologic amounts, they have an inhibitory effect on glucose-stimulated insulin secretion. When administered on a chronic basis, however, they increase insulin response to either glucose or tolbutamide administration. Studies evaluating the interaction of insulin and its receptor have been conflicting. Some studies suggest a decrease in receptor affinity (in vivo) on red blood cells after dexamethasone or prednisone ingestion. Studies using monocytes as the receptor marker suggest an increase in binding after prednisone administration, and this appears related to a rise in receptor number. Conversely, short-term infusion of cortisol in humans has no effect on insulin binding to monocyte receptors. It is thus apparent that the effect of cortisol on carbohydrate metabolism will be variable, depending on many factors.

Of patients with excessive cortisol production (that is, Cushing's disease), about 25 percent will develop overt diabetes, with as many as 75 percent developing impaired glucose tolerance. Once the primary disease is corrected, the glucose tolerance becomes normal in most instances. In patients treated with glucocorticoids for other conditions, only about 20 percent develop overt diabetes, and there is a high rate of spontaneous remission once steroids are discontinued.

In children with IDDM the cortisol production rate is normal unless significant stress or acidosis or both are present. The production rate increases markedly in these situations. Thus, although glucocorticoids may affect insulin binding, cause a degree of insulin resistance, and alter glucose tolerance, there is no convincing evidence that these hormones significantly contribute to the pathogenesis of diabetes.

Catecholamines

The autonomic nervous system exerts marked effects on insulin secretion via alpha- or beta-adrenergic receptors. Insulin secretion is inhibited by alpha-adrenergic stimulation and enhanced by beta-adrenergic stimulation. Consequently, the decrease in insulin secretion seen after epinephrine or norepinephrine administration is primarily due to stimulation of the alpha-receptor. Likewise, agents such as propranolol (a beta-inhibitor) also tend to inhibit insulin release, whereas phentolamine (an alpha-inhibitor) or isoproterenol (a beta-stimulant) will promote or augment insulin release. Disturbances in glucose tolerance following major stress (that is, surgery, burns, and so forth) may be explained on the basis of inhibition of insulin release following alpha-adrenergic stimulation. Plasma catecholamine levels have been shown to increase in response to diabetic ketoacidosis, to hypoglycemia, and even to

significant hyperglycemia. Thus, available data suggest that catecholamine secretion is the result of metabolic derangement rather than being an initiator of diabetes.

Growth Hormone

Human growth hormone (HGH) antagonizes insulin-responsive glucose transport into muscle. Thus, chronic hypersecretion or administration of HGH induces hyperglycemia and increased insulin secretion. Plasma HGH concentrations are higher throughout the day in patients with IDDM than in individuals without diabetes, and they increase to a greater degree in response to various stimuli including arginine, glucagon, and exercise. These higher levels of HGH are linearly correlated with the degree of blood glucose control. With normoglycemia, the concentration of HGH returns toward normal. Thus, as with catecholamines, the abnormalities observed in growth hormone secretion appear to be secondary rather than primary.

Glucagon

This hormone is a protein with 29 amino acids and a molecular weight of 3485 daltons and was identified as a hyperglycemia factor shortly after the discovery of insulin. Some studies have demonstrated that plasma glucagon concentrations are inappropriately high in patients with diabetes. In the nondiabetic individual, plasma concentrations of glucagon typically fall after a carbohydrate meal, but in the person with diabetes this does not always occur. Instead, the glucagon concentration most often either remains unchanged or increases. The question has been raised as to whether this abnormality of secretion is a primary alpha-cell defect or is secondary to insulin deficiency. The answer to this question is not yet available. Although glucagon levels are lower in diabetic patients who are appropriately treated with insulin, the concentrations may not be suppressed as they are in the nondiabetic individual. Thus, a primary alpha-cell abnormality is suggested by some investigators. However, it has also been argued that alpha-cell suppression can only be attained by glucose-induced paracrine secretion of both insulin and somatostatin. Since intraislet concentrations of in-

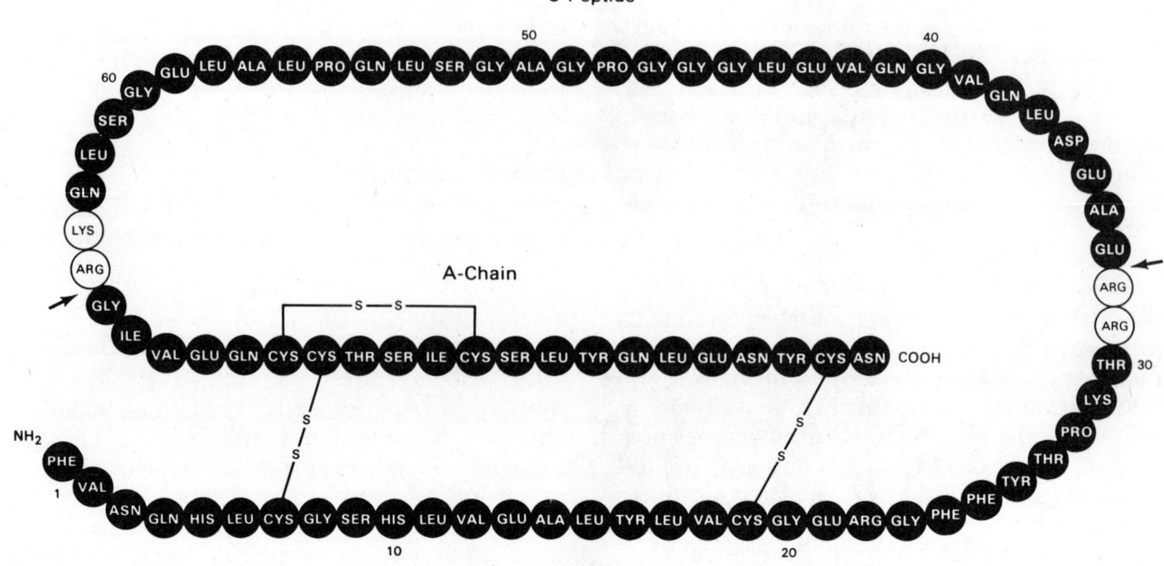

Figure 2–1. Biochemical structure of proinsulin. During processing within the beta cell, the C-peptide linkage between A and B chains is cleaved. Equimolar portions of "insulin" (that is, A and B chains) and C-peptide are then secreted in response to appropriate stimuli.

sulin bathing the alpha cell may be as high as 20,000 μU/ml, it would be impossible to correct this defect with exogenous insulin. It has additionally been argued that if a defect in paracrine secretion is responsible for the increased glucagon levels, it should take higher amounts of insulin to suppress the levels than has been shown to exist.

Another abnormality of glucagon has been identified in the diabetic and may be of much more significance. During insulin-induced hypoglycemia, nondiabetic individuals have about a threefold increase in plasma glucagon concentrations, whereas persons with diabetes often have no rise at all. Thus, one of the major counter-regulatory responses to hypoglycemia appears deficient.

Yet another bothersome aspect of glucagon metabolism concerns whether the increased levels are due to hypersecretion or to decreased clearance. Hyperplasia of alpha-cells that would presumably be seen with hypersecretion is not found either in streptozocin- or alloxan-induced diabetic rats or in humans with Type I diabetes. Thus, the pathogenesis of the glucagon abnormalities remains unclear, but there is no persuasive evidence to suggest a primary alpha-cell defect in diabetes.

Somatostatin

Somatostatin is a peptide secreted by the delta, or D, cells of the pancreas. Several substances appear to stimulate somatostatin secretion in vitro: glucose, arginine, leucine, and glucagon. Beta-adrenergic stimulation increases also somatostatin release, whereas adrenergic stimulation inhibits its secretion.

Somatostatin is a powerful inhibitor of insulin and glucagon secretion both in vivo and in vitro. The response of both hormones to all secretagogues can be inhibited by an adequate concentration of somatostatin, but the extent of inhibition depends on the character and degree of the stimulus. Certainly, the ability of somatostatin to inhibit the secretion of other islet hormones and the anatomic proximity of the secretory cells suggest that this peptide is important in regulating or modulating insulin and glucagon secretion; but its actual role is unclear. There are no data to suggest that abnormalities in D-cell function are primary in diabetes.

INSULINOPATHIES

Another pathogenesis for the phenotype of diabetes mellitus is the insulinopathies.

Biochemical studies have elucidated the synthetic pathways and structure of circulating insulin and its precursors (Fig. 2–1). Preproinsulin is composed of the A and B chains of insulin, the connecting peptide chain (C-peptide) and a prepeptide segment attached to the NH_2 end of the B chain; the latter is rapidly cleaved during synthesis. The C-peptide link between A and B chains is cleaved from the proinsulin molecule during processing in the beta cells. Intact proinsulin has less than 5 percent of the biologic activity of insulin, whereas the B chain plus the C-peptide fragment possesses 50 percent of the biologic activity. Such a defect, inherited as an autosomal dominant, has been reported in a family in whom there was no apparent abnormality in glucose tolerance. A Japanese family has also been reported in whom there was a mutation of the cleavage site between the A chain and C-peptide, thus making this peptide fragment the circulating form of insulin. This family had non–insulin-dependent diabetes, inherited as an autosomal dominant trait. Another type of insulinopathy has been described in a nonobese man with insulin-dependent diabetes. This patient demonstrated fasting hypoglycemia, hyperinsulinemia, normal levels of plasma proinsulin, glucagon, growth hormone, and cortisol. Insulin antibodies and insulin-receptor antibodies were undetected. Insulin sensitivity and insulin receptors on circulating monocytes were within the normal range. A normal responsiveness to exogenous insulin was demonstrated. Isolation and purification of the insulin suggested that the defect in circulating insulin was at the receptor-binding region.

3

The Clinical Disease

Diabetes in the young person is distinct from diabetes that commonly begins after the fourth decade. The former is virtually always insulin dependent, whereas the latter is rarely dependent on exogenously administered insulin for health restoration. Genetically, etiologically, and physiologically, the two types of diabetes appear as different disease states, and it is therefore easy to understand and accept their clinical diversity. Table 3–1 lists some of the more common differences that are observed. NIDDM is commonly associated with obesity and an associated receptor defect, whereas this combination has been observed in less than 1 percent of persons with onset of diabetes within the first 20 years of life (IDDM). On the other hand, although onset of IDDM has been observed throughout life, over 90 percent of such patients experience this during their first 20 years.

From a physiologic standpoint, the most notable difference lies in the ability of the pancreatic beta cell to produce and secrete insulin. Whereas the plasma level of free insulin is either normal or increased in persons with NIDDM, there is usually a striking insulinopenia in those with IDDM. This usually translates into the occurrence of more marked hyperglycemia and episodes of ketonemia and ketonuria, features generally missing in NIDDM. The early appearance of ketonemia in IDDM is seemingly a reflection of the more extreme deficiency of insulin action. The consequences of significant ketonemia on the body's fluid and acid-base

Table 3–1. DIABETES CHARACTERISTICS*

	IDDM (Type I)	NIDDM (Type II)
Age at onset	<40 yrs (80% >20 yrs)	>40 yrs
Sex predilection	None	Female
Nutritional status	Normal/Thin	>60% Obese
Clinical onset	Rapid (>80%)	Insidious
Degree hyperglycemia	Marked	Mild to moderate
Ketonemia-ketonuria	Present	Absent
Insulin replacement	Absolutely necessity	Often optional
Stability of disease	Labile	Stable
Response to oral drugs	Uncommon	Common

*As indicated, there are pronounced differences in the clinical characteristics of the two major forms of this disease. These differences are so great that the similarities pale in comparison.

Table 3–2. **FACTORS CONTRIBUTING TO "SEVERITY" OF IDDM DIABETES***

1. Disease Variables
   a. Etiology/Genetic (?)
   b. Degree of insulin deficiency
   c. Degree of insulin destruction/inactivation
   d. Continued beta-cell injury (? autoimmune)
   e. Receptor/Postreceptor status
2. Individual Variables
   a. Associated disease(s)
   b. Age, developmental status
   c. Growth status
   d. Psychosocial variables
   e. Hormonal variables
3. Environmental Variables
   a. Family/Support systems
   b. Stresses
4. Treatment Variables
   a. Insulin kinetics
   b. Dietary programs
   c. Exercise programs
   d. Adherence/Compliance
5. Yet Unknown Variables

*Multiply factors contribute to the interpatient variability of IDDM. This table lists a few of the more obvious factors, but other factors may be influential.

status are at least partially responsible for the more rapid onset of clinical symptoms that occur in IDDM.

Decades of investigation and clinical experience were required before the pathophysiologic differences between NIDDM and IDDM were fully appreciated. Only now is it becoming apparent that IDDM is not a homogenous entity. Table 3–2 outlines some of the factors that contribute to the observed variability of this condition. Some variables that affect the character of the clinical disease are specific to the disease itself and to the individual in whom the disease resides, whereas other variables appear to be related either to environmental or treatment variables.

Among disease variables, etiologic factors may be most important, but definitive information is only beginning to accumulate (see Chapter 2). Early data suggest that those persons with IDDM who have HLA-B8 differ from those with HLA-B15. The former have an increased frequency of islet-cell antibodies, a high clinical association with other autoimmune endocrine diseases, and possibly a greater risk of microvascular complications. Other studies suggest that the relation of IDDM to viral disease differs in these two subsets. Although some persons appear to have islet cell destruction as a direct consequence of viral invasion, the more common occurrence is felt to be virus-induced altera-

tion in the beta cell with secondary autoantibody formation, leading to a slow, progressive destruction of remaining beta cells.

Absolute insulin deficiency was once considered the sine qua non of IDDM, but it is now apparent that there is no uniformity in the degree of insulin deficiency in these patients. Serial measurements of plasma concentrations of C-peptide in patients with IDDM have demonstrated that some continue to produce small amounts of insulin for indefinite periods, while others cease production early in the course of their disease.

CLINICAL CHARACTERISTICS

Prevalence, Age, Gender, and Seasonality

The overall incidence of IDDM appears to vary with the population surveyed, the ages of the patients included in the survey, and the preciseness of the definition of insulin dependence. Epidemiologic data from Rochester, Minnesota, and from Erie County, New York, in the United States, as well as from Canada, England, and France, all suggest similar incidence rates of between 8 and 11 per 100,000 person-years. Three other studies have suggested significantly higher rates, but definitions used for IDDM were somewhat different. In the Rochester study, approximately one third of the patients with IDDM were diagnosed after age 30.

Prevalence data collected in the United States on school children have demonstrated rates of 1.6 per thousand and a linear increase with age. On the basis of sequential examinations, some studies have suggested a secular increase in incidence, but this has not been consistently demonstrated.

Data from a number of sources have demonstrated a seasonality in occurrence of IDDM. In a combined report from three centers in this country (Gainesville, Florida; Galveston, Texas; and Pittsburgh, Pennsylvania), the months of January through April represented peak onset periods, whereas the number of new cases fell markedly during the summer months. Children less than age 6 at onset demonstrated this seasonal variation in an even greater degree than did older children. This finding is compatible with the hypothesis that onset of IDDM is associated with viral disease, which varies seasonally.

Age of onset has been similar in almost all

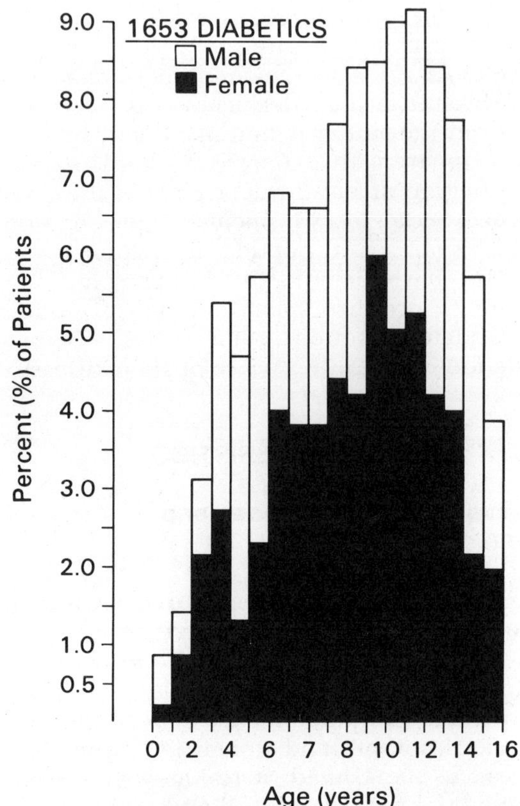

Figure 3–1. Age of onset and gender are noted for 1653 different children attending our summer camp program between 1974–1983. (See also text.)

reported studies, with the peak generally being at 9 to 12 years of age. Figure 3–1 demonstrates data on age of onset and on gender in 1653 children from our camp files, in which the peak age is 11 years. Since this camp program is free to everyone, since it accepts children from throughout the state of Texas, and since participants are limited to residents of the state, these data are probably representative of the population as a whole. Close agreement exists between these data and published studies from the United States and other countries. Sex distribution is approximately equal in most studies, although there are variances with age. Some observers have suggested a greater male incidence in early and late childhood and a greater female incidence in the peak years.

Other epidemiologic variables appear to be race, socioeconomic status, and geography. In almost all studies from the United States, there appears to be racial predilection for the Caucasian American. Blacks have the lowest overall prevalence of Type I diabetes in the United States, which may be related to their having a reduced frequency of certain types of HLA. One United States study and two studies from other countries have suggested an increased occurrence in those of higher socioeconomic status, although no explanation for this has been advanced. Regarding apparent geographic variables (that is, some communities or areas with high prevalence, others with low prevalence), some investigators have suggested differences in the composition of the soil or other environmental factors as being influential.

ONSET CHARACTERISTICS

Rapidity

It has been traditional to think of IDDM as having a precipitous onset, with a short interval between the initial symptoms and the need for medical assistance. In actuality, there are data that seem to refute this overall contention. In the experience of several large clinics, the average duration of symptoms prior to the need for medical intervention was approximately two weeks, with a range from a few days to several months. But can one equate the onset of symptoms with the beginning of diabetes? Recent information suggests that they cannot be equated. A number of patient examples have now been collected in which glucose intolerance has been observed intermittently for long periods prior to development of classical IDDM. The following case is one such example:

N. L. was one of five children from a family without known history of diabetes. At the age of 6 years, he acquired a Rhus dermatitis which was treated with a topical steroid. During this course of therapy, he developed polyuria and polydipsia and was found to have hyperglycemia and glycosuria. Six days after stopping steroid applications, a glucose tolerance test result was abnormal, and he was placed on a low-carbohydrate diet. Within one month the hyperglycemia abated, and two glucose tolerance test results were normal at 6½ and 8 years of age. At age 10 he was involved in an automobile accident in which one of his sisters was killed. He developed hyperglycemia and ketonemia, which required insulin therapy for correction. Within two months his insulin therapy was discontinued, and postprandial blood glucose values were normal.

Between the ages of 11 and 13 years, he had intermittent glycosuria, and glucose tolerance testing was either normal or equivocal. At 13.4 years of age, he developed polyuria, polydipsia, anorexia, and weight loss six weeks after having herpetic gingivostomatitis. Within one week, he developed ketosis, and insulin therapy was again started. His subsequent course has been typical of IDDM, and now at age 20 he receives 0.8 units of insulin per kilogram of body weight per day and has no measurable C-peptide response.

Data from such patients suggest that onset of diabetes may be insidious. Increasing numbers of patients with varying degrees of glucose intolerance are being identified years before becoming permanently insulin-dependent. Additionally, studies of siblings of known diabetics have demonstrated that as many as 30 percent intermittently have abnormal glucose tolerance test results. Such information has led to the conceptual model of the pathogenesis of Type I diabetes seen in Figure 3–2. This model suggests that, from conception, there is genetic predisposition and a slow progression toward the clinical disease. Occasionally, under a variety of investigative or stressful conditions, minimal glucose intolerance may be observed. With episodes of significant stress and the associated elaboration of counter-regulatory hormones, frank glucose intolerance occurs. Ultimately, as a result of (1) lessening beta-cell function, (2) associated viral illness with possible immune response, (3) significant stress, or any combination of these factors, permanent diabetes occurs. Such a model may provide an explanation for the commonly observed remissive phase of early diabetes.

Symptoms and Signs

The earliest and most consistent symptom of IDDM is *polyuria*, resulting from the for-

mation of increased obligatory urine water, secondary to hyperglycemia and glycosuria. Occasionally, polyuria may occur even in the absence of persistent glycosuria. This situation occurs as the extracellular fluid (ECF) volume increases in response to increased plasma levels of glucose. As large amounts of water are lost in the urine, the altered osmole-to-water ratio of the ECF produces *increasing thirst*, and consequential *polydipsia*. Although *polyphagia* has been traditionally listed as one of the cardinal clinical features, it is our experience that *anorexia* is more commonly observed. This is particularly true in the younger child. Although the precise mechanism for neither symptom has been defined, the anorexia seems closely associated with the appearance and presence of ketonemia. Whatever the symptom, the result is similar: *weight loss*. Consequently, by the time of disease suspicion, the child has generally lost between 10 and 30 percent of his or her original weight and is often almost devoid of body fat.

Energy supply to insulin-dependent tissues decreases, resulting in *increased fatigue* and *decreased work or exercise capacity*. Muscle cramps commonly follow minimal activity and are a consequence of both altered energy metabolism and urinary loss of various electrolytes. These muscle cramps are frequently nocturnal.

As insulin activity further decreases and stress hormone activity rises, hyperglycemia and ketonemia become more marked. Non-insulin-dependent tissues become overloaded with glucose. Common but less characteristic symptoms are noted, including personality changes, lethargy, vision changes, altered

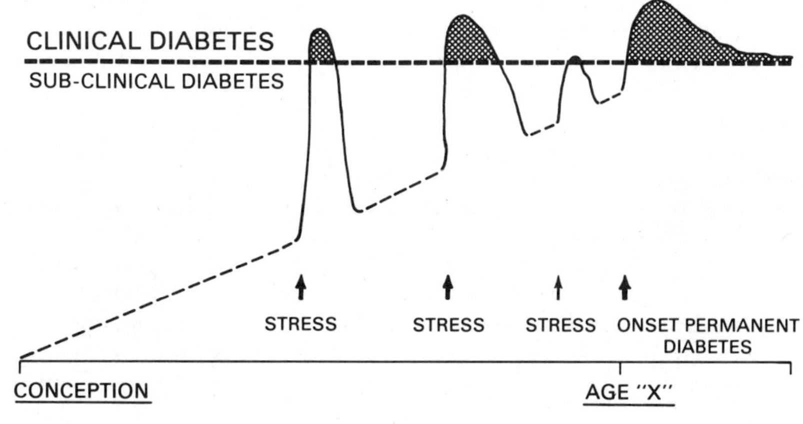

Figure 3–2. Conceptual model for the pathogenesis of Type I diabetes (IDDM). This model addresses two features: the genetic predisposition and the inciting event, the latter here depicted as "stress." Presumably, the clinical state might never evolve if the correct stimulus (incitant) were not to occur.

school and work performance, headaches, anxiety attacks, intermittent breathlessness, chest pain, abdominal discomfort and pain, nausea, and either diarrhea or constipation.

Ultimately, as the ketonemia increases, unbuffered hydrogen ion in the ECF accumulates, with development of overt *metabolic acidosis*. This produces increased rate and depth of respirations, which eventually becomes persistent (Kussmaul's respirations). Fluid loss from urination and increased respirations is cumulative, and if fluid intake is curtailed either by anorexia or by vomiting, dehydration rapidly ensues, with development of uncontrolled acidosis (diabetic ketoacidosis, or DKA). Further alterations in the level of consciousness occur, and semicoma or coma results. Occasionally, abdominal symptomatology during this period may be so marked as to suggest an acute surgical abdomen.

This sequence of symptoms may occur over a period of several months or may be compacted into a period of time of only a few days. Symptoms may be recognized so early that significant abnormalities in physical examination may be absent. If symptoms are detected later, the physical examination may then reveal weight loss, varying degrees of dehydration, tachypnea and hyperpnea, a fruit-like odor to the breath, generalized abdominal tenderness, and hepatomegaly. In this stage, the sensorium is usually depressed, and, on occasion, evidence of a cataract or peripheral neuropathy or both may be observed.

Laboratory Investigations

Studies from the laboratory usually confirm the clinical examination, with the degree of abnormality relating to the stage or severity of the clinical illness. Early in the symptomatic phase, the only abnormality observed in the laboratory may be *hyperglycemia* and *glycosuria*. The magnitude of the blood glucose elevation depends on the degree of insulin deficiency, the magnitude of glycogenolysis and gluconeogenesis, and, to a lesser extent, on earlier food intake. *Ketonemia* and *ketonuria* occur early, with the magnitude dependent on the degree of insulin dysfunction and the extent of lipolysis. Further studies to confirm the disease are not usually required, but studies of acid base homeostasis, electrolyte metabolism, and

mineral status are often obtained and reveal varying degrees of abnormality. Specifically, a glucose tolerance test is not generally necessary to confirm the diagnosis.

Hemoglobin and hematocrit values are usually increased owing to hemoconcentration, and the white blood cell (WBC) count is commonly elevated. In early phases of ketosis, the WBC is often 15,000 to 20,000 cells per cubic millimeter, but levels up to 40,000 are occasionally observed in persons with severe acidosis, even in the absence of infection. The marked increase in WBC is thought to be a reaction to stress. The urine, in addition to containing increased glucose and ketones, may also contain small amounts of protein; and pyuria without bacteriuria is common. Hyperlipidemia is commonly observed.

Laboratory studies are not often useful in either furthering the diagnosis or in benefiting management of the typical patient. On the other hand, some assessment of glucose tolerance may be necessary in the mild or early cases, in which the diagnosis is equivocal (see further on). Plasma levels of glycosylated hemoglobin (hemoglobin A_1C) are usually elevated and are often obtained as a baseline for monitoring subsequent therapy. Some diabetologists suggest that thyroid function be examined, and others feel that an assessment of thyroid antibody is useful because of the relatively high prevalence of positive results (>15 percent) and because of its association with subsequent development of hypothyroidism.

Additional studies that may be of interest but that are, at this time, of little or questionable value in management include plasma insulin levels, plasma C-peptide levels, insulin antibody studies, islet-cell antibody studies, HLA typing, and plasma levels of the various counter-regulatory hormones (glucagon, cortisol, growth hormone, catecholamines). As more information accumulates, these and other studies may take on added importance.

DIFFERENTIAL DIAGNOSES

In most instances, the diagnosis of IDDM is made on the basis of clinical presentation, laboratory studies, and absence of other conditions that could cause hyperglycemia. On occasion, however, there are problems in assigning a clinical diagnosis.

On initial examination, nonglucose meliturias must be excluded. If the urinary reducing substance is glucose, it is most likely caused by a low glucose threshold (renal glycosuria) owing to heterogeneity of the normal nephron population. Polyuria is occasionally present in patients with this condition. Renal glycosuria should not be confused with diabetes mellitus, as hyperglycemia is not a feature of this condition. The child with compulsive polydipsia may be suspected of having diabetes because of the consequential polyuria, but neither hyperglycemia nor glycosuria will be present. This is also true of the person, usually female, who has urinary frequency secondary to either vaginitis, urethritis, or cystitis.

Type II (NIDDM) diabetes mellitus can occur in childhood and may present diagnostic dilemmas for the clinician. These patients are generally obese, frequently have a positive family history of diabetes, exhibit varying degrees of hyperglycemia and glycosuria, but rarely if ever demonstrate ketonemia and ketonuria. They may have either normal or increased plasma concentrations of insulin and usually have a defect at the insulin-receptor level. Commonly, they are relatively unresponsive to exogenous insulin administration but seem to respond best to graduated weight reduction. The maturity onset diabetes of the young (MODY) has been discussed earlier. These patients are clinically similar to the person with NIDDM but are not obese and always have a strong family history of diabetes.

Type III (secondary diabetes) is the term reserved for an abnormality of glucose/insulin homeostasis that occurs in the presence of other well-recognized disorders or diseases. The designation is often arbitrary, and, whereas most patients merely demonstrate glucose intolerance, some have been associated with clinical diabetes. These have been noted in Chapter 1. Table 3–3 outlines some of the syndromes or diseases associated with glucose intolerance that have been documented in the young person.

Drug- or chemical-induced glucose intolerance must also be considered in the differential diagnoses of IDDM. Glucocorticoid administration is commonly associated with glucose intolerance and occasionally with clinical diabetes. One is often uncertain as to whether clinical diabetes has been caused by steroid administration or whether the drug has merely precipitated the appearance of the diabetes. Insulin administration may be nec-

Table 3–3. DISEASES OR SYNDROMES ASSOCIATED WITH GLUCOSE INTOLERANCE

1. Metabolic Disorders
   a. Cystic fibrosis
   b. Glycogen storage disease (Type I)
   c. Hyperlipoproteinemia (Types III, V)
   d. α-Antitrypsin deficiency
   e. Sickle cell disease
2. Obesity-Hypogonadism Syndromes
   a. Prader-Willi syndrome
   b. Laurence-Moon-Biedl syndrome
   c. Alstrom's syndrome
3. Endocrine Disorders
   a. Human growth hormone deficiency (isolated)
   b. Multiple glandular disorders
4. Neuromuscular Disorders
   a. Muscular dystrophy (Duchenne's, myotonic)
   b. Ataxia-Telangiectasia
   c. Other ataxic syndromes (Friedreich's, Huntington's)
   d. Wolfram's syndrome (DM, DI, and optic atrophy)
5. Premature Aging Syndromes
6. Lipodystrophies
7. Cytogenetic Disorders
   a. Turner's syndrome
   b. Trisomy-21 syndrome
   c. Klinefelter's syndrome
8. Miscellaneous

essary in cases of drug- or chemical-induced glucose intolerance. Ingestion of sulfa-containing diuretic agents (chlorothiazide, furosemide, and so forth) is occasionally associated with appearance of glucose intolerance. After extensive study, diphenylhydantoin has been found to produce glucose intolerance, with or without clinical diabetes, in a significant percentage of those undergoing treatment for convulsive disorders. Various epinephrine and ephedrine compounds used in the management of asthma also may precipitate mild to moderate glucose intolerance.

Various *acute poisonings* may mimic an acute diabetic state. Salicylate intoxication may be associated with hyperglycemia and glycosuria, and the initial metabolic state may mimic DKA. In general, however, the hyperglycemia is mild, and the acid-base picture is a mixed metabolic acidosis–respiratory alkalosis. We have recently seen an instance of dextroamphetamine overdosage that was associated with hyperglycemia and ketonemia in a child with a positive family history of diabetes mellitus.

IMPAIRED GLUCOSE INTOLERANCE AND GLUCOSE TOLERANCE TESTING

As indicated earlier, Type I diabetes is generally a clinical diagnosis that is merely supported by laboratory studies. Rarely is it necessary to resort to glucose tolerance testing, since the finding of fasting or postprandial hyperglycemia (or both) is sufficient to establish a diagnosis. However, there are instances when the practitioner is faced with one or more of several dilemmas: When or to whom should a glucose tolerance test be given? How should glucose tolerance be tested? How should its results be interpreted? And what is to be done with the patient once results are obtained? These questions represent valid and highly relevant concerns, for such situations are not unusual. The following example is one of many similar ones we have seen over the past 20 years:

S. R., a 7-year-old Caucasian boy was noted by his mother to be drinking more fluids than usual. The mother, having just observed an ADA commercial on TV, decided to have him checked for diabetes. Since Mrs. R. worked for a physician, she obtained blood and urine glucose oxidase strips from the office and examined the child in midafternoon. The blood glucose was estimated at between 120 mg/dl and 180 mg/dl, but the urine was negative for both glucose and ketones. She repeated the test two days later with similar results.

Mrs. R.'s employer (a physician) was consulted on a Thursday and recommended a glucose tolerance test for the following Monday. "Well-balanced" meals that excluded "a lot of starches and sugars" was recommended and given during the weekend. On Monday morning, a "standard" five-hour glucose glucose test (using 1.75 grams of glucose per kilogram of body weight) was performed, producing the following results: F–84 mg/dl, 30 min–168 mg/dl, 60 min–152 mg/dl, 90 min–136 mg/dl, 120 min–130 mg/dl, 180 min–94 mg/dl, 240 min–100 mg/dl, 300 min–82 mg/dl; with a 0.5 percent urine sugar at 60 minutes.

The boy's parents were told that the child had diabetes mellitus, and he was referred to our center for initiation of therapy and education. Additional historic interviews did not contribute significantly, and the physical examination was normal. When the blood glucose values in the fasting and postprandial states were normal on two consecutive days, the child was placed on a high-carbohydrate diet (greater than 50 per cent of calories as carbohydrates) for three days and re-examined by modified tolerance testing (see further on). The values for blood glucose at 0, 60, and 120 minutes were 60 mg/dl, 96 mg/dl, and 76 mg/dl, respectively.

Over the subsequent three years, this child has had no glycosuria on multiple testings and has grown and thrived normally; however, the diagnosis of "prediabetes" is firmly entrenched in the child's and parents' minds.

An analysis of this example will be presented later, but it is first important to lay some foundations for this analysis and to address the questions posed earlier.

Impaired glucose tolerance (IGT) is the term recommended by the National Diabetes Data Group (NDDG) for those patients who have nondiagnostic glucose level elevations found in either a fasting blood glucose test or a properly performed glucose tolerance test (GTT). Moderate abnormalities of blood glucose in the range under this heading may represent an early stage in progression toward diabetes, particularly toward NIDDM. Well-documented instances are reported in which progression to IDDM has taken place in patients over 10 to 30 years, but the frequency of this occurrence is thought to be only between 10 and 40 percent. Conversely, serial observations over 20 years have documented an absence of progression to overt diabetes in from 60 to 90 percent of patients.

The NDDG provides three other useful classifications besides IGT that enable the practitioner to label persons with glucose abnormalities more properly: Previous Abnormality of Glucose Tolerance, Gestational Diabetes, and Potential Abnormality of Glucose Tolerance. These were discussed more fully in Chapter 1.

When or to Whom Should a Glucose Tolerance Test be Given?

There is no absolute answer to this question, and a final decision must be left to the discretion of the physician. In general, the physician must assess glucose tolerance in three types of situations: (1) persons who are incidentally found to have an abnormality (that is, hyperglycemia or glycosuria); (2) the pregnant woman; and (3) members of multiplex families (that is, diabetic inheritance appearing as an autosomal dominant trait, or MODY). In the first category, a diagnosis must either be confirmed or refuted; whereas in the other two instances, there is evidence that institution of specific therapy in the asymptomatic state may prevent recognized complications.

Another situation in which the physician must contemplate an assessment of glucose tolerance is that of the sibling of a known diabetic, particularly the sibling who is found to have an identical histocompatibility haplotype. Even though such individuals are at high risk of developing diabetes mellitus, there is no evidence that the natural course of events can be altered even if the disease is recognized early. This group of children may become more important in the future.

How Should Glucose Tolerance be Tested? How Should its Results be Interpreted?

Various methods have been advocated for glucose tolerance testing, but, for routine clinical usage, recommendations of the NDDG are most useful:

The examination should be performed in an otherwise healthy person who has been free of acute illness for a minimum of two weeks and is not taking drugs known to interfere with glucose tolerance. Some examples of such drugs are: alcohol, alpha- and beta-adrenergic blockers, diuretics of the thiazide type, contraceptives containing estrogens, glucocorticoids, phenothiazides, salicylates, sympathomimetics, and theophylline. The test should be preceded by at least three days of a moderately high carbohydrate intake, since carbohydrate-deficient diets increase the likelihood of false positive results. Testing should be performed in the morning after a 10 to 12 hour fast, during which time water is permitted. The dosage of glucose recommended is 1.75 grams/kilogram of body weight, up to a maximum of 75 grams. It should be administered in a solution of glucose (or dextrose) containing a concentration of no greater than 25 grams per deciliter. Samples of blood are obtained prior to the ingestion and at regular time intervals beginning with the initiation of drinking.

Table 3–4 represents a slight modification of the recommendations of the NDDG. This modification requires only two blood samples (during fasting and two hours post-glucose-loading) as criteria for the diagnosis or exclusion of diabetes. Half-hourly sampling during the first two hours, as recommended by the NGGD, does not seem to add materially to the examination. Neither we nor the NGGD recommend testing past the two-hour period, because of variability of results and their lack of usefulness.

Reanalysis of the patient data presented earlier suggests that the early diagnosis of "diabetes mellitus" was ill advised on the basis of the results obtained and of the inappropriate preparation of the patient for examination. Based on this suggestion and on S.R.'s subsequent clinical course, it may be inaccurate even to label him as having impaired glucose tolerance.

CLINICAL COURSE

It is perhaps inappropriate even to address something as global as clinical course or natural history, for to do so implies a degree of uniformity. Figure 3–2 suggests that the natural progression of diabetes from onset is one of individual variability overlying a consistent theme. Additionally, to suggest that progression of diabetes today is "natural" would be untrue. The ordinary history of IDDM prior to the introduction of exogenous insulin therapy is in stark contrast to that influenced by current management. However, despite these forewarnings, there are some relatively consistent features that should be noted.

Period of Metabolic Recovery

The majority of patients with IDDM are symptomatic when first observed and show

Table 3–4. DIAGNOSIS OF DIABETES MELLITUS

Clinical State	Study State	Glucose Concentrations (mg/dl)		
		Venous Plasma	Venous Whole Blood	Capillary Whole Blood
Normal — Asymptomatic	Fasting	<130	<115	<115
	2 hrs pg1*	<140	<120	<140
IGT — Asymptomatic	Fasting	<140	<120	<120
	2 hrs pg1	>140	>120	>140
IDDM — Polyuria, Polydipsia Weight loss, Ketonuria	Random	>200	>200	>200
DM** — Asymptomatic	Fasting	>140	>120	>120
	2 hrs pg1	>120	>180	>200

*pg1 = post–glucose-loading, which means an oral glucose load, administered under standardized conditions of 1.75 g glucose per kilogram body weight, up to a maximum of 75 g.

**To establish the diagnosis of diabetes mellitus, the abnormal results should be obtained on more than one examination.

evidence of increased catabolism (that is, weight loss). The degree of malnutrition at this stage depends on both the severity of the disease process and its duration. Almost immediately after the introduction of insulin therapy, there is diminished catabolic activity, and a phase of anabolic activity or metabolic recovery begins. During the first days of therapy, the dosage of insulin required to initiate this reversal is variable but may be as high as 1.0 to 3.0 units per kilogram per 24 hours. In most instances, a sense of improvement or well-being is observed within the first two to three days as polyuria, polydipsia, and anorexia decrease and vitality is renewed. The young person usually demonstrates a vigorous appetite, and initial weight gain may be dramatic. Increased muscle strength is observed, but its return to preillness levels may require four to six weeks. Likewise, it is often four to six weeks before preillness weight is regained and appetite begins to diminish. By approximately six weeks after initiation of therapy, the daily insulin requirement has dropped to levels between 0.2 and 0.5 units per kilogram per day.

During the first few days of metabolic recovery, two features that are worthy of notation may occur in some persons. *Liver enlargement* with either discomfort or tenderness in the right hypogastrium may be detected. This finding is most commonly observed in patients who have had significant or prolonged ketonemia and is felt to result from the redeposition of glycogen in lipid-laden hepatocytes. *Peripheral edema* of mild to moderate degree is often noted in dependent tissues, particularly in the aftermath of treatment of ketoacidosis. Its pathogenesis is incompletely understood but results from renal sodium retention, which is felt to be related partially to earlier stimulation of the renin-angiotensin-aldosterone system by the consequences of ketoacidosis and dehydration. Variations in *visual acuity* are common, and *hair loss* is occasionally noted.

REMISSIVE PHASE

A period of significantly reduced exogenous insulin requirement occurs in 50 to 60 percent of young persons with IDDM. The first such period occurs between the second and sixth months after onset. In most instances, the dosage of insulin required to maintain euglycemia drops to levels between 0.1 and 0.4 units per kilogram per day. About 8 to 10 percent of patients may actually require little or no insulin, and there are a few reported cases in which glucose tolerance has returned to normal.

Various studies have demonstrated a return of endogenous insulin secretion as measured by the presence of plasma C-peptide concentrations, which are indicative of the pancreatic secretion of proinsulin. Precise reasons for this return of function after a period of complete absence are not completely understood. One suggestion is that there is some resolution of inflammatory changes and attendant edema within islet cells, which allows minimally injured cells to function, either partially or completely.

During this remissive phase, the patient with IDDM is usually quite sensitive to small amounts of exogenous insulin and is only partially dependent on these exogenous sources. In many instances, the beta cell seems to respond appropriately with an outpouring of insulin in response to glucose elevations following meals. Consequently, postprandial glucose surges are buffered, and "tight" control is easier to achieve. Because this phase is a time of remarkably few problems, some have referred to it as the "honeymoon" of IDDM. A number of studies have been directed toward attempts at preserving the remaining beta-cell function and prolonging the "honeymoon." The use of sulfonylureas to accomplish this has not been successful. Several investigators have reported that, by maintaining normal control of blood glucose during the first two months, they were able to extend the remission. Recently, other studies, somewhat better performed, have seemed to refute this contention, but it still remains an open question. Currently, some anecdotal reports suggest that the use of anti-inflammatory agents such as prednisone, azathioprine (Imuran), or cyclosporine in the first few weeks of diabetes may be successful in inducing and prolonging the "honeymoon." Controlled investigations must be performed prior to any routine introduction of such therapy.

In a few children who have a significant remission, the "honeymoon" is not bliss. In these patients, the secretion of endogenous insulin appears to be erratic and imprecise. This irregular pattern of insulin secretion, plus the extreme sensitivity to exogenous insulin, can cause some misery, particularly to the very young. The importance of an understanding of the possible occurrence of a remissive phase cannot be overemphasized. As insulin secretion returns and sensitivity to injected insulin is exaggerated, there is an increased likelihood of significant hypoglycemia. Insulin dosages must be reduced systematically in order to avoid this possibility.

The remissive phase lasts for a variable period of time. Based on data from C-peptide studies, a few persons with IDDM appear to continue throughout life with some, albeit minimal, endogenous insulin secretion and appear to have less difficulty with ketosis and ketoacidosis. In most patients, however, significant remission lasts only three to six months and rarely extends beyond a year. By two years' duration, the average dose of insulin has stabilized at 0.8 to 1.0 units per kilogram per day, and there are insignificant levels of C-peptide.

It has not been our practice routinely to discontinue insulin therapy in those few patients who transiently undergo complete remission. Instead, insulin dosage is reduced to its lowest possible level and maintained. These children and their families have learned good techniques, practices, and habits in the first few months of diabetes, which once interrupted, are difficult to recapture.

TOTAL DIABETIC STATE

The stage of "total" diabetes is generally thought of as that phase when endogenous insulin secretion no longer plays a significant role in glucose homeostasis. The body is then almost entirely dependent on action curves of commercial insulin and is without the benefit of a continuous glucose monitor. As expected, the ability to fine-tune such a delicate and complex system is curtailed, and the span of the undulations in blood glucose concentration increases. Because of the loss of feedback control of insulin secretion, some have labeled this stage of diabetes one of lability, whereas others have identified it as a "brittle" phase.

The increased dependence on exogenous insulin may happen gradually (over weeks to months) or there may be an abrupt changeover to dependence, usually precipitated by an infection. Figure 3–3 demonstrates this in two girls, both of whom had onsets at 9 years of age. Both girls had dramatic decreases in their exogenous insulin requirements follow-ing onset and reached levels of about 0.2 units per kilogram per day in order to maintain euglycemia. Patient L. W. had a slow and gradual increase of the need for injected insulin over a two- to three-year period, only transiently interrupted by an infection and mild ketosis after 10 months of treatment. Patient R. S., on the other hand, also had an infection at about 11 months into treatment; but following its subsidence, her dosage level remained around 1.0 unit/kg/day. Dosages of insulin in the range of 0.8 to 1.0 unit/kg/day are felt to represent the total diabetic state. At this level of exogenous insulin administration, there is virtually no C-peptide response following administration of either glucagon or a sulfonylurea.

Fluctuations in the need for insulin continue to occur, even in this total diabetic state. Some factors responsible for these variations are growth, activity, internal and environmental stresses, and the type and quantity of oral intake. Other, less well-defined factors also produce variability in the need for insulin, including insulin absorption kinetics, hepatic responsiveness, insulin antibody formation and binding, receptor binding, and postreceptor states.

Physical growth, with its attendant increase in caloric intake, is associated with increased demand for insulin. This increased need is, however, not entirely related to increased intake of food, and hormonal factors are believed to play a major role in antagonizing insulin action. At times, during the periods of rapid growth surrounding puberty, the need for insulin may reach 1.5 to 2.0 units per kilogram per day. This is most often seen in the young woman around menarche. *Activity and inactivity* also have effects on blood glucose and insulin needs. These are covered in depth in Chapter 8. Suffice it to say that in the well-controlled diabetic, there is variation in insulin demand that is often observed through differences between dosages required on weekdays versus weekends and in winter versus summer. *Stress*, both that of internal and external generation, causes elaboration of stress hormones, which antagonize insulin action. Variability in the type or quantity of *food intake* represents another common variable.

LATE NATURAL HISTORY

It is difficult to convey to the individual who has diabetes much of the group data

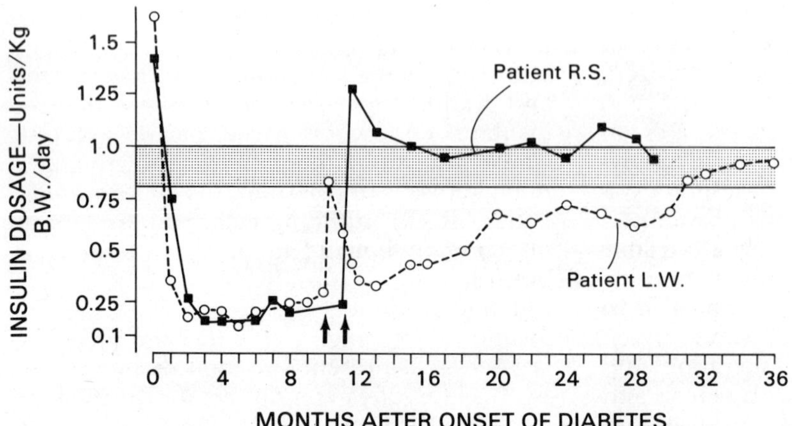

Figure 3–3. The vertical axis expresses the exogenous insulin dosage required to maintain "good" control as the number of units per kilogram of body weight. The cross-hatched area across the center depicts that level of exogenous insulin felt to represent "total replacement." This picture presents the course of two different children during their first three years of having diabetes. Both children had a remissive phase, and both eventually became total diabetics, one abruptly and the other more gradually.

accumulated over time, because many factors influence this natural chronology. Some of the elements that affect this have been alluded to earlier (that is, growth, stress, intake, hormonal factors, insulin biokinetics, and so forth); and others, such as the degree of carbohydrate control and genetic components, are discussed in greater detail in other chapters.

Based on group data, the overall outcome for patients with IDDM does not appear favorable, even though some individuals have long and uncomplicated survivals. In general, the life expectancy of the diabetic appears to be reduced by at least 25 percent compared with that of the nondiabetic. Recent studies suggest that, of those developing IDDM before age 30, only 50 percent will be alive 30 years after onset. This increased mortality appears to be true for most diabetics and is not confined only to those whose diabetes appears more serious or those who are most labile. Even those patients whose diabetes appears mild and unassociated with extreme hyperlability have a shortened lifespan when compared with the nondiabetic individual. One of the reasons why the data cannot be applied directly to the individual person with IDDM is that the degree of control of blood sugar is felt to influence longevity significantly. Other genetic factors may also play a role.

Not only the quantity but also the quality of the person's life is under assault. Complications may either directly or indirectly involve most other organ systems of the body, and derangements in organ function often lead to significant morbidity. Glucose control and other factors are felt to play a major role in the development of these complications.

4

Development of a Management Plan

Before the first patient with IDDM is seen, a most important activity must occur if care delivery is to have a reasonable chance of succeeding. The physician or team or both must decide on the general and overall management philosophy. Consideration must be given to those principles and guidelines that will be used to pilot diabetes care. An overall management plan is the desired outcome. Without such a plan, diabetes care will be erratic at best, and the patient is likely to be confused and noncompliant. Development of a plan is important even if the "team" consists only of the physician, but it becomes an absolute necessity as the size and complexity of the team increases. Nothing is more disconcerting to patients than to have their health providers disagree over issues of their health. For a more in-depth discussion, the reader is referred to Chapter 19.

What are the characteristics that all good management plans or programs have in common? Table 4–1 outlines some of the characteristics of a model management program. The plan must clearly establish operational goals and objectives. This is extremely important when there are varying opinions of current doctrine. Unless the objectives and their relative priorities are agreed on early, the team will not be able to act in harmony, thus leading to confusion and disorder. It is sufficient to say that the management program must be one that is scientifically valid

Table 4–1. **SOME CHARACTERISTICS OF MODEL MANAGEMENT PROGRAMS**

1. Identify both short-term and long-term goals and objectives.
2. Assign relative priorities to goals and objectives.
3. Provide a mechanism for addressing each goal or objective.
4. Ensure that program is based on information that is scientifically accurate and current.
5. Use technologies that are current.
6. Ensure that program is consistent, while allowing for maximum flexibility.
7. Allow for variations in response to individual patient needs.
8. Ensure that program is balanced with respect to medical needs and lifestyle demands.
9. Identify and assign responsibilities.
10. Ensure that program is reduced to its simplest components and that complexities are minimized.
11. Ensure that program has a system for self-evaluation and feedback.
12. Ensure that program is capable of change with expectation of growth.

and based on sound principles of ethical practice.

There has been an information explosion concerning diabetes and diabetes care over the past decade. It is therefore incumbent upon the physician to either possess or acquire current concepts and competencies. For example, it may have been perfectly acceptable in the 1960s or 1970s to question the role of hyperglycemia in the pathogenesis of microvascular disease. Information now exists that definitely establishes a primary association between the two. Thus, in the 1980s, it is only acceptable to debate the relative emphasis placed on the management of hyperglycemia in the overall context of diabetes. As another example, home blood glucose monitoring was not an acceptable alternative to urine testing in the 1970s. The situation is now reversed. Because of the relative infrequency of Type I diabetes, the practicing physician may have difficulty in keeping abreast of such changes in appropriate management. It may thus serve the physician well to become a member of a diabetes care team.

A management program must have a consistent theme without becoming rigid and inflexible. It is the good outcome that is important, not necessarily the method chosen. For example, although it seems apparent that a "split-mix" insulin schedule is more often associated with desired carbohydrate control than is a single dose of NPH, is it an error to continue a patient on the latter regimen if both objective and subjective monitors suggest "good" control? A management team can have a philosophy of tight control without being rigid or unyielding. Flexible schedules, geared to individual needs and desires, foster compliant behaviors.

The overall program must be one that is balanced between those needs that are predominantly medical (that is, insulin, diet, blood glucose measurements, glycosylated hemoglobins, lipid profiles, and so forth) and the lifestyle desires and demands of the patient. Attention favoring the former is often met with persistent anger, lingering patterns of denial, and, ultimately, poor adherence to medical programs. Likewise, excessive attention to lifestyle issues may suggest a lack of seriousness of the disease and lead to poor overall care. Compromises are usually necessary, on behalf of the medical team and the patient, for successful coping. The program should have sufficient scope to allow for such compromises.

CONTROL OF DIABETES

Definitions, Meanings, Inferences

The word "control," as used in the context of diabetes management, seems to have varied meanings, not only to patients but also to professionals. As the word appears to be intended, it means the regulation or direction of the diabetic state. It implies that there is an ability or power that one must, or should, possess, presumably to overcome some lack of direction or regulation. Many young persons with diabetes, particularly adolescents, resent the implication that they might be "out-of-control." "Control" in this age group is closely allied to such issues as independence/dependence or power/impotence—all very important to the adolescent. The fact that the accepted antonym of control is "freedom" lends support to this idea.

In younger children, and occasionally in older persons, there is confusion about what it means to be "in control." Many of these patients, having an external locus of control, feel subordinate to their diabetes, feel that their lives are "controlled" by their disease. Although perhaps not intended to be so, diabetes is the single focal point in the lives of many patients and their families.

In their consideration of this issue of control, professionals are often torn between what can be judged ideal and what might be deemed practical. Ideal is defined as "perfect, or exactly as one would wish," and there is no question but that the compassionate professional would desire this for those under his or her care. "Ideal" control of diabetes is not, at this time, achievable for the vast majority of persons with Type I diabetes. Although precise regulation of carbohydrate metabolism is obtainable for short periods while the patient is on a glucose-controlled, insulin-infusion (closed loop) pump and in a few patients following transplantation, could anyone be so naive as to suggest that these therapies are "ideal?" Thus, although continued search for idealized therapy is important, the technology is not at present available to offer this to patients, even as an option.

At the opposite extreme is the issue of practicality, simply defined as being "concerned or dealing realistically or sensibly with everyday activities or conditions." But who defines what is realistic or sensible? Home blood glucose monitoring would not have seemed realistic in the early 1970s, but technology has made it so today. I would not have felt it realistic in the 1960s to start all patients on two or more shots per day, would not have felt it sensible in the 1970s to suggest that teenagers may prefer blood testing to urine testing, and would not have felt it realistic in the late 1970s and early 1980s to suggest that 5-year-olds could be successfully managed by insulin pumps. Time and experience have shown that what is "practical" is ever-changing. If professionals aim only for what is felt to be currently practical, then, overall, the health of persons with diabetes will not be improved.

This then is one of the compromises that must be reached in preparing for the care of the diabetic: setting high standards (close to "ideal") and balancing these against what the patient and family find are practical. In this book, we will use the term *optimal* (that is, "the best or most favorable") to indicate this balanced pragmatism. For control to be optimal, the care delivered must be optimal.

Control of What? And Why?

Obviously, the aim of optimal diabetes care should be to restore and maintain metabolic balance to the degree that all parameters of measurement will be similar to those of the nondiabetic. Later in this chapter and in Chapter 5, we will consider goals and those parameters by which goals can be measured. In Chapter 18, we will look at specific long-term complications and their probable relations to control. At this point, however, it seems prudent to view the issues at hand in a more global fashion and, perhaps, to reach a consensus about the reasons for controlling diabetes.

That there are both acute and chronic complications of the diabetic state and that these complications contribute to diabetic morbidity and mortality are not debatable. What has been a point of some contention and controversy for the past five decades is the precise relationship of the metabolic and physiologic abnormality of diabetes to the anatomic and pathologic entity of longstanding disease. One group has been adamant that there is a cause-and-effect relationship between the two and has stated further that the degree of abnormality (as measured by blood glucose) correlates highly with the presence or absence of long-term pathologic conditions. This group became subscribers to a school of rigid management, advocating tight control of diabetes in order to modify future complications. Another group was less certain of the close correlation between blood glucose control and degenerative changes. This group felt that the many "exceptions" to such a correlation provided evidence that other factors, perhaps genetic, were involved. In the early 1960s, such evidence was pre-

sented by one of the better investigative teams in this country, which demonstrated that muscle capillary basement membrane thickening in the patient with diabetes was genetically determined and bore little relationship to glucose control. This excellent study, although subsequently proven to be in error owing to technical and methodologic problems, seemed to provide scientific validity to this viewpoint. Since it was known that the ability to control diabetes tightly was extremely difficult and it was recognized that many with diabetes fared poorly under this rigid discipline, a school of "reasonable" or "acceptable" care was born. Those caregivers were termed "loose controllers" by those of the more rigid discipline. In actuality, however, no one believed in loose control, only in degrees of "tightness."

Evidence accumulated over the past 15 years has generally tended to support the concept of a direct correlation between blood glucose control and the presence or absence of certain chronic complications: microvascular disease, neuropathy, cataracts, delayed growth. Studies in experimental animals are the most convincing, but some short-term studies in humans have also strongly suggested this association. The expected has happened: the ranks of those physicians assigned earlier to the "loose" camp have shrunk, and the "tight" controllers have become more rigid in their management philosophies. Are these outcomes justifiable?

That current evidence suggests a direct relationship between diabetic control and long-term complications is not now in contention, but there are major questions that remain unanswered. Some of these are:

1. Why do only 30 to 50 percent of persons with Type I diabetes develop clinical nephropathy?
2. Why do 20 to 30 percent of diabetics, regardless of control, not develop significant retinopathy?
3. Why do some persons with apparently good control develop early and severe microvascular complications?
4. Does the finding of limited joint mobility merely indicate patients in poor control, or is it a marker of those in whom blood glucose elevations will produce complications?

As indicated earlier, current studies seem to indicate that Type I diabetes is a syndrome, rather than a disease. If this is so, are there subtypes of the syndrome in which blood glucose elevations are uniquely pathogenic? Are there other subtypes in which the risk of chronic hyperglycemia is less? Research over the next decade will surely answer some of these questions and perhaps allow us to be more specific as to whom we treat "tightly."

For now, the only aspect of the diabetic state that appears manageable is the degree of hyperglycemia. In the absence of evidence indicating a nonharmful effect of such blood glucose elevations, the prudent physician must consider it an obligation to control diabetes as well as possible.

How Tight Is Tight?

Teleologically, it must be assumed that the extremely narrow range of glucose excursion in the nondiabetic individual is important to long-term preservation of the species. If the evolutionary process had indicated that a mean blood glucose of 200 mg/dl or a glucose excursion of 150 mg/dl were desirable, such would most certainly have occurred. Thus, although there is no evidence available to date that states that a certain level of hyperglycemia is more or less harmful than another, it does appear wise to consider the normal range of glucose as a target; an appropriate amount of pragmatism will determine the "hit" on this target.

GOALS OF MANAGEMENT

Table 4–2 outlines the overall goals used in the Childtren's Diabetes Management Center in Galveston. The items under heading I are generally short-term goals that, it is hoped, will allow those items listed later (headings II through IV) to prevail as natural occurrences. This outline thus is based on certain presumptions, the most significant of which is that control of carbohydrate metabolism will either enable certain outcomes (that is, prevent complications, allow normal statural growth) or will not interfere with the normal occurrence of other developmental processes (that is, allow normal psychosocial development). Consequently, the discussion in the remainder of this section will return to the subject of control and consider these short-term aspects.

Table 4–2. OVERALL GOALS OF MANAGEMENT

I. "Control" of Carbohydrate Metabolism, to Maximum Degree Possible
- A. Good health
  - Freedom from most symptoms
  - Feels and looks as good as most nondiabetic peers
- B. Normal functional capacity
  - Able to compete on functional level with peers
  - Normal school or work attendance
- C. Regulation of biochemical markers
  - Blood (or urine) sugars as near nondiabetic as possible
  - Blood glucose values 80 to 150 on >75% of checks
  - Glycosylated hemoglobin as near nondiabetic as possible (see text)
  - Lipid profile normal
- D. Adaptive coping pattern that is successful

II. Normal Growth, Development, Maturation
- A. Optimum statural growth
  - Normal linear growth
  - Normal height/weight ratio
  - Normal physical potential
- B. Optimum psychosocial development
  - Achieve intellectual and behavioral potential
  - Attain maturity of mind and thought
  - Preparation for "leaving home'

III. Prevention of Significant Acute Complications
IV. Delay or Prevention of Chronic Complications
- A. Microvascular disease
- B. Neuropathy
- C. Hyperlipidemia
- D. Macrovascular disease

Good Health

This is the first and most important aspect of control. Patients who feel poorly because of their diabetes are in poor control, regardless of what other markers demonstrate. Basically, the well-controlled patient with diabetes should have few symptoms that are directly attributable to the disease. On the other hand, this well-controlled patient may have and often does have symptoms that are attributable to the disease management (for example, hypoglycemia). Specifically, it should be realized that it is difficult to control hyperglycemia adequately without producing some hypoglycemia. As Service, Molnar, and associates (1970) and others have demonstrated, when one lowers the zenith of blood glucose excursion, the nadir is also lowered. It is hoped that the number and degree of hypoglycemic episodes will be minimal.

It is important for the diabetic individual to recognize that the human body is quite adaptable and that after a long period of poor control, the person may "feel well" and have blood glucose values ranging between 300 mg/dl and 600 mg/dl. Such persons may transiently feel worse when attempts are made to achieve normal glucose levels. The converse is also often seen. Young persons may say they "feel good," because of the comparatively poor way they felt just days earlier. Sometimes they recognize "poor health" only when a noticable change is effected. Only after an adjustment period will "feeling better" occur. Thus, feeling well is not *the* criterion of good control; it is *one* criterion.

Normal Functional Capacity

The person with IDDM should be able to function in a daily capacity that is equivalent to those of nondiabetic peers. School or job attendance of the person with controlled diabetes should be no different from average attendance of the healthy person. Some studies in the person with poorly controlled IDDM have suggested a significant decrease in work performance, but this appears reversible with adequate blood glucose control and proper conditioning. A feeling or expression of fatigue is common during childhood, particularly during adolescence. Thus, such a feeling may have little to do with diabetes control. On the other hand, diabetes is frequently suspected or incriminated as a causative factor, with the occurrence of almost any symptom.

Similar to the situation with healthy attitudes, the ability to perform "normally" does not by itself demonstrate adequate carbohydrate control. Some persons with chronic hyperglycemia are able to compete with nondiabetic individuals. On the other hand, a number of young persons with diabetes demonstrate improved performance when blood glucose values are normalized.

Regulation of Biochemical Markers

For persons with diabetes to be truly "in control," it is important for them to feel well, function normally, and have their biochemical monitors as near normal as is feasible. This we call optimal control. For an in-depth review of these biochemical monitors, the reader is referrred to Chapter 5. At this point, it is sufficient to discuss these only briefly.

Home Blood Glucose Monitoring

This is the best formative testing of diabetes control that is available. Patients are asked to monitor themselves two to five times per day and to keep precise records. Our objective for most patients is to aim for values between 60 to 150 mg/dl, and we consider glucose control to be successful if 75 percent of the values fall within this range. Children and their parents are taught to use consistent patterns of glucose control (that is, all blood glucose levels before lunch, or all blood glucose levels before bedtime, and so forth) to judge needs for change in treatment modalities (see Chapter 6). As will be noted later, we do not ordinarily recommend that supplemental doses of regular insulin be given to lower glucose levels unless there are associated symptoms. This seems to be treating after the fact. It seems to make more sense to observe for patterns of hyperglycemia and make alterations in the program of usual insulin doses so as to prevent hyperglycemia. Insulin doses are altered downward if the frequency of hypoglycemia becomes unacceptable.

Urine Glucose Determinations

Despite their known inaccuracies, urine sugar estimates will remain one of the formative markers in selected patients in the near future. When used, it is important for the patient to be certain of the renal threshold for glucose. Even then, it is perhaps best to use periodic blood glucose values as backups to urine testing. If the renal threshold is normal, then it seems appropriate to aim for virtually all urine determinations in the aglycosuric, or "negative," range. If unacceptable hypoglycemia occurs (unacceptable either in frequency or in degree), then reduction in the frequency of aglycosuria becomes necessary.

Glycosylated Hemoglobin (Hg A_{1C})

These determinations are generally measured at three- to four-month intervals and provide information concerning the average blood glucose concentration over the preceding 6- to 12-week period. This is an objective test that is not easily manipulated and that does provide good summative data. The values obtained are laboratory and method specific and must relate to each laboratory's individual internal controls. Our laboratory currently dialyzes the red cells to remove "sticking" of glucose to the membrane and then performs values by the microcolumn method. With this technique our mean values for the nondiabetic person are 5.2 percent (3.2 to 6.1 percent). It is our belief that "acceptable" levels for the patient with diabetes are up to 50 percent above the mean normal value: in our case, up to 7.8 percent.

A Successful Adaptive Coping Pattern

This allows incorporation of diabetes into the patient's lifestyle and increases patient adherence. Such a coping pattern is usually learned from parents but also can be taught by qualified clinicians. Early in the course of diabetes care, this is one of the major areas of importance that the diabetes team must consider. Adequate coping is one of the keys to successful management and will later be discussed in greater detail.

INDIVIDUALIZING GOALS AND OBJECTIVES

Individualization of goals and objectives is extremely important to diabetes care. All persons with diabetes are similar, but also they have distinct differences that mandate a tailoring of treatment programs to specific needs. Some factors that must be considered in individualization of care are noted in Table 4–3 and are arbitrarily divided according to those related to the child, to the family, and to the disease.

The Child

The chronologic and developmental age of the child is an extremely important factor in the individualization of diabetes care. The youth 14 years old must be considered differently from a 6-year-old or a child of 2. Whereas the 14-year-old might be effectively treated by a very tight control concept, the 6-year-old would not initially perform as well under such control, owing to differences in his or her functional level. The 2-year-old, on the other hand, would be placed at con-

Table 4–3. FACTORS TO BE CONSIDERED WHEN INDIVIDUALIZING GOALS OR OBJECTIVES

A. The Child
Age of onset of diabetes
Current age and development
Cognitive level
Emotional and behavioral development
Other illnesses or conditions (stressors)
B. The Family
Cognitive functioning
Supportiveness
Judgment
Other stresses
Prior coping abilities
C. The Disease
Its response to "standard" care
Acceptable
Unacceptable
Degree of lability
Complicating factors
Stage of the disease

siderable risk of hypoglycemia and brain injury by this same program of rigid control.

The cognitive functioning of the child is an important factor, as is the child's emotional and behavioral development. Consideration must be given to whether the child is capable of recognizing problems and of responding appropriately. Attempts at extremely tight control in the young child often fosters parental overprotectiveness, which may compromise the child's maturation.

The presence of other conditions or illnesses may also influence decisions regarding diabetes care. The two most commonly noted are asthma and convulsive disorders. The mere management of asthma may seriously compromise care of diabetes, as both the stress of the illness and the anti-insulin effect of asthma medications come into play. The presence of a convulsive disorder may cause the physician to alter plans of rigid control, for fear that hypoglycemia may trigger such attacks.

The Family

How well the family functions is a key to tailoring diabetes therapy. An extremely intelligent, well-motivated, and stable family can function in a true partnership role; but others, less endowed, cannot assume the degree of responsibility necessary for extremely tight control. Some families handle diabetes superbly and integrate it into their family life in a nondisruptive style. Others, particularly those that are dysfunctional, have considerable problems in even ensuring that the child eats well and takes the prescribed dosages of insulin. Even well-functioning families intermittently have difficulties, particularly when other stresses are present. Such things as parental or sibling illness and financial distress may transiently compromise care, thus calling for some changes in the management program.

The Disease

As noted in an earlier chapter, IDDM is not a single disease but a syndrome that comprises a relative to absolute deficiency in insulin secretion and a resulting glucose intolerance. The degree of the defect varies; thus, acceptable management must vary. The response of the body to exogenous insulin is not always the same, and variations in therapy may be dictated by alterations in the state of the disease. If the patient does not respond to standard care, other options must be explored. An example of this is seen in the following patient:

K.Q. had onset of IDDM at 6 years of age. His parents, both highly intelligent and supportive persons, immediately went through a comprehensive educational program and began to institute excellent care. During the first 18 months of disease, K.Q. was on two shots per day of NPH/Regular. His dosage initially dropped to a low of 0.12 unit per kilogram per day and then rose by 11 months to 0.76 units per kilogram per day, where it stabilized for the next seven months. Home blood glucose monitoring (HBGM) revealed fasting levels of 60 to 110 mg/dl and postprandial levels of 80 to 165 mg/dl. Glycosylated hemoglobin values ranged from 6.8 percent to 9.1 percent (normal 5 to 7 percent). At 19 months' duration, the patient developed "viral gastroenteritis," with vomiting, diarrhea, fever, and abdominal pain and was admitted elsewhere for intravenous fluids. He did not become ketotic during this episode. Following the subsidence of the virus, K.Q.'s blood sugar control became erratic, and multiple changes in insulin regimen failed to restore control. He experienced intermittent diabetic ketoacidosis (DKA) and was hospitalized twice more for its treatment. Various insulin regimens were of no apparent avail.

K.Q. was started on an external insulin pump and rapidly improved. After three weeks of this therapy, he was again euglycemic and was switched to a three shot per day regimen to mimic pump therapy. Ketosis rapidly recurred and was interrupted again with pump therapy. After three

---

Table 4–4. KEYS TO SUCCESSFUL MANAGEMENT

I. Initiate Proper Management Philosophy *Early*
  Incorporation of diabetes into lifestyle
  Establish long-term goals
  Establish short-term objectives

II. Conduct a Comprehensive Educational Program
  Personalize care to individual child and family
  Establish clear areas of responsibility
  Establish mutual respect and trust (a partnership)
  Establish ongoing educational and support program

III. Transfer Responsibility to Patient and Family
  Maintain a senior partner/junior partner relationship
  Base degree of patient and family responsibility on their attributes and abilities

IV. Provide for Emergency Consultation and Care
  Someone with similar philosophy or beliefs
  Provide 24-hour/day access to someone qualified (preferably the above)

V. Provide for Periodic Evaluation and Reappraisal
  Review successes by providing reinforcement or rewards
  Review failures by providing empathy and re-education

VI. Provide Opportunity for Program Re-Evaluation
  Based on changing knowledge
  Based on changing technology
  Based on changed lifestyle

---

other attempts to remove the pump were unsuccessful, a decision was made to continue and the patient returned to his preillness health.

Numerous studies on this young boy have failed to reveal a cause for the sudden loss of control and subsequent lability of his diabetes. Despite his young age, it was felt necessary to institute pump therapy; and its results have been spectacular, even if they still do not reveal the mechanism of the altered glucose dynamics.

KEYS TO SUCCESSFUL MANAGEMENT

Successful management of a young person with diabetes is difficult to accomplish, but with an appropriate blending of planning, skill, and providence it is achievable. Table 4–4 itemizes six major categories that we have found to be important.

Early Initiation of Management Philosophy

This is extremely important in setting the tone and tempo for long-term care. Diabetes must be incorporated into the patient's lifestyle, and the medical team must assist in this endeavor. Long-term goals are essential for the caregivers, but short-term goals are more timely for the patient. These must be negotiated goals that are shared with the patient, and they must be constantly updated so as to ensure their relative importance.

Comprehensive Educational Program

A comprehensive educational program (Chapter 10) does much more than teach knowledge and skills about diabetes care. In the early stages the program provides empathetic support and either aids in adaptive coping or teaches new strategies for dealing with life stresses, including those of diabetes. Survival skills are introduced and are ultimately followed by the learning of new knowledge and refined skills. Diabetes is gradually introduced into the patient's and the patient's family's lifestyle. Parents and children are taught, when possible, to assume a responsible role in the overall management program. As far as it is possible and reasonable to do so, patients and their families begin to make judgments on major matters of day-to-day care. Areas of patient responsibility are developed, and the child or parent or both become partners with the diabetes team they are working with.

Transfer of Responsibility

Some responsibilities are assumed by every patient and his or her family initially as they depart from the hospital. These are survival skills: How to monitor, how to give insulin, how to plan meals as they relate to insulin timing, how to recognize trouble (that is, hypoglycemia, ketonemia); how to appropriately manage hypoglycemia; and how to contact the diabetes team. For some, this is the extent of patient involvement that will be possible. But for many others, the intelligence, judgment, and willingness of the family and patient to participate can be translated into a good partnership.

The responsibilities allowed the patient and family will depend on a variety of factors such as age, cognitive and physical abilities, and the willingness to assume some personal care responsibilities. It will also depend on how willing the physician and diabetes team is to relinquish certain responsibilities and to allow the patient and family as a unit to become a partner. Some patients or families or both actively resist this role and prefer, instead, to have the physician or diabetes team act as director rather than advisor and facilitator. At one time or another, the competent physician will function in each of these roles.

In deciding on the responsibilities of the patient and family, there are certain factors that should be considered: family dynamics (strength, supportiveness); the patient's and family's overall attitudes about the illness and its management; their demonstrated abilities to carry through on assigned duties or tasks; how well other non-diabetic-related situations are going in their lives; and assessment of their skills in logical thinking and problem solving. When these are mixed with the proper proportions of intuition and luck, the outcome can be a truly rewarding united experience.

Provisions for Emergency Consultation

Unfortunately, diabetes management is a 24-hour-a-day, seven-day-a-week undertaking. The physician or full-time diabetes team member must be available to the patient and his or her family at all times. It is not sufficient to have someone to "sign out to," unless that person's philosophy of care and expertise is equal to those of the primary team. Otherwise, confusion tends to arise, and problems soon begin to occur. The 24-hour contact does not necessarily have to be in person and is often by phone, but such contact saves countless unnecessary visits and hospitalizations. It also works wonderfully to provide relief from anxiety.

Provision for Evaluation and Reappraisal

The results of the care program (the short- and long-term goals) must be periodically evaluated in a structured format. If this is not done, the patient or family or both will soon either lose interest or begin to make inappropriate decisions. Some tangible rewards must be made for successes, whereas re-education becomes the (intangible) reward for failures.

Provision for Program Re-evaluation

This is a vital part of any successful program that must continue to increase its sophistication with time and to reflect full knowledge of all new and innovative ideas or technologies or both. Also, as family lifestyles change, the program must be altered to afford practical, germane care.

SUMMARY

Planning the management program in advance of the first patient pays off with many dividends over the years of practice. But the single, most important ingredient of a good program is the ability and willingness of its professional participants to be periodically introspective and to look at its goals and objectives in the light of new information, new technologies, and changing lifestyles.

If excellent diabetes control is the target, then there must be careful attention given to all aspects of care. From a physiologic standpoint, this means (1) deliberate mindfulness of the dietary program, (2) vigilant observance of an exercise program, and (3) an orderly and thoughtful examination of various insulin regimens to determine the one best suited to the patient. Even if this is accomplished, the patient and the patient's family must also be able to modify or manipulate the various components of therapy in an effort to reach predefined goals. The next few chapters will deal with some of these individual aspects, but the real key for the patient and family will be the ability to integrate the various facets and to incorporate them into a meaningful life. Everything must be put into the context of the dual goals of management: to improve the quality of life and to increase longevity.

5

Monitoring Results of Management

Once a therapeutic management plan has been initiated, monitors must be determined to evaluate the plan's effectiveness. Regarding the child with IDDM, health providers occasionally place an inordinate emphasis on biochemical measures, even to the point of altering therapy on the basis of a single blood glucose determination. It is important to keep in perspective the concept of the "child with diabetes" versus the "diabetic child" (Fig. 5–1). The latter is dominated by shots, blood or urine tests, HbA_{1C} levels, dietary exchanges, and hypoglycemia; the former is concerned with school, friends, play, and maturation but also needs to do a few additional things in order to feel well in the presence of a chronic illness. Thus, children with good control of their diabetes may be defined as (1) those who feel well and who verbally and behaviorally convey this feeling of well-being to others, (2) those who feel that they are doing well with their personal lives, (3) those who function at the level of peers as evidenced by participation in age-related activities and appropriate school attendance, (4) those who show normal statural and emotional growth, and (5) those who show appropriate biochemical control. Too often, biochemical control is the major focus of the physician, child, and parents. Cer-

tainly, monitors of biochemical control are important but not to the exclusion of other measures of control. The child who experiences three or four hypoglycemia reactions a day (even if mild to moderate in degree) and who has normal growth and a HbA_{1C} of 6.0 percent is not necessarily in good control; this child may not feel well, because control may be too rigid. This child may not be allowed (by parents, teachers, coaches, and so forth) to function as his or her peers function, for fear of the consequences of more unrestricted behavior.

Measures that are currently used to monitor management are listed in Table 5–1. First listed are those monitors that are common to all children, followed by those specific for diabetes.

MONITORS COMMON TO ALL CHILDREN

It is important that all children have a sense of well-being in order for them to interact with their peers and have normal developmental and psychosocial growth. Data concerning healthy feelings are best obtained initially in conversations with the child and his or her parents; inquiries about

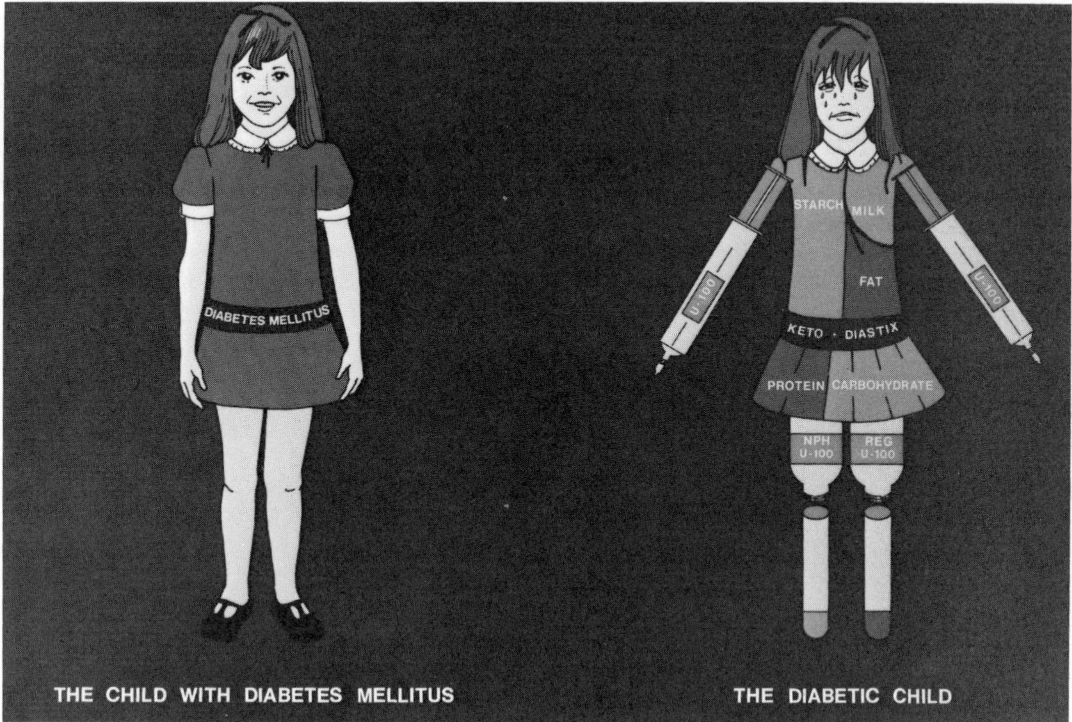

Figure 5–1. This illustration, which the author (LBT) originally designed in 1968, is still relevant today. The child with diabetes (left) represents how we wish such persons to be and to view themselves. But when professionals use the adjective "diabetic" to describe such persons, there is small wonder that many children see themselves as a composite of what they feel is the disease itself.

Table 5–1. MONITORS OF MANAGEMENT

Those Common to All Children

1. Good Health
   Feeling well
   Conveying sense of well-being
2. Appropriate Functioning
   Enjoying normal peer relations
   Participating in age-related activities
   Good school or job attendance
   Appropriate number of outpatient visits to health provider
   Few hospitalizations
3. Statural Growth
4. Weight
5. Behavioral, Psychologic, and Social Development
6. Sexual maturation

Those Specific to Children with Diabetes

1. Incorporation of Diabetes into Everyday Living
   Demonstrating age-appropriate cognition
   Demonstrating age-appropriate skills
   Demonstrating age-appropriate judgments
2. Adherence to Most Medical Regimens
3. Use of Appropriate Biochemical Markers of Carbohydrate Control
   Monitoring blood or urine sugar on a regular schedule
   Measuring glycosylated hemoglobin
   Recording results properly

school, activities, and friends not only may identify areas of potential concern but also may help establish bonding between physician and child. Problems or items of concern may or may not be related to diabetes, and it is essential that the child and parent understand and be able to differentiate between those that are and those that are not diabetes associated. The child with diabetes is subject to all the maturational problems and stresses that the nondiabetic child experiences. However, such stresses in the diabetic may manifest themselves as fluctuations in blood sugar, thus becoming a "diabetic problem." It is essential that the primary problem be identified; otherwise, management will be poorly directed. During this initial period of conversation, the skilled interviewer can also acquire some feeling about emotional and psychosocial development, learn about parent-child interrelationships, and obtain other valuable information concerning the family.

Statural Growth

A more objective clinical measure that is essential for every child is the acquiring and plotting of growth data. Linear growth is a reliable indicator of health status and may provide useful estimates of biochemical control. Growth is a complex process with numerous requirements, including a fine interplay between insulin and other growth-promoting hormones; yet the association between blood glucose control and normal growth is not clearly defined. The classic, monozygotic-twin studies conducted by Tattersall and Pyke (1973) demonstrated that the diabetic twin does not ordinarily achieve the same height as the nondiabetic twin. Anecdotal data from various clinics have demonstrated conflicting reports. Investigation of children with IDDM who have grown poorly reveals that a higher percentage have demonstrated overall evidence of maintaining poor control during critical growing years. On the other hand, initial observation of those diabetics with poor control reveals that a higher percentage will have grown normally in contrast to the few who have had significant delay. Likewise, there are some diabetic persons with significant growth delay who have exhibited excellent blood glucose control.

Evidence that poor carbohydrate control and failure to maintain normal linear growth are sometimes associated is shown graphically in Figure 5–2 and in the following case analysis:

P.A. was diagnosed as having IDDM at 6.4 years, and, at that time, was in approximately the 30th percentile for height and the 50th percentile for weight. From age of onset until approximately 8 years of age, the boy's control was rated as "good," and there were no hospitalizations. Beginning at 8 years of age, family turmoil became more intense, culminating in parental divorce when P.A. was 9 years old. Between 8.3 years and 10.5 years of age, the boy was hospitalized for DKA on 16 occasions, and he was constantly hyperglycemic and frequently ketonuric. His weight fell, and as his linear growth rate diminished his height fell below the fifth percentile.

A better degree of carbohydrate control was established at about 10.5 years of age, soon after P.A.'s mother remarried and family dynamics stabilized. Between the ages of 10.5 and 12.5 years, his growth paralleled the fifth percentile, but catch-up growth did not occur. An external insulin pump was instituted at age 12.5, and diabetic control subsequently improved markedly with HbA_{1c} dropping to 7.5 percent. Some catch-up growth was then observed.

Certainly, this boy's linear growth seems temporally related to his level of carbohydrate control. Controlled studies in several centers have suggested that an accelerated growth rate is frequently associated with excellent carbohydrate control.

In the years following introduction of insulin therapy, control of diabetes was often poor, and the Mauriac syndrome (growth retardation, sexual infantilism, hyperlipidemia, and hepatic dysfunction) was commonly seen and was felt to be the result of this poor control. In those early years of insulin therapy, one author reported that 16 percent of patients with IDDM had final heights that were greater than two standard deviations below the mean. A later study demonstrated that only 1.5 percent of children with IDDM were growth retarded at the time of school entry. Laron and associates (1977) found a positive correlation between growth velocity and normal glucose concentrations in only 5 of 25 children who had been followed for 3 to 12 years. These investigators did find an association between insulin dose and growth; catch-up growth in the prepubertal group was associated with a daily insulin dose of more than 200 units/m² (0.67 unit/kg/day) and in the pubertal group with a mean dose of more than 400 units/m² (1.3 units/kg/day). They postulated that those patients with higher insulin levels had lower blood sugars and thus were in better biochemical control.

Studies conducted in our laboratory on a number of growth-retarded children with IDDM have generally shown poor glucose control, decreased levels of somatomedin C, and elevated plasma concentrations of cortisol and growth hormone. The elevated levels of cortisol are in the range that has been shown to retard linear and organ growth in experimental animal studies. It is our assumption that this stress hormone elevation is either directly or indirectly related to retarded linear development. Rudolf and associates (1982) have reported that significant increases in growth velocity (5.3 ± 2.2 cm/year to 9.4 ± 3.9 cm/year) could be achieved in adolescents through intensive insulin therapy. The growth velocity increase has been accompanied by an increase in somatomedin C levels. These findings lend credence to the case study described previously and further suggest a direct relationship between diabetes control and growth. How this interplay works remains undefined; but it should be emphasized that normal physical growth is important to both the physical and emotional functioning of all children. It must

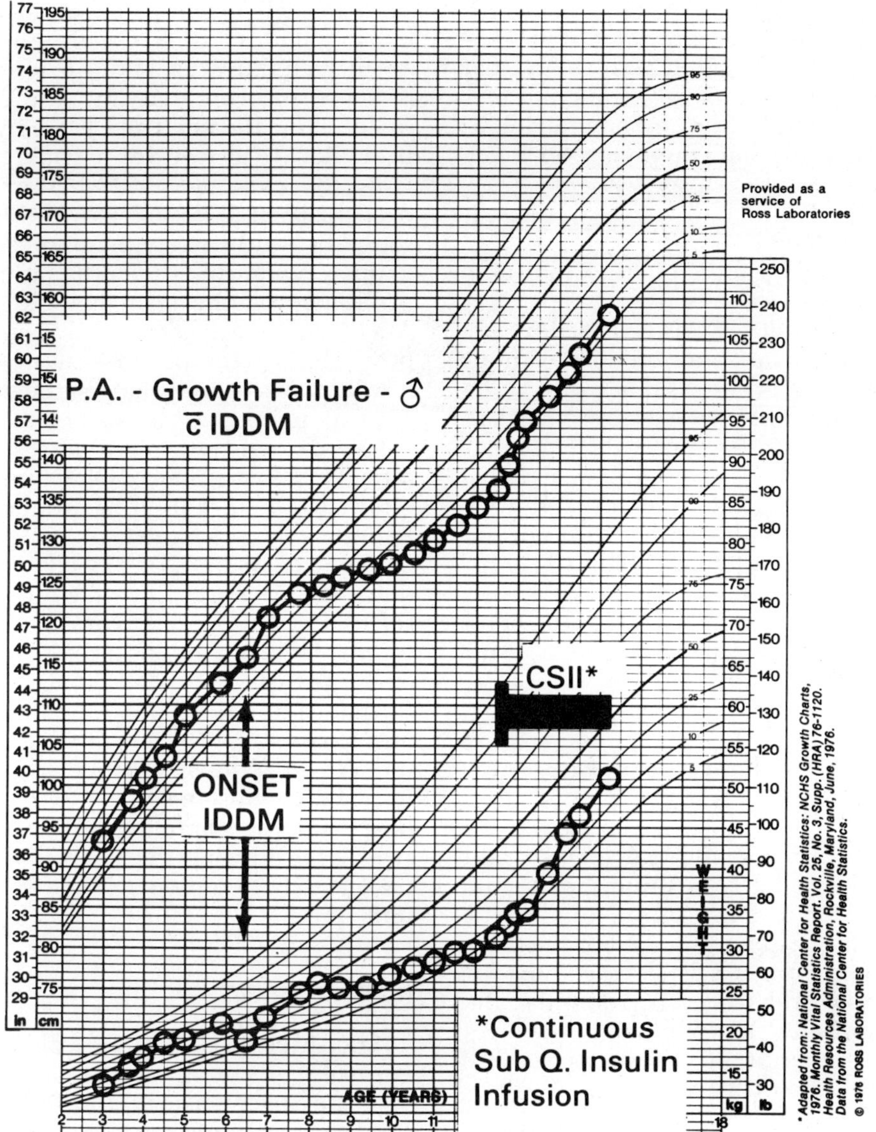

Figure 5–2. Growth chart on patient P.A. (See text for discussion of growth rates relative to diabetic control).

be one criterion for evaluating the adequacy of management.

Sexual Maturation

Sexual development must also be assessed periodically and should be found to be progressing normally. Puberty may be delayed in the individual with poorly controlled diabetes. Again, the precise mechanism in unknown, but, presumably, decreased insulin levels and hyperglycemia are either directly or indirectly involved in the pathogenesis. Laron (1975) reported that the level of insulin received was directly related to the onset of menarche in the adolescent girls he studied, all requiring more than 1.3 units per kilogram per day.

Weight

This variable represents another monitor of control of diabetes. Acute loss of weight may indicate hyperglycemia with glycosuria and be due to loss of a significant number of calories in the urine. Some teenage girls purposely undercontrol their diabetes by decreasing insulin dosage in order to achieve weight control without reduction in dietary intake. This is acknowledged by some patients only when confronted with the factual evidence of marked hyperglycemia and elevated levels of glycosylated hemoglobin. Other patients are sometimes not so lucky and thereby develop ketosis, with its consequences of abdominal discomfort, nausea, vomiting, and dehydration.

Excessive weight gain is another indicator of problems, and its causative factors must be explored. Most often, this is caused purely and simply by dietary indiscretion, without hidden meanings; but occasionally it may be symptomatic of significant stress, problems at home, depression, or even the development of hypothyroidism. At other times, particularly if the weight gain is associated with "good" blood glucose levels and with normal levels of glycosylated hemoglobin, it may indicate that the dosage of insulin is too high and that control is too tight or that the child is attempting to manage the diabetes with insulin alone.

Behavioral, Psychologic, and Social Development

Attaining normal emotional growth and stable peer relations is as important to the child with diabetes as it is to the nondiabetic child. The physician and the health team are obligated to monitor this aspect carefully, for there are powerful forces surrounding the child with diabetes that might otherwise retard normal maturation. These aspects are covered in detail in Chapter 9.

MONITORS SPECIFIC TO CHILDREN WITH DIABETES

Incorporation of Diabetes into Daily Living

If, as suggested earlier, one of the primary goals is to foster the concept of a child who merely has diabetes, rather than a diabetic who happens to be a child, then some measurement of how well the person incorporates diabetes into his or her daily life is essential. Young persons must learn to balance the demands of their personal lives with the demands of their diabetes. They must be helped to recognize that such balancing is neither easy nor unexpected—only necessary. The physician or diabetes team or both must spend conversational time inquiring about such things as: How the morning snack is being incorporated into the school program? How the child reacts when the child's peers decide to stop for a "Coke and fries?" How the child decides whether or not to participate in athletics? How the young person copes with overnight parties? And with dating? Only by methodic and emphatic prodding will the team be able to discover whether diabetes is truly being incorporated properly into the person's life. Occasionally, it will be discovered that the person is being "incorporated into" his or her diabetes.

In order for the child to integrate diabetes into daily living, he or she must have the knowledge and skills appropriate to the task. As indicated in Chapter 10, education is one of the cornerstones of diabetic care; but the outcome measurement of education is performance, and performance must be monitored. Cognitive abilities can be evaluated by either verbal or written testing, whereas performance of skills is best monitored by auditing records and by scrutinizing actual techniques. Once again, the person and his or her family must have suitable attitudes for proper incorporation of knowledge to occur. It is apparent that the degree of incorporation is partially dependent on the family unit—on its acceptance and its motivation.

Biochemical Monitoring

The three most common clinical monitors are urine glucose determinations, blood glucose measurements, and evaluations of glycosylated hemoglobin. The advantages and disadvantages of these monitors will be discussed later but are noted in Table 5–2. Some diabetologists recommend also a periodic monitoring for abnormalities in the patient's plasma lipid profile. Others include proteinuria, changes in appearance of the optic lens and retina, presence of hypertension, and deterioration of peripheral nerve function. These other monitors appear to be markers of longstanding control or of the complication of diabetes and will not be considered to any degree in this section but will be covered in Chapter 18.

Urine Glucose Monitoring

Urine glucose measurements have been the hallmark of diabetes monitoring for the past

Table 5–2. **VARIOUS MONITORS OF BIOCHEMICAL CONTROL**

Chemical Examination		Advantages	Disadvantages	Comments
Urine	*Daily Semi-quantitative*	1. Simple, easy to perform 2. Noninvasive 3. Multiple daily sampling possible 4. Inexpensive	1. Variable renal T_G 2. Glucose threshold increases over time 3. Blood glucose must be 2 to 3 times normal before "spill" occurs 4. Range is narrow 5. Other substances interfere 6. Falsification of data common	1. Some feel it is dirty or degrading 2. Better than nothing 3. Relation to blood glucose not precise 4. Bladder emptying problem
	24-Hour, or Fractional	1. Appears quantitative 2. Can be related to diet, insulin 3. Done at home	1. Gives intermittent results only 2. All disadvantages noted above 3. Compliance is often poor 4. Day-of-collection is different	1. May be more inexact than daily urines
Blood	*HBGM*	1. Relatively easy to perform 2. Quantitative data 3. Multiple sampling possible	1. Invasive 2. Expensive 3. Compliance problems 4. Possible "numbers" obsession 5. Falsification of data possible	1. Preferred method by most teenagers, young adults, and parents 2. Technique is important
	Office	1. Quantitative	1. Infrequency makes it difficult to use alone 2. Decisions based on limited data	
Glycosylated Hemoglobin		1. Objective 2. Cannot be easily manipulated 3. Outlines a goal to be reached	1. Relatively long time between tests 2. Differences among laboratories 3. 2 "bad" weeks may negate 6 "good" weeks	

half century. While recognizing their limitations, diabetic specialists found that, with proper use, the frequent measurement of urine glucose did offer an added dimension of information over merely relying on how the patient felt. Other than the intermittent office monitoring of venous or capillary blood glucose, physicians prior to the last decade had no acceptable chemical marker besides home urine glucose monitoring. Urine glucose levels were and are used to give indirect estimates of the blood glucose level. With current technical advances in blood glucose monitoring and with the universal acknowledgment of its obvious advantages, it is tempting to consider urine glucose determinations as a relic of the past and to discuss this monitor no further. We contemplated this course but considered that it would be a disservice to dismiss an "old friend" so lightly. Besides, until current technology reduces the costs of blood glucose monitoring and further lessens its discomfort, urine glucose determinations will remain more than a piece of antiquity to some patients with diabetes.

As noted in Table 5–2, there are striking disadvantages to urine glucose monitoring, the most notable of which is the variability of the renal threshold for glucose (T_G). Owing to the heterogeneity of nephron populations, the T_G may normally be as low as 110 mg/dl or as high as 240 mg/dl, with the average being about 140 mg/dl. Thus, it is nonsensical to use urine glucose monitoring to estimate blood glucose without first acquiring information about the T_G of the patient. If the T_G of a patient has been determined, then repeated testing may give the clinician some information unobtainable by noninvasive means. Studies in our laboratory have demonstrated that, in a given patient, the T_G usually remains relatively constant for 5 to 10 years, after which it tends to rise.

Several other disadvantages of urine testing are obvious. The most evident *disadvantage* is that a negative urine glucose test result

Table 5–3. URINE SUGAR MONITORING: HOW TO USE A "POOR" TEST MOST EFFECTIVELY*

1. Examine 3 to 5 urine samples per day; keep records.
2. Make changes in insulin or diet, based on patterns of spill, determined over 3 to 5 days (see Chapter 6).
3. More than an occasional 2% to 5% reading is unacceptable.
4. If the patient feels well, functions normally, and has either no hypoglycemia or few mild to moderate hypoglycemia reactions, try to achieve sugar-free urines all the time.
5. If the frequency or severity of hypoglycemic reactions becomes unacceptable, make alterations in insulin, diet, exercise, or all three.

*Renal threshold for glucose (T_G) should be estimated initially.

reveals no information relative to the level of blood glucose below the T_G. Thus, blood glucose values of 20 mg/dl, 40 mg/dl and 120 mg/dl would all have comparable urine glucose recordings. It is for this reason that an old axiom was upheld: If all urine glucose levels are negative, hypoglycemia is more likely than if some urine glucose levels show small amounts of sugar. Another hindrance to the use of urine glucose values is that the range of blood glucose encompassed by the semiquantitative urine measurement is extremely narrow. With a T_G of 140 mg/dl, the urine would presumably show a trace of glucose at 145 mg/dl, but 5 percent glycosuria would likely be seen at blood glucose values as low as 240 mg/dl. Thus, the difference between 0 and 5 percent is often only 100 mg/dl.

The urine glucose method becomes even less exact over time as bladder volume increases and incomplete emptying occurs. The occurrence of large bladders in a patient with autonomic neuropathy negates use of urine glucose monitoring.

The *advantages* of urine glucose monitoring are also noted in Table 5–2. Not only is it a noninvasive method and one that is much less expensive than blood glucose monitoring, but also it affords multiple samplings per day.

How Can Urine Glucose Determinations Be Used Most Effectively? It should first be re-emphasized that these testings will never be comparable in accuracy and reliability to blood monitoring. To use urine glucose level monitoring correctly, certain guidelines are needed, and these are noted in Table 5–3. As noted earlier, an estimation of the T_G

should be made initially and the levels are usually examined by performing the following sequence *several times daily*: (1) void completely and test urine for glucose; (2) measure blood glucose immediately; (3) revoid 15 to 20 minutes later and remeasure urine glucose; and then (4) remeasure blood glucose. Effectively using the urine sugar involves the observation of several urine samples per day over three to five days, observing for patterns of urine sugar "spill" (that is, glucose levels consistently high prior to lunch, or consistently low before bed, and so forth) and correlating the results obtained with the clinical evaluation.

If the patient is normal clinically and has either hypoglycemia or mild hypoglycemic episodes, then a reasonable goal would be to achieve an absence of glycosuria. Until such is obtained, modification of some parameter of management (for example, insulin or diet) should be made at three- to five-day intervals. If the urine becomes negative as a result of this manipulation and if neither the frequency nor the severity of the hypoglycemia increases, it would appear appropriate to decrease the "offending" insulin or to add extra food.

Considerable discussion has centered on the question of whether the first or the second voiding of urine should be used in tests of control assessment. Theoretically, the first voiding should empty the bladder of urine formed earlier, and the second voiding should give closer approximation of the blood glucose in the very recent past. Our experience at camp with 170 children suggests that there is individual variation; some children had closer approximation of blood glucose on the second urine sample, but most demonstrations showed both first and second urine samples to be identical. These findings are supported by several other investigators, and most often, a second voiding is not considered necessary.

Urine Testing Materials. These involve either strip (TesTape, Clinistix, Diastix, Keto-Diastix) or tablet methods (Clinitest, five-drop method). These methods do not offer a wide range of sensitivity (2 percent glycosuria is the maximum that can be measured) although 5 percent glycosuria can be monitored using the two-drop Clinitest method or by Chemstrip Ugk or Diastix-5. In a local comparison of three of the methods (Keto-Diastix, TesTape, and Clinitest), the two-drop Clinitest method was found to be the

Table 5–4. **SUBSTANCES INTERFERING WITH URINE TESTS FOR GLUCOSE**

Substances	Test	Effect
Antibiotics		
Ampicillin	Clinitest	Unpredictable
Carbenicillin	Clinitest	Unpredictable
Cephalosporins	Clinitest	False-positive
Chloramphicol	Clinitest	False-positive
Sulfonamides	Clinitest	False-positive
Tetracyclines	Clinitest	False-positive
Probenecid	Clinitest	False-positive
Ascorbic Acid		
<500 mg/day	Clinitest	None
	Diastix	None
>500 mg/day	Clinitest	False-positive
	Diastix	False-negative
Salicylates	Clinitest	False-positive
	Diastix	False-negative
Protein	Clinitest	False-negative
Ketones (moderate-large)	Diastix	False-negative

most consistent and therefore is preferred. All tests reasonably approximate the degree of glycosuria; but the strip methods have the greatest variability, and distinction among color changes is often difficult, particularly with TesTape. The sensitivity (expressed as a ratio of detected to actual glycosuria) is similar for all tests, whereas the specificity (capacity to correctly identify negative glycosuria) is best for Clinitest.

Results of urine glucose testing are now reported as percentages, the old "plus" nomenclature having been abandoned. The reasons for the change from a plus system to a percentage system had to do with the variability in meaning of pluses (for instance, 2 percent and 5 percent glycosuria both indicate being 4 +).

Certain ingested substances may interfere with the accuracy of readings of all methods, but in most situations the amount ingested must be substantial before the reaction is affected. Some of the tests and substances involved are listed in Table 5–4.

Twenty-four–Hour Urine, or Fractional, Collections. In an aim to obtain more meaningful information from the urine, various investigators have evaluated more quantitative measurements of urine. Urine samples are collected over a designated period, and an excretion of glucose per unit of time is calculated. As noted in Table 5–2, there are few real advantages to this process. The physician or diabetes team is often led to believe that this analysis is more quantitative than is standard urine testing. However, conditions attendant to the test make it likely that results are also less reliable: (1) the test can be done only intermittently; (2) a "missed" urine sample gives an erroneous impression of better control than exists; and (3) the day of collection will always be different (in terms of diet, and so forth) than usual days, as the child soon learns to "please" the caregivers. Our studies suggest that this is not a worthwhile addition to ambulatory care, even though it may have some uses in the hospitalized child.

Home Blood Glucose Monitoring (HBGM)

The ability for individuals to monitor blood glucose at home has been with us since 1964, when Dextrostix were introduced. However, the difficulty encountered in visually reading the color changes on these strips limited their use to highly selected patients. Ames Laboratories introduced the first reflectance meter in the early 1970s, and with it, the era of true HBGM began. Even then, the use was primarily limited to selected patients or groups of patients (pregnant diabetics, those with high or low glucose thresholds, and so forth). Our first experiences with HBGM occurred in 1974 when two children with low T_Gs and frequent episodes of severe hypoglycemia were given such monitoring. The ability to maintain control without frequent occurrences of hypoglycemia was dramatic in both children, and there are a few such recorded anecdotes attesting to the use of HBGM.

But the real age of HBGM was actually launched in the latter portion of the 1970s. The impetus for its widespread enthusiasm and use came from several directions. There was an accumulation of information that seemed to demonstrate the advantage of tight control in altering chronic complications: (1) several studies pointed out the significant inaccuracies of urine glucose testing; (2) a method for accurate assessment by a visually read technique, Chemstrip bG (Boehringer Mannheim) was introduced; (3) better optical systems for measurements (Dextrometer, Glucometer, Stat Tec, Accu-Chek, and so forth) were developed; and (4) perhaps most importantly, the introduction of a new breed of stylets that created "pinholes," rather than the "knifecuts" created by the older stylets. All of these factors have led to an unexpected acceptance of HBGM and have probably influenced diabetic control more than any other element in the last 20 years.

Both the visually read Chemstrip bG and

the Dextrostix/Dextrometer-Glucometer system have been shown to correlate with blood glucose as measured by the AutoAnalyzer (Technicon Instruments Corporation). For values between 50 and 400 mg/dl, the correlation coefficient between the Dextrometer and the AutoAnalyzer is 0.98, and good accuracy has been confirmed for samples in the range of 10 to 90 mg/dl (r = 0.903). The correlation between Chemstrip bG and the AutoAnalyzer is 0.996 when the blood glucose is between 50 and 400 mg/dl. The Chemstrip bG may also be read optically on the Accu-Chek, with comparable results. Another strip method, Visidex I, has been shown to have greater variability and a broader range of error, but Visidex II appears comparable to Chemstrip bG.

Results obtained by HBGM are highly dependent on technique, and this begins with application of the specimen of blood to the reagent pad. The time of contact (number of minutes) with the reagent must be precise. With the Dextrostix method, the blood must be washed off with a stream of water and the pad blotted and immediately read. This wet method introduces two potential error points (washing and blotting) that are critical to its accuracy. When using either the Chemstrip bG or the Visidex II, the blood sample is removed at one minute by dry wiping, and actual reading is delayed for another one to two minutes. The color change in both these latter methods is easily read and is stable for several days.

Cost is a significant factor in considering HBGM. The cost for either the Glucometer, the Accu-Chek, or other comparable instruments is currently less than $200.00 and is often covered by third-party payers. Both Dextrostix and Chemstrip bG have costs that vary from $0.40 to $0.65 per strip. This is significant when from two to seven tests per day are necessary. Patients have found that both Chemstrip bG and Visidex II can be cut lengthwise into either two or three strips, thereby decreasing their cost.

Routine Use of HBGM. This method is strongly recommended for nearly all patients, as indicated in Table 5–5. Absolute indications are for those in whom the use of HBGM has been shown to effect major changes in patient morbidity. Almost added to this list of absolute indications is the child under 4 years of age, in whom wide fluctuations are common and the necessity of preventing significant hypoglycemia is real. Even

Table 5–5. **HOME BLOOD GLUCOSE MONITORING**

A. *Absolute Indications for Routine Use*
  1. Low or high renal glucose threshold
  2. Extreme hyperlability
  3. Pregnancy
  4. Patients on pump or multiple-injection programs
B. *Strongly Recommended Routine Use*
  1. Everyone who can afford it financially
  2. Children under 4 years of age
  3. Hyperlabile states
  4. During stressful states
C. *Recommended as a Back-up to Urine Sugar Determinations*
  1. Everyone who cannot afford it as a routine
  2. Those who refuse it as a routine

those who either cannot afford this routine use or who refuse to use it as a routine monitor should be taught the techniques and should use them during periods when diabetes is out of control.

Patient acceptance of HBGM has indeed been remarkable, and this includes children. Teenagers have generally chosen this method in preference to urine testing, the latter not being as socially acceptable. It is our feeling that patient compliance among adolescent users is better than that among teens expected to check urine sugars. Parents readily accept its use in the very young child, and there have been no major problems with the child's eventual acquiescence. Even the child between 6 and 13 years has seemed to accept the role of HBGM in management. Recently, at a camp of 220 children between the ages of 6 and 13, about two thirds were using HBGM at the beginning of camp and almost 100 percent were doing so by camp's conclusion. The parents of children in this age group varied widely in their degree of acceptance. In general, physicians who are not in fulltime diabetic practice have been the most reluctant to accept this change.

Regular usage schedules vary from child to child. At the beginning of attempts at control, we recommend four to five tests per day and generally schedule these before each meal, at bedtime, and around 3:00 AM.. Once control has been established, we recommend only two tests per day. The first of these tests is regularly scheduled before breakfast. The second test time is varied: sometimes at one of the other times previously noted, depending on which insulin dosage is being addressed. For a while, the second test may be before lunch, as the action of the morning regular test is assessed; later, this test is moved to before supper, as the morning isophane insulin suspension (NPH) or insulin lente is assessed and so forth. Once control is established, we also attempt to have one measurement per week taken at 3:00 AM.

Acceptable levels of glucose control vary with the opinion of each diabetologist writing on the subject. While recognizing that significant fluctuations in the hyperglycemic range are undesirable, most diabetologists also appreciate the risks of serious hypoglycemia when control is extremely tight. Thus, most programs arrive at compromises situated between blood glucose profiles that are ideal and those that are considered practical. Such compromises have been made in each of the multicenter trials investigating the relationship of glucose control to the incidence of complications. Most of these studies have set goals for their intensive control groups at preprandial glucose levels between 60 mg/dl and 110 mg/dl and 90- to 120-minute postprandial glucose levels less than 160 mg/dl. It should be noted that these values appear easy to achieve in those patients treated either with the insulin pump or with multiple insulin-dose injections but difficult to achieve consistently with two injections per day.

Our goals are for most children to obtain blood glucose values between 60 and 150 mg/dl on 75 percent or more of their preprandial specimens. Prebreakfast objectives are a little higher than ordinary, with 80 to 110 mg/dl being felt to be safer than lower levels. Values when tested at 3:00 A.M. should always be above 80 mg/dl.

The physican must decide, for each patient, whether these goals are reasonable. Factors to be considered in making such decisions are age of the child, compliance on other therapeutic measures, and frequency of appropriate monitoring.

Glycosylated Hemoglobin (HbA$_{1C}$)

The routine use of this test has been one of the more valuable additions to diabetic care. HbA$_{1C}$ is the most abundant minor component of hemoglobin in normal red cells and is elevated as much as threefold in diabetic red cells. HbA$_{1C}$ is the component of HbA that has a glucose attached to the N-terminus of the beta chain by ketoamine linkage (Fig. 5–3). Biosynthetic studies in vivo indicate that HbA$_{1C}$ is formed nonenzymatically, slowly, and continuously, throughout the life of the red cell. Thus, levels of HbA$_{1C}$ provide an integrated measure of blood glucose levels over the preceding two to three months. The kinetics shown in Figure 5–3 bear directly on interpretations of reported results. Pre-A$_{1C}$ may comprise about 10 percent of total A$_{1C}$ if it is not eliminated. Pre-A$_{1C}$ can be eliminated by two methods: (1) use of prolonged column procedure (rather than a rapid column method) that measures only HbA$_{1C}$ and not A$_{1A1}$, A$_{1A2}$, A$_{1B}$, or pre-A$_{1C}$; and (2) dialysis and/or saline incubation of the red cell before application to the column. More recently, a chemical analysis has become available that is more stable than earlier methods of this sort. These considerations become important when comparing results among laboratories.

As noted earlier, normal results vary from technique to technique and from laboratory to laboratory, even when similar techniques are used. Additionally, the reaction is not stable, and results become highly suspect if the room temperature time exceeds a few hours or if the time at 4°C exceeds one week. Consequently, how does the physician intelligently use a commercial laboratory to assess his/her patients' control? These principles and thoughts should be considered: (1) the laboratory should have a good reputation for quality control; (2) the laboratory should have its own normative data, not just that supplied by the manufacturer of "the Kit;" (3) the physician should ascertain what is being measured—HbA$_1$ or HbA$_{1C}$; (4) the laboratory should run control or normal blood samples with each "abnormal" run; (5) duplicate samples should be the rule; (6) blood samples should be appropriately collected, usually in heparinized or EDTA tubes and placed either in the refrigerator or freezer; and (7) blood samples should then be shipped to the laboratory as expediciously as possible.

Normal values in our laboratory have varied as our techniques have evolved. Our current normal range is 3.2 to 6.1 percent with a mean of 5.2 percent. Our patients are uniformly told that the closer they approach this normal range, the less the likelihood of degenerative complications. We find that we are able to achieve normal values in only a few persons; notably, those in the "honeymoon" and those on intensive insulin regimens (either multiple injection or pump therapy). Thus, we have established an "acceptable" level that we feel is achievable in most patients on a two-shot per day program. This level is 50 percent above (1.5 times) the

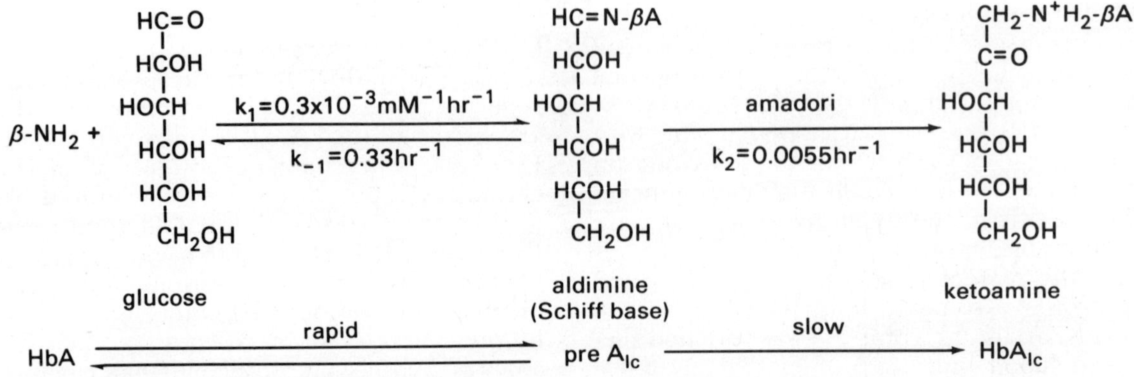

Figure 5–3. Chemical reaction converting HgbA to HgbA$_{1C}$ in presence of glucose. (See text).

mean normal value. We believe the physician can use this same factoring in establishing acceptable levels with a commercial laboratory and in relating values from different reports.

Early studies demonstrated that the concentration of HbA$_{1C}$ correlates closely with mean serum glucose concentrations. In a hospital setting, HbA$_{1C}$ can be returned from high to normal levels in four to six weeks; whereas on an outpatient basis, this process may take longer. Numerous studies have documented declines of HbA$_{1C}$ with improved blood sugar control, and levels of HbA$_{1C}$ are positively correlated with fasting blood sugar

(Fig. 5–4), urinary sugar, and various other numeric scores relating to degree of diabetic control. Glycosylation of other proteins occurs just as with hemoglobin. Because of the shorter half-life of proteins like albumin or transferrin, their levels of glycosylation may give the physician some markers that are intermediate between blood glucose monitoring and HbA$_{1C}$. Although HbA$_{1C}$ has not been found to consistently correlate with serum levels of triglyceride or cholesterol in insulin-dependent diabetics, a recent study on a large series of patients (N = 566) did show a weak but significant correlation between HbA$_{1C}$ and serum cholesterol or triglyceride. As a measure of control, HbA$_{1C}$ offers a more objective monitor than any other assessment. It minimizes the problems of multiple sampling errors attendant with blood glucose measurements and the unreliability of urine glucose tests. It serves as a check on the accuracy, reliability, and thus, compliance of the child and of his or her records, while also providing feedback.

In the Children's Diabetes Management Center, we obtain HbA$_{1C}$ values at three- to six-month intervals and report these to the child and parent and to their local physician. Figure 5–5 is a sample record from one of our patients, noting the results over time. Such reporting serves as feedback on prior performance and also helps the patient to establish overall goals.

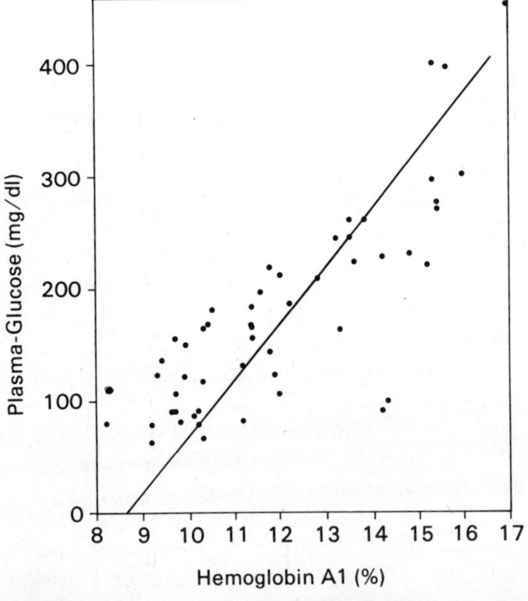

Figure 5–4. Correlation of Mean Plasma Glucose. Values obtained from multiple glucose testing over several months and hemoglobin A$_1$ levels. (Adapted from Gonen B et al.: Haemoglobin A$_1$: An indicator of the metabolic control of diabetic patients. Lancet 2:734–736, 1977.)

RECORD KEEPING

Monitoring without maintenance of records detailing the results appears ludicrous, and yet it appears to be a frequent happening among persons with diabetes. Even some of those patients who do keep records do so in

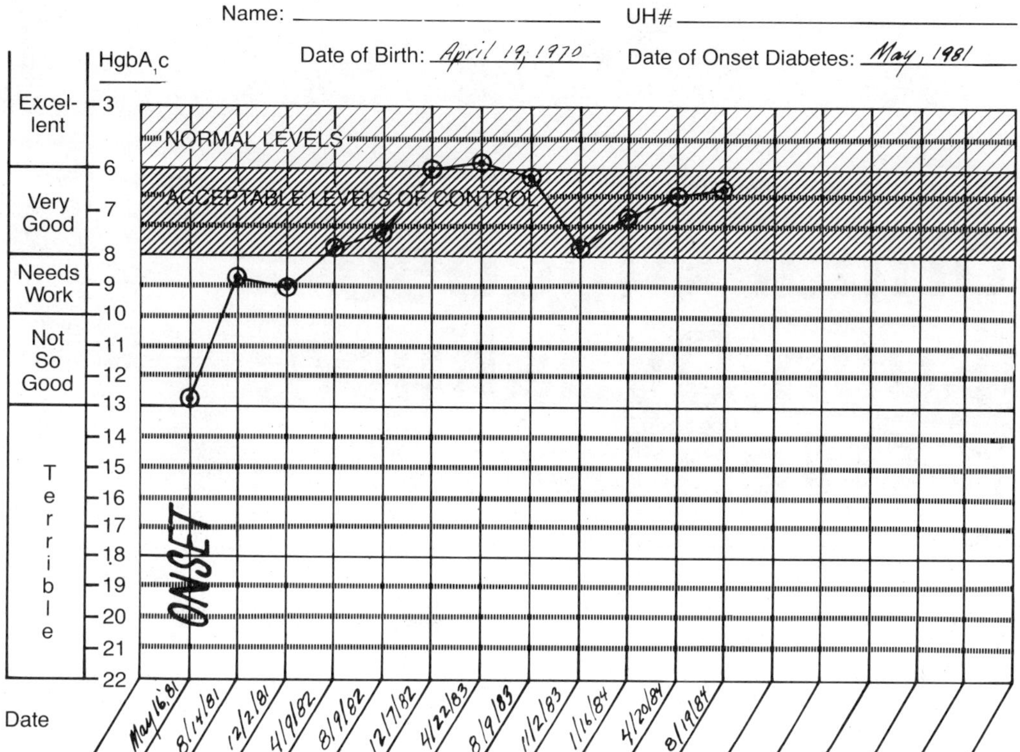

Figure 5–5. Graphic representation of diabetic control (hemoglobin A_{1C} results) over time. This graph, with new data applied, is photocopied and sent to the child and family following each visit.

such a disorganized fashion that the usefulness of these data are questionable.

The reason one monitors diabetes care is presumably so that alterations can be made in that care if control is determined to be less than optimal. Persons with IDDM are often more compliant in monitoring than they are in recording. Often, young persons fail to record results, for they do not consider it more than a necessary chore to be completed. People tend to perform tasks for which they can see benefit; and if the reasons for recording results are not understood, then the likelihood is great that records will not be maintained. Why is monitoring required? To enable the person to make appropriate alterations in dosages of insulin or in diet. Why is recording required? Because individual memory of events in the past is limited. The ability to remember exactly more than a day or so of blood test results would be unusual, but changes in insulin dosage must be made on the basis of patterns established over several days.

We do not have an answer to the question of how to ensure the maintenance of adequate records. However, by demonstrating to the young person how the data are to be used and by allowing the patient some freedom to make appropriate alterations in care based on the data he or she collects may be one approach. Changes in insulin dosage based on collected data are discussed in Chapter 6.

SUMMARY

In evaluating methods to be used in monitoring, all types should probably be employed at one time or another. Many measures should be used to judge the adequacy of control. A scoring system that incorporates several methods has been found successful by some, with each component of the scoring system providing some exclusive bit of information not provided by another component. Each parameter has a place in management. Daily blood (or urine) sugar determinations are necessary if one is to make formative adjustments in management with insulin or with diet, or both. HbA_{1C} values can provide summative data of an objective nature, whereas growth measurements can indicate long-term control patterns. Thus, all measures need to be integrated into a program of long-term care.

6

Normal Glucose-Insulin Dynamics: An Overview

Carbohydrate metabolism is a tightly regulated system in the nondiabetic individual. The integral parts of this system (gastrointestinal system, nervous system, and various hormonal regulators) are intricately woven into a process of interdependent and intradependent functions, all working to incorporate intake, use, and disposal of metabolic fuels. Despite the complexities of the system, the degree of individual uniformity in carbohydrate balance from one day to the next is spectacular. Under most conditions, the normal blood glucose profile demonstrates that the mean amplitude of glucose excursion rarely exceeds 50 mg/dl, even in the postprandial state. Additionally, when meals and activity are held constant, the variation in blood glucose concentration at a given time of two consecutive days is less than 10 mg/dl. Although multiple hormones play a role in this glucose homeostasis, insulin is the major regulator in tissues that are insulin dependent.

An exhaustive and comprehensive treatise of normal carbohydrate metabolism and insulin dynamics is beyond the scope of this book. More importantly, such would not be in keeping with our objectives in writing it. For more comprehensive information, the interested reader is referred to several excellent texts and review articles (see Selected References). Thus, although no in-depth discussion will take place, it seems appropriate to present a broad overview of some of the physiologic and biologic aspects of this system. This is proper, because the correct insulin regimen for any person with diabetes should be one that simulates normal metabolic activities as closely as possible.

NORMAL INSULIN SECRETION

Table 6–1 and Figure 6–1 outline the most important aspects of insulin secretion. Insulin output from the pancreatic beta cell is continuously secreted in a low concentration that maintains plasma levels in the range of 10 mU/ml (basal insulin secretion). The stimulus for this basal insulin release has not been fully delineated, but the fact that it does not disappear during hypoglycemia suggests that the level of plasma glucose is not the only factor governing secretion. On the other hand, basal levels of insulin do rise significantly in response to sustained glucose loading. There are also diurnal variations in basal secretion, with the lowest levels being ob-

Table 6–1. SOME PHYSIOLOGIC FACTORS THAT REGULATE INSULIN SECRETION*

I. Persistent basal insulin secretion
II. Diurnal variations in basal secretion
III. Substrate-mediated secretion
    Gut hormone stimulation
    Neural (parasympathetic) factors
    Elevated blood glucose
IV. Substrate-related cessation of secretion
V. Secretion into hepatic portal circulation
VI. Variation in secretion in response to stress
    Neural (sympathetic) factors
    Catecholamines
    Other factors

*Only the most important factors are listed. See also Figure 6–1 for more graphic representation; for details, see text.

served in the late morning and early afternoon and the highest in the early morning hours (usually between 4:00 and 8:00 AM). This predawn or dawn effect corresponds to similar increases in secretion of stress or counter-regulatory hormones.

Superimposed on this basal level are bursts of insulin secretion that correspond to food intake or hyperglycemia or both. These episodic outpourings are regulated by neural factors, gut hormones, and elevated blood glucose concentrations. The regulation is such that, even prior to a rise in blood glucose from gastrointestinal absorption of food, there is a rise in the level of blood insulin. This fact enables glucose use to commence early and prevents significant postabsorptive hyperglycemia. As glucose concentrations reach their zenith and then begin to fall, the normal beta cell ceases its insulin release by mechanisms that are still not fully understood. This feedback loop probably relates to intraislet autoregulation involving somatostatin and glucagon. A protracted or late fall in blood glucose is thus prevented.

Endogenous insulin is secreted directly into the hepatic portal circulation, and in the post ingestion period, insulin levels in this circulation are almost threefold greater than in the systemic circulation. Thus, the hepatic actions of insulin may be presumed to be primary. However, the insulin is exposed to the liver insulinase system early, and this may merely be another mechanism for limiting the amount of insulin seen peripherally.

Another primary feature concerning endogenous insulin is the effect that other hormonal and neural systems have on its release. Sympathetic neural activity, catecholamines, serotonin, prostaglandin E activity, somatostatin, and perhaps cortisol all inhibit pancreatic insulin secretion. During stress of almost any description, the secretion of these hormones blunts insulin release, allowing glucose concentrations to rise.

It is apparent that the loss of normal beta-cell function, as it pertains to reduced insulin release, causes a significant problem for the

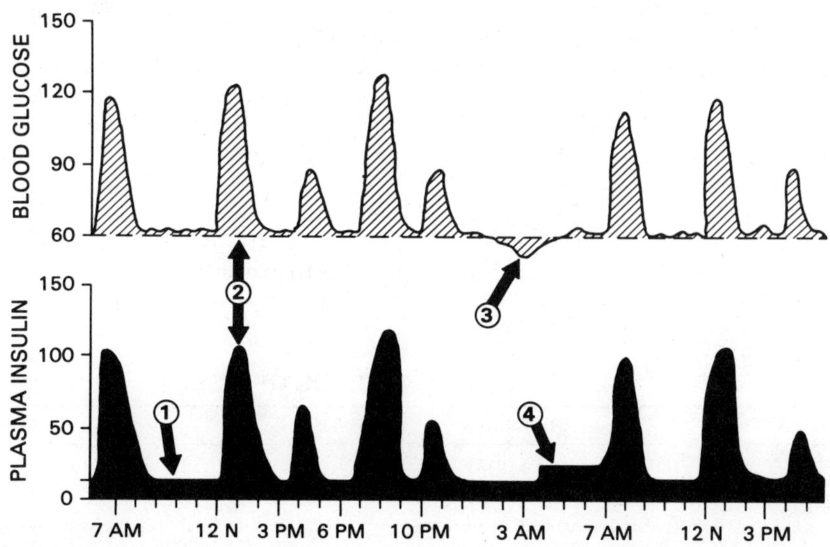

Figure 6–1. Normal glucose-insulin relationships are demonstrated. Four points are indicated (*arrows*): (1) there is a basal secretion of insulin that is persistent and independent of intake or fluctuations in blood glucose; (2) there is a substrate-related release of insulin, as well as substrate-related cessation of secretion; (3) the lowest point in the blood sugar curve is ordinarily around 2:00 to 3:00 AM; and (4) the basal secretion of insulin normally increases in the predawn time period. (See text for more information.)

body, but the entire story may be much more complex. There is growing evidence that the beta cell is not just the site of insulin synthesis and secretion but also the precise glucose sensor and metabolic integrator of various neural and hormonal signals and of glucose.

PHYSIOLOGIC ACTION OF INSULIN

Insulin is the major hormone in the body responsible for overall fuel metabolism. Although the action of insulin in relation to carbohydrate metabolism is more commonly considered, particularly in relation to diabetes, insulin also influences major functions related to protein and fat metabolism. Overall, insulin should be considered as both an anabolic and an anticatabolic hormone as it has both stimulatory and inhibitory effects. Some of these effects are noted in Table 6–2 and in Figures 6–2 and 6–3.

As suggested in Figures 6–2 and 6–3, the extracellular concentration of glucose is primarily determined by the balance that exists between its delivery (gastrointestinal absorption plus hepatic production) and its use by both insulin-dependent and non-insulin-dependent tissues. In the basal or postabsorptive state, the relative absence of insulin (except for the small basal secretion that persists) allows accelerated hepatic glucose production and lipolysis to occur. This keeps the plasma glucose within a range in which sensitive non-insulin-dependent tissues, mostly the brain and nervous system, can carry on their metabolic functions unimpeded. Glycogenolysis occurs in the liver, accounting for about 75 percent of glucose production, whereas gluconeogenesis from amino acids and glycerol accounts for the remaining 25 percent.

In the postfeeding state (Fig. 6–3), glucose utilization is the primary activity, and insulin is a major factor in its disposal. Insulin inhibits glycogenolysis, gluconeogenesis, and lipol-ysis. Insulin also stimulates glucose transport into muscle and fat cells. Glucose transport into the liver is not insulin dependent, but insulin stimulates two intrahepatic enzymes: glycogen synthetase and glucokinase. Insulin is also responsible for the increased amino-acid uptake by muscle, for increased triglyceride uptake by the adipocyte, and for significant protein synthesis.

Insulin is also important in many other factors of body metabolism, which will be discussed in subsequent sections. It is a major growth factor and is influential in electrolyte and mineral fluxes.

INSULIN THERAPY IN PATIENTS WITH IDDM

From the foregoing discussion, it is obvious that insulin deficiency as seen in the patient with IDDM produces major metabolic problems. The degree of insulin deficiency, as well as the magnitude of any concomitant stress, determines the severity of the problem. With insulin deficiency, hepatic glucose production, protein catabolism, and lipolysis all go unchecked. Ketogenesis is accelerated. Glucose use by the liver, muscle, and fat cells decreases, and the plasma concentration of glucose subsequently rises. This overloads those non-insulin-dependent tissues in which transport is by mass action of the substrate. The situation within insulin-dependent tissues can be likened to the condition of starvation.

Although it is obvious that appropriate therapy is the physiologic replacement of the deficient hormone, the intricacies of glucose-insulin homeostasis are virtually impossible to mimic with present-day therapy. Precise metabolic control can be achieved for short periods by the use of the glucose-controlled, insulin-infusion system (closed-loop pump) or following pancreatic or beta-cell trans-

Table 6–2. **PHYSIOLOGIC ACTIONS OF INSULIN**

Substrate	Stimulates	Inhibits
Carbohydrates	↑ Glycogen synthesis (liver and muscle) ↑ Fatty acid synthesis (liver and adipocyte)	↓ Glycogenolysis (liver) ↓ Gluconeogenesis (liver)
Fats	↑ Fatty acid synthesis (adipocyte) ↑ Glycerol synthesis (adipocyte)	↓ Lipolysis (adipose tissue) ↓ Ketogenesis (liver)
Proteins	↑ Amino acid uptake (muscle) ↑ Protein synthesis (muscle)	↓ Protein catabolism (muscle) ↓ Amino acid output (muscle) ↓ Amino acid oxidation (muscle)

Figure 6–2. In the basal or post-absorptive state, the body is generally in balance. Glucose needs, predominantly for use by non-insulin-dependent tissues, are derived from glycogenolysis and gluconeogenesis. Plasma glucose levels are quite stable for long periods.

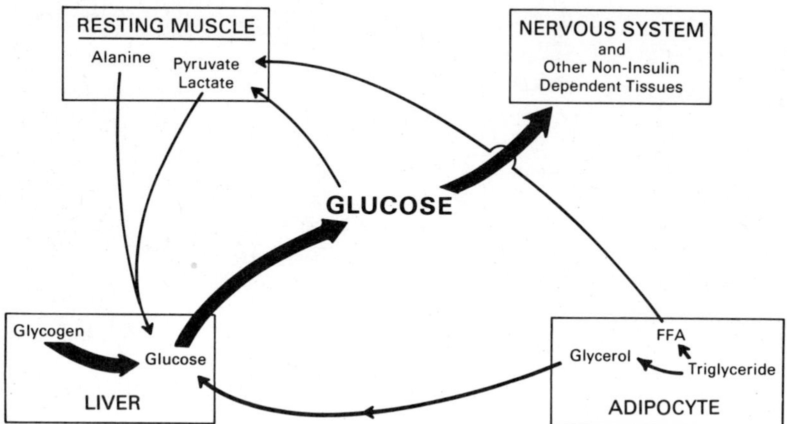

METABOLIC STATE—BASAL, POST-ABSORPTIVE

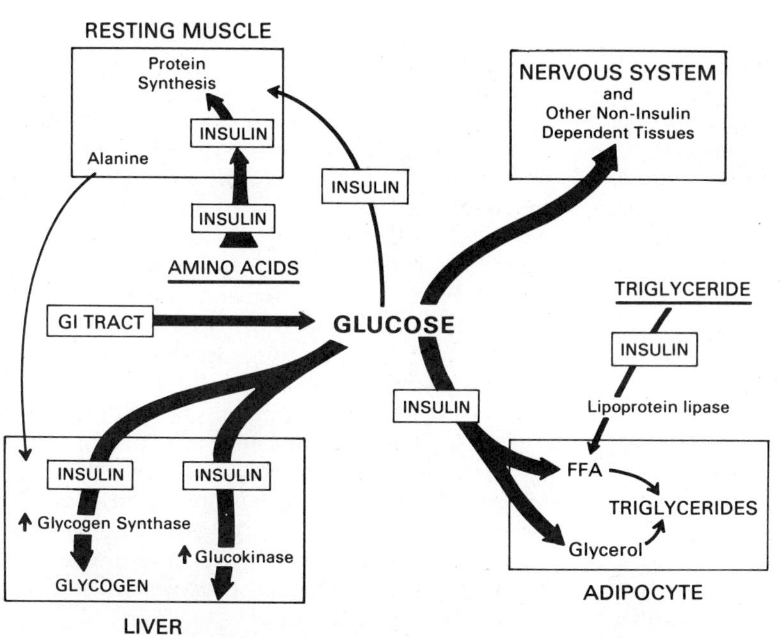

Figure 6–3. Following food ingestion, plasma levels of glucose rise and insulin facilitates its metabolic utilization by those insulin-sensitive tissues. Once again, blood glucose values are maintained close to normal.

METABOLIC STATE—NORMAL POST-FED

plants. However, these entities are not yet practicable for the masses of persons with IDDM, and other potential methodologies are still experimental. Consequently, the reality is that all control is less than ideal and all therapies merely degrees of poor control.

Objectives of Insulin Therapy

It should be obvious that insulin therapy is only one facet, albeit the most important, of diabetic therapy. For precise regulation of the level of blood glucose and for the return of metabolic abnormalities to normal, attention must be directed to all aspects simultaneously. These include insulin, dietary intake, exercise, and stress management. For purposes of this chapter, unless otherwise addressed it will be assumed that aspects other than insulin are being held constant or stable.

The specific goal of insulin therapy is to normalize carbohydrate, fat, and protein metabolism and to return both postprandial and postabsorptive states to normal. To do so precisely is not currently feasible, but to attempt to achieve this goal is not only possible but a requirement of good practice as well. A re-examination of Table 6–1 will help the reader grasp the magnitude of the problem that the insulin-deficient patient faces. Which of these normal secretory functions can we expect to achieve with the exogenous administration of subcutaneous insulin? Which goals are practical for most persons with IDDM? We will now consider them in more detail.

Persistent Basal Insulin Levels with Diurnal Variations

The persistent basal insulin levels in the nondiabetic person are relatively low (approximately 10 to 15 μU/ml) and relatively constant, except for diurnal variations. Such basal levels are achievable either by continuous, subcutaneous insulin infusion (external pumps, or CSII) or by one of the three-shot per day or four-shot per day regimens to be described later. These basal levels are not readily achievable by either of the two most common methods of insulin delivery (the one-shot per day or two-shot per day regimen). In both of these methods, free insulin levels fluctuate markedly and are not in synchrony with the diurnal pattern.

Substrate-Mediated Secretion and Substrate-Related Cessation

Obviously, these factors are not currently achievable by any of the present ambulatory treatment programs. Exogenous insulin is delivered from its depot site into the circulation at a rate based on the character of the insulin preparation and kinetics at the injection site. The best a clinician can do to handle this situation is to attempt to match the peak activity of the insulin injected with the delivery of glucose from the gastrointestinal system. As will be discussed later, this may be accomplished with Regular insulin because of its relatively predictable absorption, but it is much more difficult with intermediate- and long-acting insulins because of their relatively unpredictable delivery from the depot site.

Although it is difficult to duplicate the preciseness of insulin delivery that occurs in the nondiabetic person, it is even more difficult to shut the system off as the blood glucose level falls. The person with diabetes has no internal control to accomplish this, so the absorption of insulin from a subcutaneous site will continue despite hypoglycemia.

Secretion into the Hepatic Portal System

With the exception of those few patients who receive their insulin directly into the peritoneal cavity, insulin is first delivered into the diabetic patient's systemic circulation, producing a concentration either equal to or greater than that in the hepatic portal circulation. Thus, the 40 percent extraction of pancreatic insulin that normally occurs on first passage through the liver does not occur in these patients until later. The overall significance of this difference in initial exposure is uncertain for the vast majority of patients. However, one might suggest that the all-important inhibitory functions of insulin on glucose production and on triglyceride breakdown would be delayed or diminished, whereas the actions on glucose utilization would be accelerated.

A few studies of diabetic patients undergoing peritoneal dialysis, as well as studies by Eaton and Schade (1983) of patients in whom intraperitoneal insulin delivery is supplied via an open-loop pump, suggest that glucose control and normalization of fat metabolism are more easily attainable by these methods

Table 6–3. SOME FACTORS AFFECTING INSULIN BIOAVAILABILITY*

A. Insulin preparation
    Source
    Composition
    Purity
B. Insulin regimen and dosages
C. Absorption of insulin
    Site and depth
    Techniques
    Local factors
D. Degradation of insulin
E. Inhibitors of insulin action
    Antibodies
    Stress factors
F. Exercise

*Action of insulin in normalizing glucose.

than by subcutaneous injections. More studies will be required to document this theory.

Variation of Secretion in Response to Stress

The inability of depot insulin to vary according to demand is one of the factors leading to lability in patients with Type I diabetes. In the management of the person with diabetes, the physician and patient must anticipate either exaggerated or diminished needs for insulin and make appropriate adjustments. If such is not done, then compensatory adjustments must be made during stress periods. This will be discussed subsequently.

Bioavailability of Injected Insulin

Table 6–3 lists some of the factors that affect the bioavailability of injected insulin and that are therefore significant factors in determining its control.

Insulin Preparation

Source. Commercially available insulin is derived from either animal (beef, pork) or synthetic sources (human, by biosynthetic enzymatic substitution). Animal-derived insulins are either pure (beef or pork) or mixed (beef-pork). It appears that for most persons there are only minimal differences in absorption characteristics among the animal-derived insulins. On the other hand, biosynthetic human insulin appears to be absorbed more rapidly and thus may have a shorter biologic half-life. Beef insulin is more dissimilar to human insulin than is pork insulin, and is consequently more immunogenic and creates higher titers of inhibiting antibody. Thus, pure pork insulins seem to be biologically the more potent. The same is obviously also true for the synthetic human insulins.

Composition or Type. Unmodified or crystalline (Regular) insulin has a reasonably consistent absorption and a more uniform pattern of action. The longer-acting insulins have been modified either by the addition of protamine or by physical-chemical alterations in their molecular configuration. These additions or alterations retard absorption of insulin from subcutaneous sites and thus delay onset, peak, and duration of action.

Purity. All insulins, with the exception of biosynthetic human insulin, have some impurities; but the degree of impurity is now of more importance to marketing than it is to the patient. The relatively impure insulins of several years ago are no longer around, and all commercial insulins in the United States contain less than 20 to 25 ppm of proinsulin; the ones labeled "purified" contain less than 5 ppm. From a purity standpoint, the bioavailability of insulin is therefore no longer a problem. Additionally, current insulins are very stable at room temperature and no longer require refrigeration.

Insulin Regimen and Dosages

The precise insulin regimen and dosages used influence the circulating levels of free insulin. Whether the insulin comes premixed (crystalline plus a longer-acting insulin) or is mixed in the syringe immediately before use influences the rapidity of onset, peak and duration of action. Crystalline insulin that is premixed with either isophane insulin suspension (NPH) or Lente insulin has a variable amount of binding to the longer-acting forms. Dosage does not generally affect the time of onset of activity but does affect the peak of action, which, in turn, affects the duration, as the insulin decay curve is lengthened.

Absorption of Insulin

This is the most variable of all other factors. Multiple factors are responsible for the variations in delivery, some of which have already been noted. Galloway and his associates (1981) have reported that there are "marked intra- and intersubject variations in serum insulin concentrations and blood glucose responses to Regular, NPH and Lente insulins." This has been the clinical experience of most diabetologists. Here we will briefly record some of these factors.

Site, Depth, and Technique of Injection. Absorption from the deltoid and abdominal areas is more rapid than from either the anterior thigh or the buttocks. Numerous studies have demonstrated that insulin absorption from areas of lipohypertrophy is very erratic. Regular and modified insulins both demonstrate the effects of these site differences. The magnitude of the difference is significant with respect to serum insulin levels but is insignificant in relation to changes in blood glucose levels.

The depth of insulin injection, whether given subcutaneously, superficial intramuscularly, or deep intramuscularly, produces insignificant differences in both serum insulin levels and blood glucose level responses. Most studies show that the use of the air-pressure method produces a more rapid peak and a shorter duration of insulin action.

Local Factors. Increasing the temperature at the injection site increases insulin absorption markedly, whereas decreasing the temperature has the opposite effect. The most significant local factor influencing absorption is site massage, which greatly enhances delivery of insulin from the depot. Other factors may be volume and temperature of injected insulin.

Degradation of Insulin

Subcutaneous insulin degradation occurs at the injection site to some degree in all patients, but in a few reports the degree of such degradation has been remarkable. Studies have demonstrated increased peptidase (insulinase) concentrations at the site. These patients require remarkably high dosages of insulin when administered subcutaneously but normal amounts when administered either intravenously or intraperitoneally. The addition of a protease inhibitor, protinin, to the insulin has been reported to aid in overcoming the syndrome.

Elsewhere in the body, most notably in the liver and kidneys, insulin-degrading substances (for example, insulinase) can be detected, but they do not appear to cause significant clinical problems, except in end-stage renal disease. The decreased insulinase activity present in this condition may produce a prolonged insulin half-life.

Inhibition of Insulin Action

Transient inhibition of insulin action occurs commonly and usually results from the presence of other neural or hormonal factors. True insulin resistance, on the other hand, is relatively uncommon in the young person and is characterized by a patient who requires greater than 2.5 units per kilogram per day, or over 200 units per day.

Insulin Antibody Formation. Insulin antibodies form in a high percentage of patients treated with beef- or pork-derived insulins. The antibodies are often first detected after about 6 to 12 weeks of insulin therapy. Insulin antibody formation interferes with the action of insulin when in high titers by binding the hormone initially and then releasing it later, thus increasing the half-life of insulin and prolonging its effect. A few patients seem to have true insulin resistance owing to antibody formation, but this appears to be an unusual situation.

Stress Hormones. These will be discussed in detail in Chapter 11. It is sufficient here to state that stress hormones often interfere with the actions of insulin and that they contribute to variations in its effectiveness.

Exercise

This subject will be discussed in greater detail in Chapter 8. Suffice it to note that exercise increases a patient's rate of absorption of depot insulin, particularly if the extremity in which the insulin is placed is exercised vigorously. This shortens the injection-to-peak volume and decreases the half-life of the insulin.

INSULIN THERAPY—YOU DO THE BEST YOU CAN!

Review of the previous two sections may lead to the pessimistic conclusion that IDDM cannot be controlled. Nothing could be further from the truth. Diabetes can be controlled, but not in all patients and not often to the degree that the medical caregivers would like. The point of the foregoing discussion was intended to be more realistic than pessimistic. It is difficult to tune a watch with a pitchfork. There are perhaps some who can, but most would fail. Just the same, it is equally difficult to "tune" diabetes when the primary tuning agent, exogenously administered insulin, has so many drawbacks to its effective action.

But the clinician must provide the best care possible with the tools at hand. We will now begin a consideration of the specific ways of handling insulin therapy and will review more closely the tools that are available and the numerous ways in which they may be used.

Insulin Preparations and Characteristics

Three companies currently manufacture insulin for distribution in the United States. All are high-quality products, and favoring the use of one over another depends on several factors, including availability, cost, and clinical experience. The insulins comprise pork, beef, beef-pork, or human types. Standard marketing for all are in the U-100 concentration, although U-40 and U-500 insulins are also available. Despite differences in trade names and in the manufacturers' slight variations in stated action curves, these insulins are amazingly similar in actual usage. They will be categorized primarily in the following groups: fast-acting, intermediate-acting, and long-acting. A few comments will also be directed toward the biphasic insulins, Mixtard and Initard. Table 6–4 outlines the overall characteristics of these insulins, based on manufacturers' data, published investigations, and our personal experience. Within groups, there is no convincing evidence that one product is superior to another. The question of whether to use pure pork or human insulin and when to use each will be covered later in this chapter.

Fast-Acting Insulins

Regular insulin is marketed as Iletin-R (Lilly), Velosulin (Nordisk), and Novolin-R (Squibb-Novo); these are the three primary insulins of this group. They are all pure crystalline insulins and appear water-clear. Semilente is a cloudy insulin and is similar in onset of action but may have a slightly later peak and longer duration of action.

Action Characteristic. Onset of action in lowering blood glucose is stated to be approximately 30 minutes after subcutaneous injection, with the peak activity occurring 1.5 to 3.0 hours after injection. The duration of measurable insulin in the serum following injection is variable, but the effective blood glucose–lowering action is complete by four hours.

Clinical Usage

Singular Use. Because of the rapid onset of action and rapid disappearance, these insulins are rarely used alone except in insulin-infusion systems. They are often used as supplemental doses during periods of acute hyperglycemia and ketonemia. All Regular insulins may be given intravenously.

Combination Use. The most common usage of these agents is in combination with standard doses of either intermediate-acting or long-acting agents. When used either in com-

Table 6–4. **CHARACTERISTICS OF UNITED STATES INSULIN PREPARATIONS**

Class/Name	Manufacturer*	Species**	Approx. Action Curves (hrs)		
			Onset	*Peak*	*Duration*
Rapid-acting					
Regular	L, S/N	B, P, B-P, H	0.5	2–4	4–6
Velosulin	Nd	P	0.5	1–3	4–8
Semilente	L, S/N	B, B-P	0.5–1.0	5–10	4–10
Biphasic					
Mixtard	Nd	P	0.5–1.0	3–4/4–8	16–24
Intermediate-acting					
NPH	L, S/N	B, P, B-P, H	1.5–2	6–12	16–24
Lente	L, S/N	B, P, B-P, H	1.5–2	6–12	16–24
Insulatard	Nd	P	1.5–2	4–12	16–24
Long-acting					
PZI	L	B, P, B-P	4–8	14–24	36+
Ultralente	L, S/N	B, B-P	4–8	18–24	36+

*L = Lilly Laboratories, S/N = Squibb-Novo, Nd = Nordisk-USA
**B = Beef, P = Pork, B-P = Beef-pork, H = Human

bination or alone, they are most effective in preventing postfeeding hyperglycemia when given 30 to 45 minutes before the meal.

Intermediate-Acting Insulins

Such insulins either have protamine added to crystalline insulin (for example, NPH) or the crystalline structure is altered (for example, Lente) to bring about a delay in subcutaneous absorption. For practical purposes, the protamine-type insulins and the Lente-type insulins are interchangeable. All are somewhat cloudy in appearance, and a precipitate will form when the insulin is allowed to remain at room or storage temperature. This is the most commonly used group of insulins.

Action Characteristics

Onset of action is often delayed from 1.5 to 3.0 hours following injection. For this reason these insulins when given alone are not usually effective in preventing the postprandial glucose surge, particularly that which occurs after breakfast. The peak action occurs generally about 6 to 12 hours after injection. Our clinical experience suggests that the average peak is at about 8 hours. Free insulin activity is still usually found at 24 hours after injection, but the effective phase of blood glucose lowering seems to pass at about 16 to 18 hours in most persons. On the other hand, some persons appear to get more than a 24-hour biologic effect. Mixtard is said to have 70 percent NPH and 30 percent Regular insulin, but its free insulin content is closer to 15 percent. Consequently, this biphasic insulin acts similar to a 3:1 mixture of NPH:Regular.

Clinical Usage

These are the most commonly used insulins and are usually given in either a single morning injection (usually in combination with a fast-acting insulin) or in a two shot per day regimen, with the second injection usually either at the evening meal or at bedtime. There appears to be no advantage to the mixing of insulins from within the same groups (such as NPH and Lente). Premixed Mixtard should theoretically be a better product than other intermediate insulins alone, but this combination offers little advantage over that produced by mixing the insulins immediately prior to injection, except in those persons with limited vision or those for whom mixing insulins is beyond their capability.

Long-Acting Insulins

Action Characteristics

The two insulins in this group (protamine zinc insulin, or PZI, and Ultralente) act similarly. Their onset of action is quite slow, and the peak action is widely variable, ranging from 10 to 30 hours. The duration of action is equally variable, with reports usually ranging from 36 to 48 hours. As such, when given daily, there is an overlapping curve, producing a cumulative effect. When these insulins are used as primary therapy with a single injection in the morning, serious nighttime and early morning hypoglycemia is a potential consequence.

Clinical Usage

Recently there has been an interest in the use of these insulins in combination with preprandial Regular insulin, in several intensified regimens. In such programs, the long-acting insulin, given in small amounts once or twice daily, acts in a fashion similar to those of the basal infusions given during pump therapy.

Sources of Insulin and Their Uses

As noted earlier, commercial insulin derivatives are either pure beef, pure pork, beef-pork (70 percent:30percent) mixture, or human (biosynthetic or semi-synthetic).

Beef Insulin

This insulin (either USP or purified) is available on request and is priced slightly higher than the beef-pork mixture. Beef insulin is slightly more dissimilar to that inherent in humans than is pork (a three-amino-acid difference versus a one-amino-acid difference). Consequently, beef insulin is more immunogenic; and overall, insulin antibody titers are higher with this insulin than with pure pork insulin. The only indication for its routine use would be an allergy to pork insulin; but with the current availability of human insulin, there may be no future market for this product. In addition, persons who are markedly allergic to pork insulin often develop similar reactions to beef insulin.

Pork Insulin

Pork insulin differs in only one amino acid from human insulin and is thus less immunogenic than are insulins containing beef. Compared with beef or beef-pork insulins, less of the injected pork insulin is bound to high-affinity circulating antibodies, and there is more uniform action and a slightly reduced total dosage required to maintain comparable blood glucose results. In most clinical trials, the dosage of insulin has dropped by about 20 percent when a change has been made from beef-pork insulin to pork insulin. Whether there are other overall advantages is not certain. Pure pork insulin should be given a trial when there are local or systemic allergic reactions that persist; in instances when insulin resistance is associated with high antibody titer; and when there is lipoatrophy at the sites of insulin injection. Pure pork insulins cost the patient from 20 to 50 percent more than do beef-pork mixtures.

Beef-Pork Insulin

This has been the most commonly used source of insulin in the United States. It is highly purified but does contain both a beef peak (70 percent) and a pork peak (30 percent). Overall, it is the least expensive insulin on the commercial market. Most patients seem to do exceedingly well on this insulin. In our experience, there are fewer local skin reactions due to this mixture than with beef-insulin alone and antibody titers of both beef and beef-pork insulins seem to be in the same range. The antibody titer with beef-pork insulin is higher than with pure pork insulins.

Human Biosynthetic, Semisynthetic Insulin

Biosynthetic human insulin was introduced to the commercial market in 1983 by Lilly Laboratories after several years of clinical testing. This type of insulin is made by recombinant DNA techniques using certain strains of the bacterium *Escherichia coli*. Its safety has been ensured in multiple studies, and its biologic actions are almost identical to those of pure pork insulin. Early studies of human-derived insulin have suggested more rapid absorption from depot sites and a shortened half-life when compared with those of other insulins. If this is borne out in subsequent studies, then sound clinical usage may mandate a three shot per day program of this insulin to ensure good control. Semisynthetic human insulin (Squibb-Novo) was also introduced in 1983. It is made by chemical substitution of the variant amino acid from pork insulin, so as to make it chemically identical to human insulin. There have been no side-by-side comparisons of the two insulins.

At this time both biosynthetic and semisynthetic insulins are competitive with pure pork insulins in price, and indications for their use are similar to those noted earlier: insulin allergy, insulin lipoatrophy, and high titers of insulin antibodies with a degree of insulin resistance. Although on a unit-per-unit basis these insulins produce a greater fall in blood glucose than does beef or beef-pork insulin, on a general basis they appear comparable to pork in this regard. Because of the possibility of shortened half-life, their use should be in concert with careful monitoring of blood glucose.

SELECTION OF AN INSULIN PROGRAM

In this section, the discussion primarily will consider the selection of insulin programs useful to the patient with diabetes. The readers can clearly recognize that there is no single correct way to use insulin, despite the rhetoric and protestations of some diabetologists. It is not necessarily malfeasance for a clinician to suggest a single injection of intermediate-acting insulin per day if control parameters demonstrate normal or near-normal values. It would be inconsistent with good medical evidence, however, to believe that more than a few patients with IDDM can be appropriately managed by such therapy. As noted earlier, the outcome is more important than the process. Therapy must be individualized so as to achieve desirable end results.

The selection of an insulin program is not a static feature or a once-only aspect of diabetes care; it is the most appropriate management at the beginning, based on ideals of

Table 6–5. INSULIN PROGRAMS IN COMMON USE

I. One injection per day (usually in AM before breakfast)
   A. Intermediate-acting insulin *alone*
   B. Intermediate-acting and Regular insulin *together*
   C. Long-acting, intermediate-acting, and Regular insulin *together*
II. Two injections per day
   A. Intermediate-acting insulin before breakfast and supper
   B. Addition of Regular insulin to one or both of IIA
   C. IC plus intermediate-acting insulin at bedtime
III. Three (or more) injections per day
   A. Long-acting insulin in AM; Regular before meals
   B. Long-acting insulin before breakfast and supper; Regular before meals
   C. Intermediate and Regular insulin before breakfast; Regular before supper; intermediate before bedtime
   D. Regular insulin before meals; intermediate-acting before bedtime
   E. Long-acting insulin at bedtime; Regular before meals
IV. Continuous subcutaneous insulin infusion (CSII)
     Various methods

"best medical practice" and on the lifestyle issues of the patient. If the system or plan works, then minor modifications alone will tailor the program to the person. If the program does not meet expectations, then significant alterations in the management protocol may be necessary.

Specific Insulin Programs

This chapter cannot possibly discuss all programs that have been designed. Thus, a few of the more common have been chosen. Table 6–5 lists the more common insulin programs and includes those to be discussed here. The order of the methods to be discussed does not necessarily indicate our priorities of therapy. There is, however, utility in starting in an order that is the reverse of that noted in the table. It seems appropriate for the reader to return to Figure 6–1 to once again visualize those things we hope to accomplish.

Continuous Subcutaneous Insulin Infusion (CSII)

An overall and detailed consideration of external or open-loop insulin infusion systems will be discussed in Chapter 23. At this point, brief mention will be made concerning a few aspects of such therapy.

Characteristics. Figure 6–4 graphically outlines the common characteristics of CSII; these are favorably compared with the pattern of nondiabetic insulin delivery. Although there are individual differences in pumps and pump programs, all have two common characteristics: the ability to give a continuous or basal infusion and the ability to administer boluses or pulses of insulin that correspond with eating and stress. Some machines can also administer from one to five predetermined alterations in the basal rate, a feature that is particularly important with relation to an increased predawn need for insulin. The hardware, once large, cumbersome, and ugly, is now small, convenient, and relatively attractive. It is likely that this will be further accomplished with future technical advances.

Advantages. CSII, coupled with a detailed educational program, home blood glucose monitoring, and high motivation, has been shown to dramatically improve diabetes control and to return most patients' metabolic abnormalities to normal. Fasting and postprandial glucose levels are controlled, and the concentration of glycosylated hemoglobin has been shown to return to normal. Additionally, some chronic features (exercise-induced proteinuria, nerve conduction velocity, and plasma amino acid and lipid profiles) appear reversible if ideal therapy is initiated early. A single-needle injection every one to three days is an added advantage. A lifestyle that is less constrained and restricted is a possible outcome. Many patients feel better once diabetes control is established and once an accelerated rate of physical growth is possible.

Disadvantages. A high degree of motivation on the part of the patient, the family, and the physician is necessary if maximum benefit is to be obtained. Although the degree of flexibility in lifestyle that CSII permits is greatly increased (that is, more flexibility in timing and content of meals and snacks, one injection only every 24 to 72 hours, less rigid schedules, and so forth), this only accrues for the patient after considerable education and experience. At first, the degree of effort can and should be extraordinary. The pumps, even the smaller third-generation microprocessor units, are a constant reminder of diabetes. To some teenagers and most young adults, who have a mature self-concept and are motivated, this serves as an advantage. In the younger child and in adolescents who

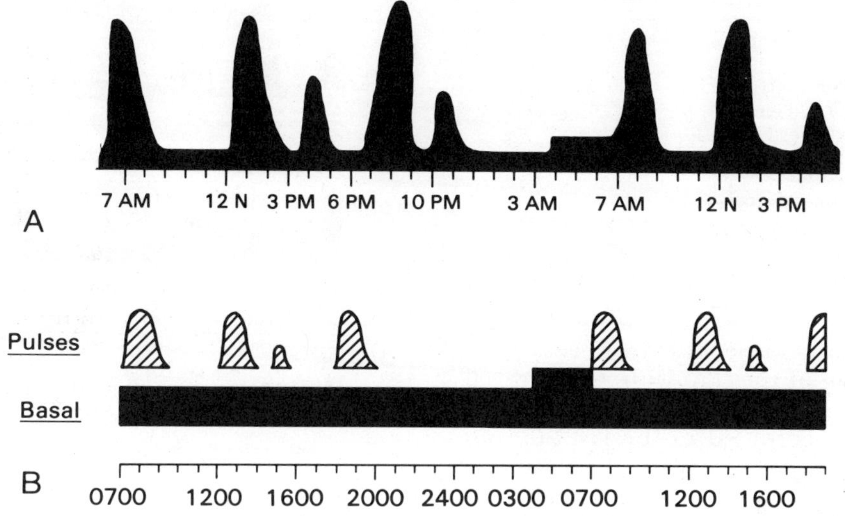

Figure 6–4. This picture contrasts the normal pattern of insulin secretion (*A*) against that which can be programmed and administered by most of the external insulin pumps (*B*). A basal secretion with a diurnal pattern is achievable, and individual pulses are comparable to substrate-mediated secretions.

are struggling with self-identity and desperately wanting to be like peers, the pump's presence may produce more stress and be a disadvantage. These children often have an external locus of control, and their own motivation is rarely sufficient to sustain them. This creates problems with adherence to proper use of such devices and can lead to frightening consequences.

Several other areas of concern should be noted, including severe hypoglycemia as a consequence of attempts at too rigid control; sudden development of ketoacidosis as a consequence of lack of insulin (catheter comes out or becomes plugged, or pump malfunctions); and the possibility of subcutaneous skin infections.

Hypoglycemia becomes more common as the rigidity of the control management increases. Several studies have demonstrated that the frequency of hypoglycemia increases in direct proportion to the reduction in the zenith of blood glucose fluctuation. One study also demonstrated that the severity of hypoglycemic episodes is directly related to the tightness of control (for example, the nearer the glycosylated hemoglobin value is to normal, the more likely the occurrence of severe hypoglycemia). One other factor also seems to be important and must be addressed. The closer the mean blood glucose value approaches normal (as measured by HbA_{1C}), the less likely it is that any resultant hypoglycemia will be characterized by "rebound symptoms" (for example, shakiness, hot or

cold feelings, pallor, sweating, and tachycardia) and the more likely it is that initial symptoms will be primarily the type that affect the central nervous system (for example, personality change, confusion, disorientation, and somnolence). It is therefore imperative that the person receiving pump therapy be able to recognize the primary symptoms of hypoglycemia and to regularly monitor blood glucose at home.

The sudden development of *diabetic ketoacidosis* is usually due to unexpected and unrecognized cessation of insulin delivery. This usually occurs when the needle or catheter dislodges from its subcutaneous site but occasionally is seen with catheter blockage or pump failure. Since there is no depot insulin on which to depend, the person rapidly becomes underinsulinized, and ketoacidosis is a consequence. This should be suspected whenever blood sugars unexpectedly rise or the person becomes sick quickly, or both. In such cases, proper assessment includes checking for the presence of urinary ketones and careful inspection of the pump, catheter, and injection site.

Skin infections are more common with CSII than they are with traditional insulin therapy, owing to the presence of an indwelling needle or catheter. Most such infections appear to be due to improper cleansing technique or to less frequent changing of sites than is recommended. Our experience with 29 children receiving pump therapy suggests a frequency of skin infection of around 15 percent

Table 6–6. **PRIMARY INDICATIONS FOR CSII***

Failure to grow normally	12
Hyperlabile	7
Desire for better control	4
Proteinuria (<1 g/day)	2
Nephropathy/Hypertension/Retinopathy	2
Seizure disorder	1
Painful neuropathy	1

*These data from our Center are for the first 29 children given an external infusion device.

but most of these occurred during the first year of patient experience. We now recommend cleansing of the skin with antibacterial agents, rather than just with alcohol. No infections have occurred in the last 200 patient-months.

Clinical Use. Chapter 23 will further outline the use of pump therapy and will give details of our experience in 29 children. Table 6–6 outlines the primary indications for CSII use in these children and encompasses the reasons for CSII in most clinical studies. Overall, we have had a reasonable degree of success with pump management. Some success has been obtained in overcoming growth retardation due to diabetes (seven of 12 patients), in hyperlabile patients (five of seven), in highly motivated adolescents desiring better control (three of four), in adolescents with minimal proteinuria (one of two), and in reduction in number of seizures (one patient only).

Prescription of an external insulin pump, although no longer considered experimental, should be made only if availability of a 24-hour per day team is ensured. Most of the finer diabetes centers and all of the reputable manufacturers of pumps have such "call-in" capabilities. Pumps are designed to aid the patient in normalizing blood sugar and therefore have the capability of producing significant hypoglycemia. The patient needs careful supervision in this area. Additionally, pumps do malfunction, and both medical and service representatives must respond to the need thus generated. The actual prescription for CSII is made after a brief hospitalization, during which the patient's glucose and insulin profiles are investigated. This is done either by hourly blood glucose measurements or by attaching the patient to a constant glucose monitor (Biostator). We prefer the latter method. A basal infusion rate (usually between 30 and 40 percent of the total glucose monitoring in the preprandial and postprandial periods) is then established.

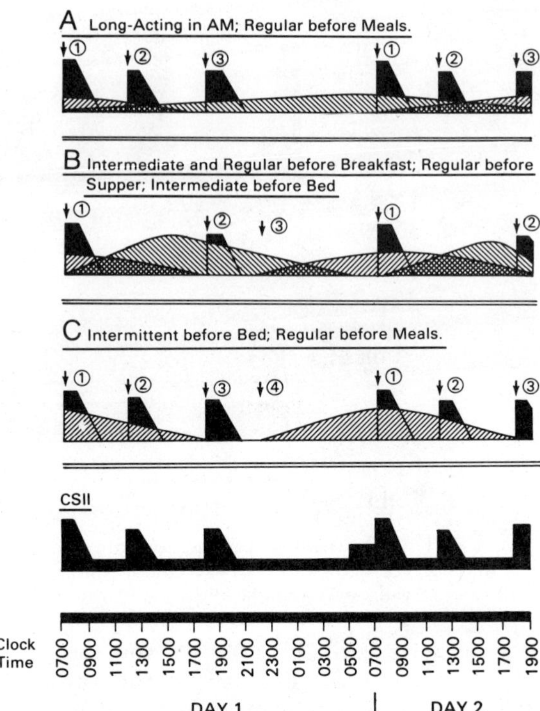

Figure 6–5. Regimens of three shots per day with Ultralente and Regular (*A*), three shots per day with NPH/Lente and Regular (*B*), and four shots per day (*C*) are noted. All give comparable results when coupled with other aspects of treatment. CSII therapy schedule is given at the botton for comparison. See text for discussion.

Three (or More) Insulin Injections Per Day

There are many programs in which multiple insulin injections are prescribed. Some physicians have used such programs for decades with apparent success, but there has also been a recent resurgence of interest in such therapy. Part of the reason has been the increased understanding of normal insulin delivery. In addition, such programs have been proposed as alternatives to CSII. The most frequently used regimens have been listed in Table 6–5 and will be briefly discussed. All give results comparable to those of CSII when the same monitoring and adjustment parameters are used. Some programs are shown in Figure 6–5.

Long-Acting (Ultralente) Before Breakfast; Regular Before all Meals (Figure 6–5A). Long-acting insulin is designed to act much like a basal infusion, and Regular insulin boluses are given prior to each meal. Although the graph in Figure 6–5 suggests that the "peak" of Ultralente occurs at the time of pre-dawn needs, variability in this absorption may prevent this pattern from being consistent. Occasionally, this regimen produces significant hypoglycemia in the 2:00 AM to 4:00 AM period. To counteract this, some have divided the Ultralente dosage into two equal parts taken before breakfast and before supper. This gives a smoother basal level, but the predawn need for a higher insulin level is absent. Some have solved this by adding Lente insulin to the night dosage.

Intermediate-Acting and Regular Before Breakfast; Regular Before Supper; Intermediate Before Bed (Figure 6–5B). This is the most popular of the three shot per day programs for children who are in school. In the main, it merely involves moving the intermediate-acting insulin at the evening meal to a prebedtime dosage. This maneuver is designed to prevent a significant drop of blood glucose between 2:00 AM and 4:00 AM and also to provide for the increased predawn needs. Problems with this regimen are hypoglycemia in the late afternoon (before supper) and in the early evening (after supper).

Intermediate Before Bed, Regular Before Meals (Fig. 6–5C). This four shot per day program is designed to provide for the increased predawn needs, while minimizing 3:00 AM hypoglycemia. Our experience in only a few patients has demonstrated that in the majority the 2:00 AM to 4:00 AM problem with hypoglycemia is magnified with this program.

Other multiple-dose regimens are certain to follow, as persons attempt to mimic the CSII routine further. The actual pattern used must be adjusted to the patient and to his or her needs.

Two Insulin Injections Per Day

The two shot per day regimen is perhaps the most popular of current options for Type I diabetes and comes close to being the standard to which other regimens are compared. Some investigators have demonstrated that control is not necessarily improved when the treatment regimen is changed from one injection per day to two per day. Improvement in one study was judged on the basis of glycosylated hemoglobin levels, and determinations were made a relatively short time following the change. The results were not surprising, since the patients were not specifically instructed to modify dosages to achieve designated blood glucose values. Several other studies have tended to show similar pictures: no significant improvement in overall biochemical control when the only change was from one to two shots per day. Contrast this for a moment with the following study, conducted by one of us (LBT) several years ago.

UTMB Study: Twenty-five teenagers (11 males, 14 females) between the ages of 14.1 and 17.5 years of age constituted the study group. All had been diabetic for more than one year, and all were on a single AM dose of insulin (NPH/Regular). All were selected because they had demonstrated compliant behaviors, and all were interested in obtaining better control. Twenty-one individuals stated verbally and on a detailed written questionnaire that they felt well and that their ability to function was equal to that of nondiabetic peers. Four individuals said they felt poorly but, other than increased fatigue, could not define this further. All patients were presented with "evidence" suggesting that two shots per day improved control and might lessen the rate of long-term complications. Verbal and written information was given concerning this, and the patients were asked to indicate decisions by initiating a phone call to the study center one week after returning home. All 25 called, and 23 decided to move to a two shot per day program. The patients' mean glycosylated hemoglobin was 10.6 percent (range of 6.8 to 13.6 percent, normal 5.2 to 7.0 percent) prior to the study.

Six weeks later, all 25 individuals were given a repeat health assessment. Two of the four who had felt badly on the initial evaluation (glycosylated hemoglobin value of 9.1 and 11.0 percent) felt "better," despite no change in their HbA_{1C}. More surprising, eight of the 19 who had said they felt "well" initially (and who changed to a two shot per day regimen) spontaneously remarked that they felt "better," had more energy, more stamina, and so on. The other 11 claimed to feel no different. The average HbA_{1C} was 11.0 percent (range 6.2 to 12.1 percent).

Twenty-one of the original 23 who changed to two shots per day stayed on this program over the one-year study period. The other two dropped out, because they "kept forgetting their second shot." Of those staying on the two-shot program, the most common reasons for doing so were: (1) less rigidity in meal schedules, (2) more flexibility, (3) more energy. At the conclusion of the year, the mean HbA_{1C} for the whole group had not changed; but for the six-week evaluation, their mean HbA_{1C} had dropped from 10.6 percent to 9.0 percent (ranges, 8.1 to 13.0 percent; 6.4 to 11.0 percent). The two youngsters who discontinued the study eventually returned to two shots per day voluntarily, because with this regimen they "felt better."

This study, particularly when coupled with

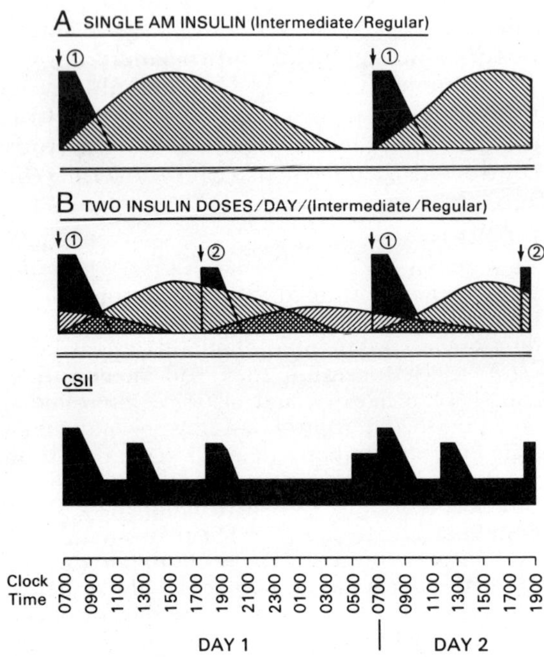

Figure 6–6. Regimens of single injection therapy with NPH/Lente mixed with regular (*A*) and classical split/mix program with two injections per day (*B*). CSII therapy is noted as a baseline. See text for discussion.

those investigations that report identical control on either regimen, suggests that there may be therapeutic subsets among patients with IDDM and reinforces the concept of individualized care. Seven of the initial group felt that their control was worse during some periods of the study. Four of these admitted to intermittent noncompliance in administration of the second shot, claiming to have forgotten it on the average of once per week. Although these data are very "soft," none of the rest of the group admitted to this type of nonadherence except on rare occasions. Those diabetologists who rigidly advocate a two or three shot per day routine for everyone must recognize that there are some who will adhere and some who will not. Those in the latter group may be worse off on a twice a day assignment than they would be on a single daily injection.

Regimen Specifics. The usual regimen for two shot per day insulin is noted in Figure 6–6*B*. The first injection of combined intermediate-acting and Regular insulin is given 30 to 45 minutes prior to breakfast; the second, 30 to 45 minutes' time prior to the evening meal. With a smaller morning dosage than would be given with a single daily injection, there is no high peak of insulin activity in the late afternoon. Consequently, we allow

Table 6–7. **USUAL SPLITS AND STARTING PLACES FOR TWO-DOSE/DAY REGIMEN**

	Usual Split of Daily Dose	Usual Distribution of NPH/Regular
Before-breakfast dosage	2/3 to 3/4	NPH—2/3 to 4/5 Reg.—1/5 to 1/3
Before-supper dosage	1/4 to 1/3	NPH—1/3 to 3/4 Reg.—1/4 to 1/2

the child some flexibility in timing of the evening meal, as long as the insulin injection is always given at the same period of time before the meal.

The usual distributions of insulin dosage between morning and evening is seen in Table 6–7. These distributions represent "starting places" for adjustments made in an effort to individualize care. This table also points out the range of distributions of the two injections. The ratio of NPH:Regular is usually higher in the morning than in the evening. The morning ratio varies from about 5:1 to 2:1, whereas in the evening it is not uncommon for children to receive a 1:1 ratio. In the evening, we try to obtain the insulin effect prior to bedtime and thus reduce the incidence of severe nighttime hypoglycemia, which seems more common when higher doses of intermediate-acting insulin are given.

Advantages. Control is improved with two shots per day for many youngsters, and more persons seem to feel well on this regimen than with a single dose per day. In our experience, 70 percent to 90 percent of children are benefited in one way or another by a two shot per day regimen. Many families describe an increased flexibility on a two shot per day regimen (for example, timing of meals does not need to be as precise); this is a major factor in young persons staying on the two shot per day program.

Disadvantages. The second injection is rarely desired. Even in those patients in whom two shots per day are initiated at onset, the evening shot is more likely to be "forgotten" than is the morning shot. This can lead to serious underinsulinization and worse metabolic control. Most children do not seem to be troubled by the two shots. Parents seem more concerned about two shots per day, and physicians often appear even more troubled than either, the reasons being complex and not fully understood.

When to Initiate a Two Shot Per Day Regimen. This is a matter of individual preference, and there is no correct answer for all situations. The options are (1) to initiate a two shot per day program at onset in all patients or (2) to convert from one shot per day to two per day if and when control worsens. By making the first choice, the physician automatically excludes that group of patients who might be controlled with a single injection. However, by making the second choice, the physician is often caught in a struggle with the child and parents concerning the issue. To be forced to go from one shot to two shots per day is a clear message to adults and children that "the diabetes is getting worse." No matter how often one repeats the statement that such is not necessarily the case, the act speaks more loudly than the words, as evidenced by this brief vignette:

K. G., a six-year old girl, was started on one shot per day insulin (NPH/Regular) at onset of her disease (five years earlier) by one of the senior authors. Mr. and Mrs. G., bright and well educated, were told repeatedly at that time and later that two shots per day would most likely be required and would be determined by the degree of control. For the first year K. G.'s control was excellent, with HbA_{1C} values close to normal. As she emerged from the remissive phase, the insulin requirement rose and she began experiencing afternoon hypoglycemia. In order to achieve 24-hour coverage, she was changed to two injections per day and the parents were again told that this was the expected course of events.

Despite this, a maternal great-aunt, and close friend of the other senior author, was told by the parents that K. G.'s diabetes had grown worse. She called this author in a panic, under the belief that K. G. had little hope of ever doing well.

In our experience, the foregoing is not an uncommon occurrence. Consequently, it is our general practice to initiate a two shot per day regimen at onset of the patient's disease.

One Injection Per Day

A single morning injection of insulin per day is still among the more commonly used regimens today. It is probably the treatment of choice for the patient with Type II diabetes who requires insulin. Some diabetologists still advocate the use of this method as primary therapy in the Type I diabetic, although the number advocating this regimen seems to decline every year. In the main, one shot per day therapy generally consists of a single morning dose of an intermediate-acting insulin, usually with Regular insulin in the same syringe. Figure 6–6A demonstrates the usual action curves of such a program. The major disadvantage of this regimen is that, in order to get a 24-hour action curve, the dose must be so high that the peak of action (early to late afternoon) is often too high, with resultant hypoglycemia. In addition, there is a period of time early in the morning when the person appears underinsulinized. This time coincides with that period of increased predawn need.

Our experience indicates that only about 10 percent of patients with IDDM can be effectively treated with a single daily injection. In the main, these are patients with residual endogenous insulin, as measured by plasma C-peptide levels. Even in these children, however, there is a great need for rigidity of diet, particularly as this relates to the timing of meals. Otherwise, significant hypoglycemia tends to occur. Many patients who attempt to use this method and control diabetes continue to experience 2:00 to 4:00 AM hypoglycemic reactions.

Regular insulin in the morning is virtually always necessary to achieve some desirable effects. This is generally mixed in the same syringe with distribution ranging between 5:1 and 2:1 (intermediate:Regular). We do not advocate *premixing* insulins regularly for the following reason; although there is some binding of the Regular and intermediate-acting insulins, the degree of binding is not consistent; and premixing limits some of the options for dosage alterations that are available to those who do not premix.

Some persons have advocated mixing of several types of insulin to achieve desired effects. One combination that has been advocated by some is the mixture of UltraLente, Lente, and Regular in a single morning injection. There are some patients who seem to do well on this regimen, but in our experience, it appears to afford no more advantages than do other single-injection methods.

INITIATION OF INSULIN THERAPY

Although it is obvious that initiation of insulin is important, the primary objective is not to be precise in the correct dosage but merely to approximate it. Subsequent adjustments will allow the clinician to tailor the dose to the patient's needs. There are a number of methods for "guessing" at the initial dosage. We will consider just two: one for the hospitalized patient (inpatient use) and the other for ambulatory patient use.

Hospitalized Patient

There may actually be two subgroups of this category: patients with diabetic ketoacidosis (DKA) and those without DKA. Those with symptomatic DKA and those still recovering from it have relative insulin resistance owing to the higher circulating levels of stress hormones. They may require more insulin to bring about a change in glucose-fat homeostasis. With either subgroup, we believe it easier to initiate therapy with multi-injection Regular insulin because (1) the action curve of Regular insulin is more predictable, (2) the insulin half-life is short and consequently prompt adjustments in dosage can be made, and (3) techniques of administration are more easily taught when several injections are given per day than when only one or two are given.

Ketotic or Post-DKA Patients

Regular insulin in a dosage of 0.05 to 0.1 units kilogram per dose should be given either every six hours (if the glucose intake is equally divided) or before each meal. The response to the insulin (and glucose intake) should be monitored by blood glucose measurements obtained two or four hours later or at both times. The next dose is then determined based on response to the previous dose. Obviously, subsequent doses may either be lower, the same, or higher than earlier ones. This is called a *prospective sliding scale* in that it requires the physician to make a decision on each dose, based on the patient's response. It should not be confused with the traditional retrospective sliding scale in which a clinical judgment is not actually made as to whether or not the next dose should be given.

Some physicians prefer to give a separate shot of Regular insulin at bedtime, but our preference is to give a small dose of NPH, usually about 0.025 unit per kilogram. This may maintain euglycemia during the night and blunt the predawn glucose surge. After two to three days, the daily dose of Regular insulin required is totaled and the sum divided into a two shot per day regimen using the guidelines indicated earlier.

Table 6–8. **KEYS TO SUCCESSFUL INSULIN THERAPY**

A. Relative stability of other factors (diet, stress, exercise)
B. Appropriate insulin regimen
   Individualized
C. Home blood glucose monitoring
D. Patient/Family understanding of:
   1. Goals of insulin therapy
   2. Meaning and use of "pattern control"
   3. Algorithms for altering insulin dosage
E. Patient/Family willingness to undertake the responsibility for D.

Ambulatory Patients

In most instances, we believe it desirable to admit the newly diagnosed patient for a short hospitalization. This admission aids the family in initial adjustment and allows for survival skills to be more easily taught. At times, however, it may be best to keep the child out of the hospital and to initiate insulin in an outpatient setting.

Regular insulin can be given in the manner noted previously for the hospitalized child. On the other hand, two doses per day of a mixture of insulins is usually best and, in our practice, an NPH/Regular mixture is generally chosen. The total daily dose is estimated at 0.2 and 0.3 unit per kilogram body weight, with two thirds given in the morning and one third at supper. Adjustments are then made according to the following program schedule.

ALTERATIONS IN INSULIN THERAPY

The key to appropriate insulin therapy is neither the type of insulin nor even the initial regimen or dosage chosen, but the willingness and ability of the patient to make alterations in dosage depending on need. This and other important aspects of successful insulin management are listed in Table 6–8. There should be some stability in other factors, particularly diet and stress. There is often a tendency among some to believe that diabetes can be controlled with insulin alone. It helps if the initial selection of insulin dosage is approximately correct. Home blood glucose monitoring is an essential feature of successful insulin therapy. But, despite the importance of these aspects, the items listed in sections D and E of this table are of the highest priority.

The patient or family or both must fully

understand the goals and objectives and must be in accord with them. These goals must be expressed in both clinical and biochemical terms, but in the context of alterations in insulin dosages the biochemical aspects must appear primary. Patient and family must understand "pattern" control and be supplied with some sample algorithms so that dosages may be altered. Most importantly, the patient and family must be willing to make alterations based on the observed patterns and needs. These aspects have been previously discussed but will be reviewed briefly here.

Biochemical Objectives of Insulin Therapy

Obtaining blood glucose values as close as possible to those of the nondiabetic, while maintaining a healthful feeling, is the goal of therapy. Our patients are taught that they should attempt to maintain at least 75 percent of their blood glucose values between 80 mg/dl and 150 mg/dl.

"Pattern Control"

The concept of pattern control involves serial observations of blood glucose, assumptions based on these observations, and a knowledge of insulin action. There are so many variables that affect isolated blood sugar values that adjustments made on the basis of single determinations are discouraged. On the other hand, one acquires some insight into control if the before-breakfast blood glucose level is either consistently high or consistently low. Similarly, one might observe blood glucose profiles at other selected times during the day or night: before lunch, before supper, before bed, 3 AM, two hours after meals, and so forth. The patient then addresses the question of whether there is a recurring sequence, or pattern, of blood glucose levels at a specific time over several days' of observation. For instance, consider the following sequence of blood glucose values in several different children and decide which represents a generally recurring pattern:

	Patient	Sample Time	Blood Glucose						
			S	M	T	W	T	F	S
1.	L.C.	Before Breakfast	78	261	288	48	136	315	200
2.	R.A.	Before Breakfast	62	110	44	80	84	56	48
3.	O.L.	Before Lunch	310	250	195	260	304	185	230
4.	M.S.	Before Supper	204	116	300	260	145	60	284
5.	S.B.	Before Bed	165	130	110	304	260	80	135

Obviously, the patterns seen in samples 2 and 3 are consistent; there is a pattern of sequence to the blood glucose levels. Patient R. A. (sample 2) has consistently low blood glucose levels, while Patient O. L. (sample 3) has consistently high blood glucose levels. But what of the others? Glucose levels in four of seven days in sample 1 are high, one is low, and two are normal. Therefore, a recurring pattern is not evident. The problems of interpretation in samples 4 and 5 are both real. Overall, these patients' values suggest that there is persistent hyperglycemia, but in both there are values that are normal. Our practice is to ask the child or parent to find at least three consecutive days of consistent results before labeling such a pattern. In neither sample 4 nor sample 5 is there this consistency.

Once the patient is skilled in identifying patterns of results, there are certain assumptions that are necessary in order to make alterations (Fig. 6–7). Although it is recognized that the morning dose of intermediate-acting (NPH) insulin maintains some effect all day, its major influence is on the before-supper blood glucose levels. Thus, if the before-supper blood glucose values were inappropriately high for several days (a pattern), an appropriate response would be to increase the morning dose of NPH insulin. Likewise by consulting this figure, the informed and willing patient should be able to select and modify the correct insulin dose in

PRIMARY INSULIN ACTIONS

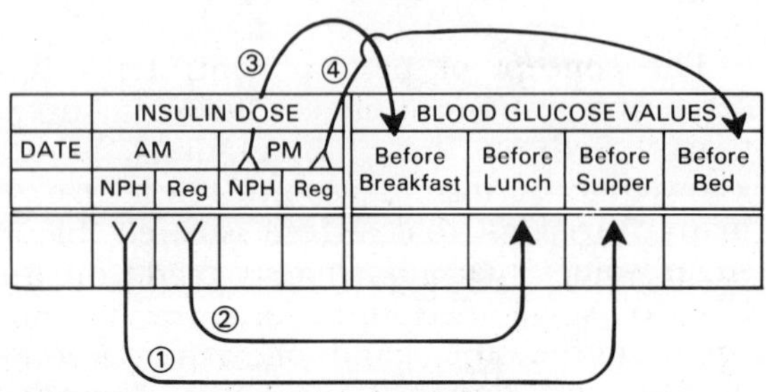

① Morning NPH has major or primary influence on before-supper blood glucose.

② Morning REGULAR has major or primary influence on before-lunch blood glucose.

③ Evening NPH has major or primary influence on before-breakfast blood glucose.

④ Evening REGULAR has major or primary influence on before-bedtime blood glucose.

Figure 6–7. When insulin doses are changed, certain assumptions must be made. These are demonstrated here and in the text.

order to alter abnormal patterns of blood glucose.

Algorithms for Insulin-Dose Alterations

The essential algorithms for modifying insulin dose are noted in Table 6–9, with some special rules governing these changes given in Table 6–10. Alterations such as these are aimed at preventing persistent abnormalities.

Table 6–9. **ALGORITHMS FOR INSULIN-DOSE ALTERATIONS**

I. *Before-Lunch blood glucose values*
  A. If pattern in over 150 mg/dl:
    raise dose of AM-Regular by 1 to 2 units
  B. If pattern is under 80 mg/dl:
    lower dose of AM-Regular by 1 to 2 units
II. *Before-supper blood glucose values*
  A. If pattern is over 150 mg/dl:
    raise dose of AM-NPH by 1 to 3 units
  B. If pattern is under 80 mg/dl:
    lower dose of AM-NPH by 1 to 3 units
III. *Before-bedtime blood glucose values*
  A. If pattern is over 150 mg/dl:
    raise PM-Regular by 1 to 2 units
  B. If pattern is under 80 mg/dl:
    lower PM-Regular by 1 to 2 units
IV. *Before breakfast blood glucose values*
  A. If pattern is over 120 mg/dl:
    raise PM-NPH by 1 to 3 units
  B. If pattern is under 80 mg/dl:
    lower PM-NPH by 1 to 3 units

Table 6–10. **RULES FOR INSULIN DOSE ALTERATIONS**

1. Use patterns of blood glucose.
2. Use algorithms to achieve objectives.
3. Make no more than a single alteration every 2 to 3 days.
4. Changes in a given dose of insulin should be approximately 10% of that dose.
5. If the before-breakfast blood glucose level is consistently below 80 mg/dl, or if the before-bed blood glucose level is consistently lower than the before-breakfast one, measure 3 AM blood glucose level.
6. Once a change is made, this change is the *new* standard insulin dose.

Once a change has occurred in one of the doses, the change becomes the new standard for that dose. Changes should generally be made no more frequently than every two to three days, and it is ill advised to change more than one dose per 24-hour period.

Some patients and families will readily accept such an active role in insulin-dose adjustment. Others will be hesitant to do so because of their fright at being placed in such a responsible position or because it is not their nature to accept medical partnership. Still others may refuse to make such alterations, even when understanding is present and indications are clear. All will require team support on the first few occasions.

MODIFICATIONS TO STANDARD INSULIN THERAPY

These temporary supplements are covered in greater detail in Chapter 11. Supplements of Regular insulin are administered when there is both hyperglycemia and ketonuria, usually during infections or other stress. In such situations, the action of the standard insulin appears insufficient and a supplement is necessary. We usually recommend giving about 20 percent of the total morning dose of insulin (0.1 to 0.2 units per kilogram body weight) as Regular insulin. Results (blood glucose and urine ketone levels) are then monitored after two to three hours. Repeated doses of Regular insulin are then given at two-hour intervals for as long as both hyperglycemia and ketonuria persist. This, coupled with an increase in fluid intake, is one of the most effective means of preventing hospitalization for DKA.

Some diabetologists recommend supplements of Regular insulin on the basis of alterations in blood glucose values alone, without concern for the presence or absence of either symptoms or ketonuria. This type of "sliding-scale" is difficult for us to comprehend and impossible for us to agree with. Such modifications, or supplements, are based on single blood glucose determinations and on past events; they are "after-the-fact" dosage adjustments. In our experience, there is often more harm than good to be derived from such actions.

An exception to this philosophy might be when the well-informed diabetic in excellent control is faced with prospects of eating a meal that is significantly different from the patient's usual meals. If this person has been adequately trained and is so motivated, small alterations in the standard insulin regimen can be made to compensate for the anticipated change:

K. S., a 17-year-old, highly motivated young woman with well-controlled diabetes, usually takes an evening dose of 10 units NPH and 10 units Regular insulin. On this particular evening, she is attending a dinner party at which she anticipates eating more carbohydrate than usual. She elects to take 10 units NPH and 14 units Regular rather than her usual dose in anticipation of the higher carbohydrate intake.

Occasionally, in the patient with well-regulated diabetes, unanticipated events may cause sudden rises in blood glucose and produce acute symptoms. Again, the well-informed person with diabetes may be able to make an appropriate adjustment, as this example and the following one indicate.

J. C., a 19-year-old, compliant young man with well-regulated diabetes, took his usual dose of evening insulin (12 units NPH/7 units Regular) at 6.00 PM and later had an extra feeding consisting of about four starch or bread exchanges. By 10:00 PM he felt somewhat listless, and his blood glucose level was 280 mg/dl. He took an extra 3 units of Regular insulin, and a recheck of blood glucose at midnight was 180 mg/dl. His pattern the following day was normal.

Neither of these two examples represent a routine sliding-scale but are based on thoughtful decisions about particular situations. Through such mechanisms, the person with diabetes can have a more flexible lifestyle. Another somewhat more complex but frequently seen situation is noted by this example:

L. M. is a 16-year-old young woman with a five-year history of diabetes. Her diabetes is very well controlled. Her history over the past three years has shown that, beginning on the first day of her menses and continuing for three days, she has hyperglycemia and feels unwell. She learned that she could eliminate the hyperglycemia by raising her total dose of insulin on these days. Through trial and error, she found that a 20 percent increase in each dose was necessary to effect this change. She now regularly makes this alteration before her blood glucose level begins to rise.

This example clearly shows a major value of record-keeping, for this allowed L. M. to make her own appropriate alterations.

Temporary Reductions

These are also discussed later in Chapters 8 and 13. When there is an anticipated decrease in insulin need, it is appropriate to make such alterations. The following example is illustrative:

D. S. is an 11-year-old whose diabetes of four years' duration is tightly controlled on two shots of insulin per day. His usual insulin dose in the morning is 24 units NPH/6 units Regular. On Saturday mornings he has soccer games, either from 9:00 to 10:00, 10:00 to 11:00, or 11:00 to 12:00. D. S. tried to take added carbohydrate and protein for breakfast on these days but this made him feel unwell and sluggish. He and his parents now electively decrease the Saturday morning doses of both NPH and Regular insulin. This maneuver plus the ingestion of a simple carbohydrate at breaks has allowed him to maintain control during his activity without significant hypoglycemia.

These types of alterations in either morning or evening doses of insulin have allowed many children to participate actively in intermittent activities without the worries that parents so often have about hypoglycemia. Preparatory to employing these temporary reductions, there is a need for patients to "know" their diabetes and to understand how their personal metabolism is likely to react to such changing situations.

PROBLEMS WITH INSULIN THERAPY

Insulin therapy can produce a number of problems, some that are merely side effects of its physiologic action and others that seem to represent changes brought about through an abnormal interaction between the host and the therapy. The problems of hypoglycemia and chronic overtreatment will be discussed in Chapters 13 and 14, respectively.

Lipohypertrophy

Lipohypertrophy, or an increase in subcutaneous fat, is quite common and is caused by an accumulation of fatty tissue at the insulin injection sites. Children often come to prefer one injection site over others (probably because of local decreases in neurosensory pain perception), and areas of hypertrophy accumulate as the number of injections in those areas increases. These sites are commonly found on the anterior thighs, on the abdomen, and on the deltoid regions of the arm. Lipohypertrophy appears also to have become more frequent as insulin has become more purified.

Since these areas represent a local response to a known physiologic action of insulin (fat deposition), lipohypertrophy represents a consequence rather than a complication of treatment. Some persons appear more likely to develop hypertrophy than others, and boys seem more likely to develop this than girls. The areas may be unsightly; but the major concern is that insulin injected into these fatty tumors is absorbed more erratically than usual, causing difficulty with control.

At each patient visit, the physician should carefully inspect the injection site or sites. The most profitable treatment is prevention of further lipohypertrophy through a proper schedule of site rotation. Areas of lipohypertrophy already present will spontaneously subside if insulin is injected in sites away from these areas, but this resolution process may take months.

Lipoatrophy

Lipoatrophy, or loss of subcutaneous fat, occurs predominantly at the site of insulin injections (Fig. 6–8). This more frequently occurs in girls, and its cause is multifactoral. One of the major factors involved appears to be an allergic response to injected insulin. Other suspected causes include cold and refrigerated insulin and minute amounts of alcohol that are carried into the tissue. The dramatic decrease in the frequency of lipoatrophy associated with the more widespread use of purified insulins supports the contention that the immunogenicity of insulin is a significant factor.

Mild lipoatrophy requires no therapy. If the area becomes more marked, then a switch to either pure pork or human insulin may be appropriate. Severely lipoatrophic areas that are disfiguring may be converted to lipohypertrophic areas by injection of pure pork or human insulin directly into the sides of the atrophic crater. Gradual filling of the crater usually occurs but may take a long time and may be initially painful.

Insulin Allergy

Insulin allergy is caused by local or generalized antibody formation. In most instances, the insulin is the immunogenic factor, but occasionally either protamine or zinc is the factor. The allergic reaction may be immediate or delayed; IgE antibodies are responsible for the former and higher titers of IgG antibodies cause the latter. The response may be local, generalized, or anaphylactoid.

The *local* response or reaction has been reported in from 6 to 12 percent of patients treated but appears to occur less frequently with the purified insulins. There is usually only a cutaneous irritation and inflammation at the site of the injection, which then subsides in from 1 to 24 hours. Sometimes it may progress and persist for days. On occasion, the site of previous days' injections will become transiently inflamed.

A *generalized* reaction occurs in less than 1 percent of cases. In most cases, this occurs in atopic individuals who have been exposed to insulin and then have had it discontinued for a while (as in the "honeymoon"). When the insulin is reinstituted, the generalized response occurs and is mostly an urticarial reaction with or without angioneurotic edema.

An *anaphylactoid* response is rare and occurs in previously sensitized individuals who are highly allergic. Most of these severe reactions are reported in adults, and we have yet to see the first incidence in a child despite the fact that we have observed several thousand children with IDDM.

Treatment for all is similar: change over to the use of purified insulins. In most instances, the course of allergy is benign and transient; but occasionally an allergic response to protamine is the culprit, in which case Lente insulins are useful. We believe that insulin should rarely be discontinued

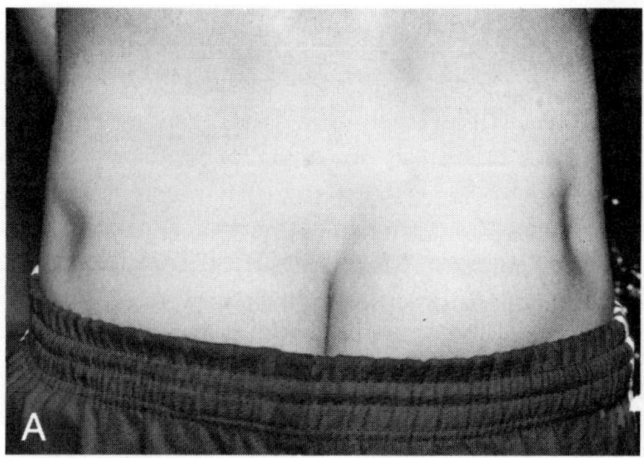
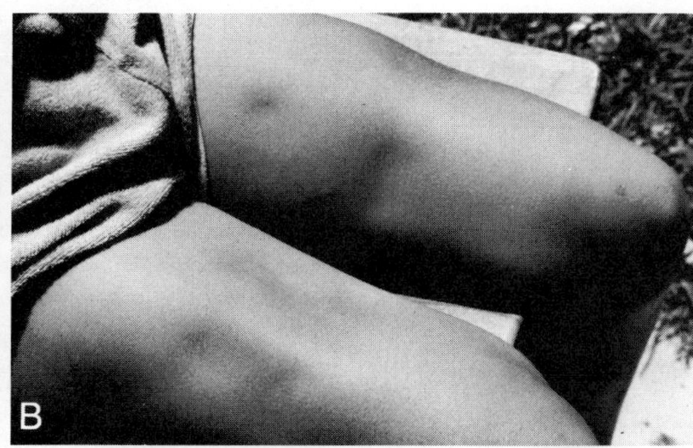
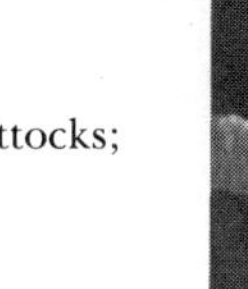

Figure 6–8. Lipoatrophy in three individuals: *A*, buttocks; *B*, legs; and *C*, arm. See text for discussion.

during the honeymoon, since allergic responses appear to be more severe when insulin is restarted. The very small doses given during the remissive phases seem to act as a desensitization program. Occasionally, we have found cyproheptadine to be beneficial in patients with persistent generalized reactions.

Insulin Resistance

True insulin resistance (that is, a requirement greater than 2.5 units of insulin per kilogram per day, continuously) is rare in those who have Type I diabetes; it occurs with a frequency of approximately 1 in 1000 to 2000 patients. Transient insulin resistance secondary to stress is quite common and is discussed in Chapter 11.

In general, insulin resistance may be categorized as an antagonism to circulating insulin (prereceptor) and as a defect in the target organ (receptor or postreceptor). Although there are a few cases reported of abnormal insulin synthesis and of incomplete conversion of proinsulin, these will not be discussed.

Prereceptor resistance is mostly related to elevated levels of counter-regulatory hormones as seen in stress but also as seen in patients with Cushing's syndrome, pheochromocytoma, and acromegaly or gigantism. A similar situation is seen in association with high titers of anti-insulin antibodies, but there is no close correlation between the two. Many patients with insulin resistance have normal antibody titers, and conversely, many persons with high antibody titers have no evidence of insulin resistance. As noted earlier, the possibility of prereceptor resistance should be considered in those patients with an accelerated destruction of subcutaneous insulin.

Insulin receptor defects are seen in several conditions that may be associated with IDDM, exogenous obesity and oral contraceptive therapy, to mention two. One might also place in this category those patients in whom it is suspected that injected insulin does not block glucose and ketone production in the liver. These patients presumably have normal peripheral action of insulin.

Postreceptor defects may be relatively common, but the ability to define these is not as precise. After insulin has bound to the receptor, one or more signals ("second messengers") are generated, which interact with other intracellular effectors to mediate the biologic actions of insulin. Abnormalities in this sequence may lead to insulin resistance. In effect, there is a decreased response in such circumstances to all concentrations of insulin. There is some evidence at present that persistent hyperglycemia itself may produce a post receptor effect, which may be reversed with better control.

Insulin-Induced Edema

Significant edema may occur when the person who has been under poor control is restored to a euglycemic state. To a modest degree, this always occurs following treatment of DKA, but the edema is generally subclinical. In some, however, fluid retention may exceed 5 percent of body weight, which constitutes clinical edema. We have seen a few patients in whom the extracellular volume was expanded to almost 10 percent of body weight. Hypertension may be simultaneously present, but this resolves as diuresis occurs, usually four to eight days after development. These patients generally do not have reduction in glomerular filtration rate and are not hypoproteinemic. The sodium and water retention here is felt to be the result of the hypovolemia that occurs during periods of poor control, with attendant increases in antidiuretic hormone and aldosterone. The effects of these hormones on salt and water retention by the kidneys persist after the cause has been removed. On occasion, the use of a thiazide diuretic may be desirable.

7

Dietary Management

Before the introduction of insulin in 1921, the only method of management for IDDM was by diet coupled with an exercise program. Dietary management was exceedingly rigid, with a meal plan consisting primarily of meats and fats. There was little incorporation of such things as potatoes, rice, pasta, or other starches. In addition, the meals were often intentionally made unpalatable, so that the person would eat less. There are, of course, times when the hospitalized patient feels that this philosophy is still in vogue. Despite this perception on the part of some, the current diet for a person with diabetes has become a well-balanced meal plan that is both nutritious and palatable and one that should be attractive to the whole family. "Well-balanced" means that the diet must contain a certain quantity and quality of essential nutrients—specifically, carbohydrates, protein, fats, vitamins, minerals, and water.

Dietary therapy has now taken on a role of secondary importance in the management of diabetes, but unfortunately some physicians and many patients have interpreted this as meaning "no importance." Although there is no question about the fact that persons with IDDM can often feel well and function acceptably while managing diabetes with insulin alone, they can rarely be "in control" of the biochemical aspects without simultaneous attention to the diet or meal plan. When one considers again the physiologic aspects of insulin therapy as outlined in Chapter 6, it is apparent that some balancing must be made between the main ingredients of diabetic control: food intake and insulin administration. To exclude diet as a factor of control is folly. On the other hand, to place undue emphasis on its relative importance would be imprudent.

BASIC ASPECTS OF NUTRITION

Dietary management of IDDM, like all other aspects of therapy, is constantly in a state of change. In addition, there is a seemingly endless stream of food fads to which the public is exposed. The physician, even though using the services of an experienced dietitian, must have a basic knowledge and understanding of nutrition in order to handle the many inquiries directed by patient and family. In this section, we will briefly discuss some of the areas in which such knowledge is required.

Basic Nutrients

Proteins

Proteins consist of amino acids that contain carbon, hydrogen, oxygen, and nitrogen. After ingestion of large protein molecules, individual amino acids are absorbed into the bloodstream and are transported to the liver, where they are sequenced for ultimate transport to the cell for specific protein manufacture. The primary function of protein is to promote growth and maintenance of tissues. Energy requirements of the body also have a high priority, and in times of such need protein will provide about 4 kilocalories per gram (kcal/g). If such were a regular occurrence, growth and tissue maintenance would be compromised. In order to spare proteins for tissue repair and maintenance, a sufficient intake of carbohydrates and fats must be consumed. Almost 60 percent of ingested protein can be converted to glucose, but when the supply of other nutrients is adequate the percentage is closer to one half this amount. Thus protein intake has significantly less immediate effect on blood glucose than does an equivalent amount of carbohydrate.

People of all ages require protein to replenish tissues that are constantly being broken down. Stress factors, such as those which occur with illness, injury, fever, and immobilization, increase this need. Most importantly, in childhood and particularly during years of rapid growth, there is a need for additional protein to synthesize new tissue. In order for the body to acquire the greatest benefit from protein in the diet, protein should be consumed intermittently throughout the day: at breakfast, lunch, and dinner. Protein taken in this manner increases the food satisfaction or satiety value and decreases hunger feelings. About 12 to 20 percent of the calories should normally be obtained from protein, and the child's diet should contain at least 2.0 grams per kilogram (g/kg) body weight.

Fats

Fats, or lipids, are made up of fatty acids (containing carbon and hydrogen) and glycerol (containing carbon, hydrogen, and oxygen). In order to be digested and absorbed, fats are emulsified with bile in the small intestine and transported via the lymphatic system, with liver and adipose tissues controlling their ultimate metabolism. When fatty acids are detached from glycerol, the glycerol is then metabolized in a way similar to that of carbohydrates.

Fats function as concentrated sources of energy, providing almost 9 kcal/g. Other functions of fats are the provision of essential fatty acids and the transport of fat-soluble vitamins. Stored fat is useful in insulation and padding of vital organs and in the maintenance of normal body temperature. Fats also give palatable and pacifying qualities to food and add to satiety. Most nutritionists generally recommend that approximately 30 percent of total caloric intake be in the form of fat and that this be equally balanced between polyunsaturated and saturated fats. This seems to lessen the atherogenic characteristics of fats in the nondiabetic and presumably in the diabetic as well.

Carbohydrates

Carbohydrates consist of carbon, oxygen, and hydrogen; and, depending on their complexity, they are classified as monosaccharides, disaccharides, and polysaccharides, or as being indigestible forms of cellulose and pectin. Monosaccharides are absorbed without enzymatic breakdown, whereas disaccharides and polysaccharides are converted to monosaccharides prior to absorption. Ultimately, most monosaccharides are converted to glucose, which functions either to provide immediate energy needs through oxidative metabolism or to be stored in liver and muscles as glycogen. Some glucose is also converted to fatty acids, which are preserved in adipose tissue. Carbohydrates provide approximately 4 kcal/g of energy.

Energy Needs

Proteins, carbohydrates, and fats are the basic nutrients that provide the body's energy needs. Each one is either completely or partially converted to glucose: carbohydrates, 100 percent; protein, 30 to 58 percent; fat, 0 to 10 percent. The amount of energy available from foods and the energy utilization that takes place in the body is measured in units of heat called calories. The amount of energy utilized at rest is termed the *basal metabolism* and varies from one individual to another based on a number of factors. Influencing the rate of metabolism are age, sex, rate of growth, sleep, body temperature, state of nutrition, and the endocrine glands' activity levels. Infants and young children thus have a different (and higher) basal metabolic rate than do adults. In the older child and in the adult, one may estimate the number of kilocalories needed daily for basal metabolism by multiplying the ideal weight (kg) for height by 24. As will be seen later, this formula is not appropriate for the younger child.

Energy is also required for daily activities, which is a significant variable. Even though young children and adolescents may appear to be quite active, the level of activity varies from individual to individual and from day to day. A broad pattern of energy needs can be assimilated by careful study of a child's daily schedule. The various activities in which young patients participate are presented in Table 7–1. These activities are expressed as the average number of kilocalories expended during sustained activity. Smaller amounts of energy are also needed for digestion and absorption of foods and for the stimulating effect of nutrients on metabolism, known as *specific dynamic effect*. In this aspect, one must consider factors such as age, sex, body size, and activity level. The Recommended Dietary Allowances for energy needs are noted in Table 7–2, and it is worthy of note that the ranges for a given age and sex are quite broad. Thus, the average or mean caloric value may be meaningless when applied to an individual child. The highest caloric level required for men occurs between ages 14 and 18, whereas with females it occurs usually between the ages 11 and 14. Basal metabolism and physical activity gradually decline at the start of adulthood, and this is when energy needs also decline.

An adequate and appropriate caloric intake is an important factor contributing to the maintenance of a normal growth rate by children. One of the most important criteria in assessing the adequacy of caloric intake is the routine charting of height and weight measurements on a longitudinal growth record. In this manner, under- or overnutrition can be easily recognized before it becomes an established problem.

Most children with IDDM will be at or near their ideal body weight, as the period of metabolic recovery is completed. If physical activity is average, a simple method for estimating a child's caloric requirement is: 1000 kilocalories baseline plus 100 kilocalories for each year of age up to 12 years of age or until puberty. To provide for growth, development, and increased physical activity and to meet the needs and individual desires of the patient, the caloric intake should be assessed semiannually. Boys require a frequent caloric adjustment until about 18 years of age, whereas girls stabilize at about age 14.

Minerals

There are recommended daily allowances for most minerals, and these are usually read-

Table 7–1. **ENERGY REQUIRED FOR SELECTED ACTIVITIES**

Activity	Kcal/kg/hr	Activity	Kcal/kg/hr
Bicycling (rapidly)	7.6	Playing ping-pong	4.4
Bicycling (moderately)	2.5	Reading aloud	0.4
Boxing	11.4	Rowing in a race	16.0
Dancing	3.8	Running	7.0
Dressing and undressing	0.7	Sawing wood	5.7
Driving	0.9	Singing loudly	0.8
Eating	0.4	Sitting quietly	0.4
Exercise		Skating	3.5
Very Light	0.9	Standing relaxed	0.5
Light	1.4	Studying	0.4
Moderate	3.1	Sweeping with broom	1.4
Strenuous	5.4	Typing rapidly	1.0
Very strenuous	7.6	Vacuuming carpet	2.7
Fencing	7.3	Walking (3 mph)	2.0
Horseback riding		Walking (4 mph)	3.4
Walk	1.4	Walking (5.3 mph)	8.3
Trot	4.3	Walking downstairs	*
Gallop	6.7	Walking upstairs	**
Playing piano slowly	1.4	Washing floors	1.2
Playing piano rapidly	2.0	Writing	0.4

Adapted from Taylor CM, et al.: *Foundations of Nutrition*, 5th ed. New York, Macmillan, 1956.
*Allow 0.012 kilocalorie per kilogram for an ordinary staircase with 15 steps, without regard to time.
**Allow 0.036 kilocalorie per kilogram for an ordinary staircase with 15 steps, without regard to time.

Table 7–2. **MEAN HEIGHTS AND WEIGHTS AND RECOMMENDED ENERGY INTAKE***

Category	Age (years)	Weight (kg)	Height (cm)	Energy Needs (with range) (kcal)
Infants	0.0–0.5	6	60	kg × 115 (95–145)
	0.5–1.0	9	71	kg × 105 (80–135)
Children	1–3	13	90	1300 (900–1800)
	4–6	20	112	1700 (1300–2300)
	7–10	28	132	2400 (1650–3300)
Males	11–14	45	157	2700 (2000–3700)
	15–18	66	176	2800 (2100–3900)
	19–22	70	177	2900 (2500–3300)
Females	11–14	46	157	2200 (1500–3000)
	15–18	55	163	2100 (1200–3000)
	19–22	55	163	2100 (1700–2500)
Pregnancy				+300
Lactation				+500

*From Committee on Dietary Allowances: *Recommended Dietary Allowances,* 9th ed. Washington, DC: National Academy of Sciences, 1980.

ily obtained in a well-balanced meal plan. Only small amounts of these non-energy-producing nutrients are needed, and charts may be consulted regarding usual requirements. In planning dietary programs for children, special attention should be given to calcium, iron, and iodine. The roles of zinc and cadmium in the diet are under debate.

Vitamins

Vitamins are subdivided into those that are water soluble (B group and C) and those that are fat soluble (A, D, E, and K groups). Vitamins all have distinct functions yet maintain the characteristic of being complementary to other vitamins. Thus, a deficiency of any one can interfere with the function of another. A variety of nutritious foods are needed to ensure consumption of adequate vitamins, but if a well-balanced diet is supplied, supplementation is not needed. An adequate complement of vitamins are not generally found in "junk foods."

DETERMINANTS OF GOOD NUTRITION

Family Influences

Good nutrition, not only for the child with diabetes but for any siblings as well, begins with the development of good eating habits and principles by the parents. It is not realistic to expect a child to consistently eat differently than the remainder of the family. Nutritional habits for a significant portion of the adult population in the United States do not conform with good health practices. This is greatly emphasized when both parents work outside the home. In such cases, meals are often erratic in timing and inferior in nutritional composition. Since regulation of the timing and content of meals is extremely important for the well-being of the diabetic member of the family, it is imperative that the physician or dietitian or both obtain an assessment of the eating practices of the family. If they are not concordant with good diabetic management, then attempts to alter the habits of the entire family are in order.

Food and eating practices are major areas of noncompliance in the young child and adolescent with diabetes. Our studies, as well as those of others, have shown a close relationship between diabetes control and family togetherness and supportiveness. Since food consumption is common to all members of the family, it is an arena in which this bolstering of one another can occur naturally. The attitudes of the other family members greatly affect the child's acceptance of the condition of diabetes and its limitations. Several short vignettes from our practices are illustrative of the problems in this area of management.

M. B., a 17-year-old girl with diabetes and hypothyroidism, had attempted to treat IDDM purely by manipulation of insulin dosage. As a result, her weight had increased markedly and was now at 85 kilograms. She had developed a relative resistance to insulin therapy and was referred to us. Her mother weighed 92 kilograms and her father 106 kilograms. Multiple attempts to have her lose weight were unsuccessful, primarily because we were never able to convince the entire family that their eating practices were unacceptable as a model for their daughter.

R. L., an 11-year-old with a two-year history of diabetes, was in poor carbohydrate control. Investigations suggested that this was due to poor dietary compliance. The girl's parents seemed to recognize the importance of diet and "nagged" her constantly about food and her eating practices. It was then discovered that the house was always full of candies, cookies, and colas for the other three children, who consumed these indiscriminately. R. L.'s willpower was not strong enough to withstand these temptations and the sibling pressure.

V. S. was referred to us for additional education because of poor control. Her history indicated that she was on a "rigid" diet, which was weighed and measured. No "sweets" were allowed, and all foods had to be broiled. "Dietetic" foods were used regularly. The parents and siblings had continued their normal eating practices. In order not to "tempt" her with "bad food," they allowed her to eat at a separate table.

In each of the instances above, the family failed in their demonstration of support for the child. Also, in each case, this led to problems with dietary adherence and to poor carbohydrate control.

Throughout the life of the child, particularly during the growing years, there is a need to promote the concept of the benefits of good nutrition and to assist in the development of healthy eating patterns. The parents should be assisted in their thinking about food; to the diabetic, the meal plan is part of the therapeutic program, and the understanding of its use is almost as important as is that of insulin's use. Initially, most mothers are greatly intimidated by the thoughts of food and their perceptions of the "diabetic diet." Some never seem to get over this problem. Others seem to place undue emphasis on meals and meal planning, with this aspect of care being viewed out of the context of growing and living. In some of these instances, mealtimes become battlegrounds, and this eventually leads to major problems.

Physician's Role

Most patients and family members look to the physician as the principal director of diabetes care, even regarding diet, but this feeling is often not supported in actual practice. The physician often gets involved directly with other areas (insulin, monitoring, exercise, and so on) but for diet refers to the dietitian, whose experience and philosophy may be different from those of the physician. The physician thus fails to give proper perspective to dietary management. For nutritional management to be effective, the physician must aid the person with diabetes and the family in learning to cope appropriately with the stresses inherent in dietary management. Unfortunately, sometimes there is an unwillingness on the part of the doctor to even discuss diet. This reluctance may be due to insufficient training, lack of time, or frustration. On many occasions the meal plan consists merely of a sheet of previously prepared dietary instructions that is handed to the patient or family without individualization, discussion, or explanation. It is important that the physician assist the patient in putting diet into the overall framework of diabetes. At least, the practitioner should work with the dietitian in coordinating goals and objectives and in incorporating diet into the whole management program.

Dietitian's Role

The effective dietitian must simultaneously play several roles: nutritional expert; diabetes dietary consultant for the young; innovative educator; and counselor, confidante, and friend. Although the dietitian is expected to possess the first prerequisite, it is seemingly just as important that he or she possess the others also. Most dietitians have had little educational or practical experience with children and even less with those who have diabetes. Some are only vaguely aware of the differences between IDDM and NIDDM, or between diabetes in children and diabetes in adults. Being thus unsure of their own competency, such dietitians often approach diet in a more traditional and dictatorial manner. A "diet" is given, often without consideration of the likes or dislikes of the child or of the eating patterns of the family. Some dietitians have considerable depth of knowledge about nutrition but little concept about the interrelationships among food, insulin, exercise, and stress. Likewise, these persons may not even have a dietary philosophy that is compatible with that of the physician.

Adherence to a lifelong dietary program is difficult. An effective dietitian must be able to educate the person and family and to motivate them continuously. Influencing a young person to remain on a program that is the antithesis of the usual agenda of peers requires all the skills of a magician. Counseling must be carried out in a nonadversarial manner, and the adroit practitioner of this discipline must help the person define appropriate incentives. This often demands a degree of flexibility that only the self-confident and experienced nutritionist is likely to possess.

Patient and Family Roles

For the dietary program to be successful, active participation by the young person is essential. The patient must have some investment in the program, and this is usually best gained by enlisting the child's participation in development of the diet. The concept of a diet as meaning "to give up something one likes" must be addressed. Complexity must be eradicated and a simple meal plan adopted. The patient should feel as if the diet were truly his or hers alone and should be given a feeling of having played an active role in the process of its development. The patient must be encouraged to explore acceptable methods by which to fit the diet to the lifestyle, but without deceiving himself or herself and without producing undue harm to diabetes control. The patient should also understand that the diet prescription is a working or changing document that needs to be periodically evaluated.

DEVELOPING A NUTRITIONAL PLAN

Acquiring Intake Information

The initial task, which is best accomplished by the physician but may later be delegated to the dietitian, is to take a dietary history. After a rapport is established, this procedure may take only minutes. The main goal is to have the patient feel comfortable with and accepted by the physician and dietitian, thereby further ensuring an honest dietary history.

The dietary history should begin with a fast assessment of the patient's cognition of, compliance with, and feelings or emotions toward dietary management. The questioning should be conducted in a nondirective and nonjudgmental manner. This history may be retrospective, consisting of a spontaneous recall of the past two to three days'

intake, or may be obtained prospectively by asking the child and family to record intake for the succeeding two to three days. If time has permitted it, then the family may have been asked to bring in a catalogue of intake over the past several days that was collected formatively. All techniques are useful and may sometimes be used in parallel. For the newly diagnosed diabetic, the practitioner should try to relate this history of intake to the time prior to onset of initial symptoms. In this manner, the therapist will obtain valuable information, such as family preferences. For the diabetic of some duration who is having a dietary adjustment, the information should relate to current interests and desires.

When the dietitian obtains a more detailed evaluation, food models and standard measuring cups will be useful in identifying serving sizes of both foods and liquids. Along with the amount and type of food consumed during the course of the day, information on time, location, activity, socioeconomic status, and special needs should be obtained. What time are meals and snacks eaten? Is the timing different on weekends? Is exercise performed on a regular or sporadic basis? Are "fast-food," gourmet, or ethnic restaurants used? Who buys or purchases the food? Is the child overweight or handicapped? Special needs items that should be included are allergies, food choices, food prejudices, and a general outline of the child's and family's lifestyle.

Dietary Assessment

After the data are acquired, the physician or dietitian should estimate the appropriate caloric, protein, carbohydrate, and fat intake needed, and compare this to accepted norms for age and size. The meal pattern is then established with the assistance of the patient and parent. Most children under age 7 will be on a three-meal, three-snack plan, as the majority of first- and second-grade classes routinely schedule midmorning snacks. Children older than age 7 will generally receive three meals and two snacks (after school and before bedtime). Our general belief is that there should be some proportional distribution of carbohydrates throughout the day, rather than stacking these at any one time. Therefore, we usually estimate the total grams of carbohydrate and divide by 10. We then attempt to distribute one fifth (two tenths) of the carbohydrate at breakfast, one fifth at lunch, one tenth at the afternoon snack, two fifths (four tenths) at supper, and one tenth at bedtime. These distributions are not based on any preconceived belief, but they do reflect the fact that most of our patients have a larger meal in the evening than at other times. On the other hand, some families have a different distribution and attempts should be made to adjust to this accordingly. We attempt to make only minimal changes in the individual's desired eating pattern. Allowing for the child's desires seems to increase compliance and demonstrates to both child and family that diabetes need not drastically alter their lifestyle. If adjustments must be made, owing to inadequate calories or nutrients, it is important that both patient and family understand that the meal plan prescribed is for the entire family and is consistent with the needs of the nondiabetic as well as the diabetic. In order to arrive at a diet that is both consistent with needs and acceptable, some negotiations and compromises are often necessary.

The Education and Counseling Processes

Just as the meal plan must be individualized, so must the educational program and process. The dietary educational program must be integrated into the overall educational program (Chapter 10). Its content will be dependent on the cognitive abilities of the child and family and on their willingness and ability to learn. As with other educational aspects, the timing is important. Early in the postdiagnosis period, neither parent nor child may be psychologically prepared to receive dietary information. Only after some initial period of adjustment is it reasonable to begin a consideration of diet as a therapeutic modality.

The most effective teaching format for diet instruction is the individual discussion and conference. There should be a verbal explanation of the complete meal plan with written guidelines for home use. Ample time must be allowed for both child and parent to ask questions and receive answers. Our experience indicates that this process is best accomplished by several 45- to 60-minute sessions over a two- or three-day period. Other methods of educating are complementary and include group counseling, audiovisual aids, and reading materials. Visual aids are numerous and may include food models, scrapbooks of labels, flashcards, video- or audiotapes, slides, games, and illustrations. Realism is an important part of the dietary instruction. If the child is able to relate the instruction to specific areas of his or her own life, then more will be remembered.

After the initial dietary instructions are completed, it is prudent to check the parents' and child's understanding of the program. Upon discharge from the hospital, the "real world" situation of home may prove intimidating to some, and new issues will frequently arise. The competent and concerned dietitian will often have routine telephone contacts at intervals during the first six weeks, or until the first posthospital visit. At this time, the metabolic recovery is usually complete, and appetite has stabilized. This is an appropriate time for a reassessment, followed by a "setting" of the basic meal plan.

Balancing Diet and Insulin

Two of the main goals of the meal plan are to increase the ease with which blood glucose concentrations can be brought to levels as close to normal as possible and to prevent wide swings in the day-to-day levels. A number of studies have demonstrated the difficulty in attaining normal blood glucose values when insulin is not in balance with the meal plan. It seems sufficient to say that these two major variables cannot be changing simultaneously if control is to be established. One strategy often used is to keep the meal pattern constant and adjust the insulin regimen; another is to keep the insulin dosage constant and adjust the meal pattern. Our experience suggests that the former strategy is the more easily accomplished; thus, it is the one used in our center. With either strategy, however, consideration must be given to both diet and insulin needs. Insulin's duration, starting, and peak action times should be kept in mind, along with the injection site and timing of insulin administration. The amount and the kind of food consumed at each meal and snack is related to peak action times and durations of insulin. Whether the person takes one, two, or more injections per day is important, as are other aspects such as exercise periods and daily schedules.

DIETARY PHILOSOPHIES FOR IDDM

To totally patronize one dietary philosophy at the expense of all others is to disregard the concept of individualization of therapy. Almost every dietary management plan has the same goal: to provide adequate calories and nutrients so as to attain normal growth, while striving to keep the blood glucose as near normal as possible. Consequently, one might deduce that there is only a single dietary philosophy. On the other hand, it is readily apparent that some diabetologists place great emphasis on diet, others little; some use easy methods for reducing the dietary content of simple sugars, others use complex formulations; some attempt to keep all dietary components fixed, others concentrate primarily on carbohydrate. Are these truly differences in philosophy? Probably not, but there is a feeling among both patients and doctors that there is a wide divergence of opinion regarding such matters. Suffice it to say that there are diabetologists who are rigid in their approach to diet and others who are more liberal.

Adding to this confusion about "philosophy" is the fact that methods of estimating dietary content and quantity differ. Some programs utilize a standard exchange diet approach for purely educational and practical purposes. Others use this same diet plan in its very strictest literal sense. Some believe that knowledge of the carbohydrate content and caloric amount of food or food groups should be an educational goal. Others have their own methods of viewing foods, food groups, and education. We have found the exchange system of approximating the caloric and carbohydrate contents of food to be very useful and, generally, easy for children and their parents to master. One of the nice things about the exchange system is the ease with which the uninitiated can learn it; another is its easy adaptability to those who wish to be more precise. Consequently, before further discussions of several dietary concepts currently in vogue, a brief overview of the exchange system seems appropriate.

The Exchange System

Regardless of the dietary philosophy, the dietary exchange system (DES) is a valuable-tool for the physician, dietitian, and patient. It has the advantages of being used universally and of having the seal of approval of both the American Dietetic Association and the American Diabetes Association. Current exchange lists are obtainable from either of these organizations as well as from most hospital dietetic departments.

The DES is divided into six food groups (Table 7–3), one of which is a "free" food category. The other five groups are separated according to their relative content of carbohydrates, proteins, and fats. Within a group, the caloric content and the nutrient composition per serving of different foods are relatively constant. The reference food within the starch exchange list is a slice of white bread with a caloric content of 68 and containing 15 grams of carbohydrate and 2 grams of protein. All other foods within the starch group can be treated as being equivalent to that slice of bread (i.e., approximately 70 calories), and a designated serving size of one food in this group can therefore be exchanged or traded for another. Although it is obvious that there will be some variations in the compositions (for instance, the composition of a small Idaho potato differs slightly from a similar-sized Maine potato in both caloric content and amount of carbohydrate), this dietary system is designed for approximations. It is questionable in the minds of most whether one needs ever to be

Table 7–3. **DIETARY EXCHANGE SYSTEM**

	Approximate Content/Serving			
Food Exchange	*Calories (kcal)*	*Carbohydrate (g)*	*Protein (g)*	*Fat (g)*
Fruit	40	10	—	—
Starch (bread)	68	15	2	—
Milk (whole)	170	12	8	10
Protein (meat)	73	—	7	5
Fat	45	—	—	5
Free	negligible	negligible	—	—

more specific than this diet when there are so many other variables in diabetes management. Some problems exist, however, which are noted in Table 7–4.

Each of the other food group exchanges is similar, in that comparably sized portions of foods within a group may be traded or exchanged for other foods within that group. Foods usually included within the various groups are listed in the appendix. We have used a variation of the standard exchange diet that was developed in our center and which enables us to teach the DES on the basis of symbols and colors (Fig. 7–1). This chart, available through the American Diabetes Association, Texas Affiliate, allows the child to understand visually some aspects of trading within groups. For instance, a child might not understand why a starch should not be traded for a protein, whereas it is easier for the child to see that a diamond and a square are different and therefore not exchangeable.

Dietary Concepts

As noted earlier, virtually all dietary programs are uniform in their desire to provide an adequate energy source of balanced composition to ensure optimum growth, good health, and satisfaction while attempting to maintain a normal blood glucose. The following discussion will deal with three slightly different programs under the nomenclature by which they are commonly known: the free diet, the rigid diet, and the constant carbohydrate diet. As will be noted, all are misnomers.

"Free Diet"

This dietary program is sometimes known as the "unrestricted" or "liberal" diet, and modern diabetologists who use this concept prefer these synonyms for they are more precise. In early days of its usage, the free diet was more true to its name, but today its intent is different. Most foods are allowed in unlimited amounts, but those containing concentrated carbohydrates are limited in amount. Consistency of intake is prescribed along with regularity of eating time, the main objective of which is the avoidance of hypoglycemia. The essential parts of a well-balanced meal plan and insistence on good basic

Table 7–4. **MEAN GLYCEMIC INDEX—SOME ESSENTIAL ELEMENTS***

BREAD, White	100
BREAD, Whole Wheat	99
BREAD, Wholegrain—Rye	58
RICE	96
SPAGHETTI	66
POTATO, Russett, Baked	135
POTATO, Sweet	70
BEANS, Baked	60
BEANS, Soya	22
APPLE	53
BANANA	80
ORANGE	66
HONEY	126
GLUCOSE	138
ICE CREAM	52
YOGURT	52

Data from Lancet 2:388, 1984, with permission.

*It has been noted that the exchange system has built-in defects, and this has led to development of this index. If a standard amount of white bread is consumed, a predictable glucose excursion occurs, and this is assigned a value of 100%. Other foods in comparable amounts can then be related to this index and expressed as percentages. For example, a standard serving of spaghetti produces only ⅔ (66%) as much glycemia as does the slice of bread.

nutrition relative to age, sex, and activity are included.

Advocates of the free diet believe that such a dietary program is more in keeping with normal family patterns and will produce less psychologic or behavioral problems than will other systems. There is also a belief that significant fluctuations into the hyperglycemic range are preventable by proper manipulation of insulin dosage. However, since starches and other foods containing carbohydrate are unlimited and since the amounts consumed will vary from day to day, there will be considerable fluctuation in levels of blood glucose. Unfortunately, most advocates of the "free diet" are also proponents of single-dose insulin therapy. Our experience with referred patients suggests that two or more injections of insulin coupled with frequent dosage manipulations are essential if one is to control unwanted hyperglycemia (Fig. 7–2).

Another problem with the "free" diet is a misinterpretation by parents and children of the term "free." If the diet is free, this leads to the misconception that some concentrated sugars might be allowable. Our feelings are that these mixed messages are difficult for

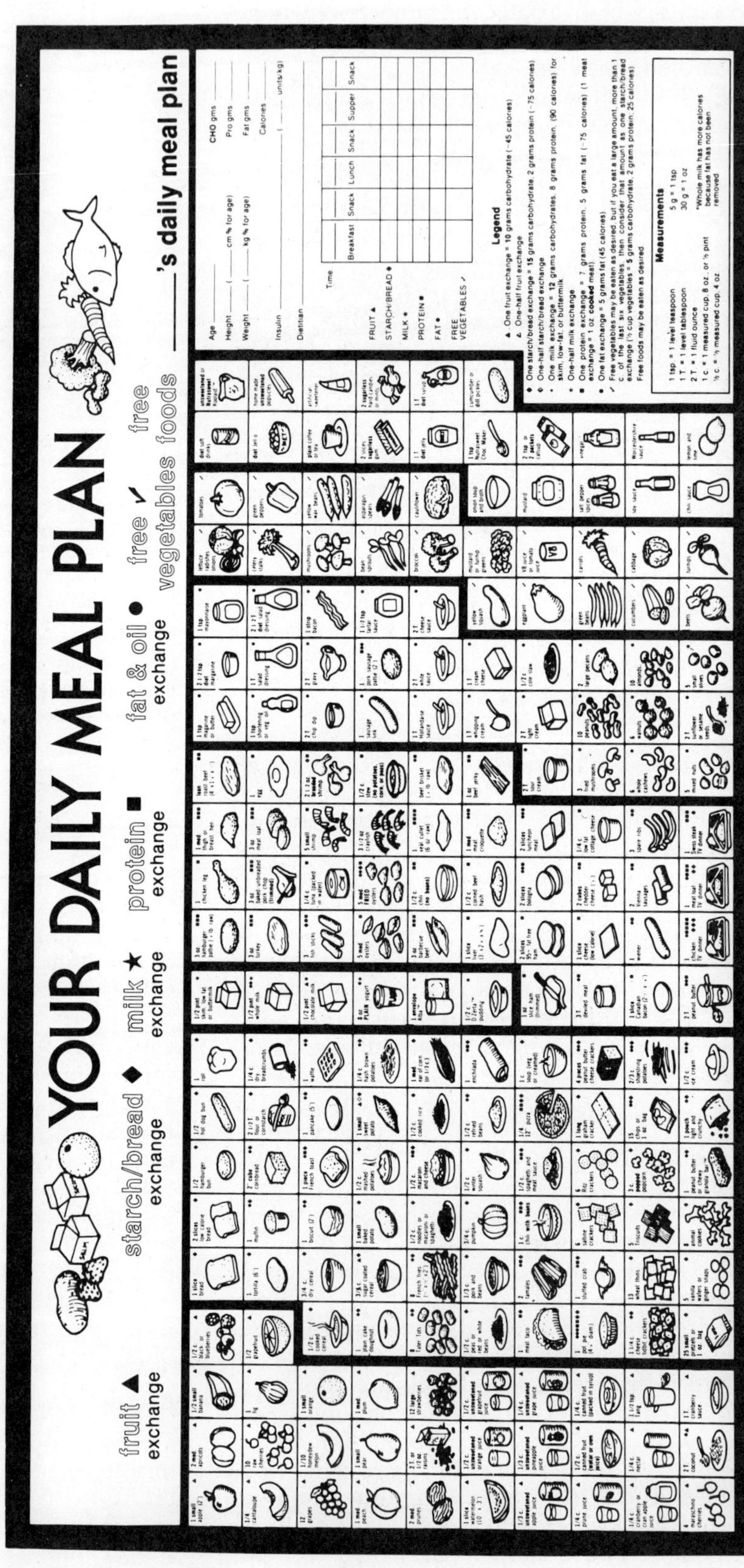
YOUR DAILY MEAL PLAN
fruit ▲ exchange
starch/bread ◆ exchange
milk ★ exchange
protein ■ exchange
fat & oil ● exchange
free ✓ vegetables
free foods
______'s daily meal plan
Age
Height
Weight
Insulin
Dietitian
CHO gms
Pro gms
Fat gms
Calories
Time
Breakfast Snack Lunch Snack Supper Snack
Legend
FRUIT ▲
STARCH/BREAD ◆
MILK ★
PROTEIN ■
FAT ●
FREE VEGETABLES ✓
Measurements

general instructions

"How to live a healthy, normal life with diabetes"

1. Let your dietitian decide the food allowances you should have at each meal and snack, taking into account your life-style, age, sex, body build, and amount of activity you do, and whether or not you are a young child growing rapidly.

2. The meal plan for the diabetic is really a well-balanced diet which the WHOLE FAMILY can follow.

"Well-balanced" means the meal plan contains certain nutrients as follows:

A. PROTEIN, which is any food on the chart with a "■" by it. Protein is important for growth, tissue maintenance and repair. Approximately 58% of protein turns into sugar.

B. FAT, which is any food represented by a "●" on your chart. Fats are a second source of energy (carbohydrates are your first). Fats also function to aid in utilization of fat-soluble vitamins. Approximately 35% of fats turns into sugar. But remember, if you want to lose weight, you may want to stay away from any of the foods that have a "●" by them.

C. CARBOHYDRATES are our best energy source. The food groups which contain carbohydrate are FRUIT ▲, STARCH/BREAD ◆, and MILK • (the first three food groups on the chart). Even though 100% of these carbohydrates turns into sugar, each does it quite differently.

1. FRUITS or anything else on the chart with only a "▲" by it, will raise the blood sugar right away, when eaten alone. Keep this in mind in the case of a low blood sugar (which is less than 80). Sugar from liquids enters the bloodstream faster than from solids.

2. STARCH/BREAD (◆) is broken down more slowly and lasts longer in the blood stream than fruits (▲). It is composed primarily of carbohydrate plus a small amount (2 grams) of incomplete protein.

3. MILK (•) is the "slowest acting" carbohydrate and has the best sustaining effect of the three carbohydrates. One serving supplies approximately an equal amount of carbohydrate as fruits (▲) & starch/breads (◆). However, milk (•) is also high in protein.

Whenever protein (■) or fat (●) is added to these carbohydrates it takes even longer to raise your blood-sugar level but will last longer.

3. Since diabetes is a family affair, there is no need to cook any differently for the child with diabetes. Beware of dietetic foods! "Dietetic" does not necessarily mean "for the diabetic," it only means that one of the ingredients has been removed and is replaced by another ingredient. Sometimes the ingredient removed is salt and Type I diabetics do not need to restrict their salt intake. Therefore, get into the habit of reading labels! (Anything ending in 'ol will eventually raise your blood-sugar level.)

4. Reading labels is important for two reasons:

a. To figure out how the serving size can be worked into your meal plan.

b. To find how nutritious the food product is.

5. There are many diet philosophies; one of those philosophies is the "constant carbohydrate" meal plan. Since 100% of carbohydrate (▲◆•) raises the blood sugar, it is important to eat the SAME AMOUNT of carbohydrates around the SAME TIME each day. By doing this, we hope to form a schedule/pattern of sugar levels. We will then know how much insulin to give to turn these foods into energy without running into problems of hypo- or hyperglycemia.

Therefore, there are three things to remember:

a. AMOUNT is the most important—that is why you see an amount in bold print by each food item. Measure your foods initially until you know visually how to measure your foods. Then remeasure every three months just to make sure you are still consuming the right AMOUNT of food to control diabetes and weight.

b. TIME is also important so that the food is there when the insulin is working. It is not a good idea to save a portion of your carbohydrates from one meal to eat at the next meal. You have more flexibility in timing of meals & snacks when on two shots per day or even three shots.

c. KIND. Even though fruit ▲, starch ◆, and milk • all raise the blood-sugar level, they do it quite differently, as stated earlier!

Besides keeping carbohydrates constant to get an even better control of your diabetes and weight, also keep your protein ■ and fat ● intake constant. Large quantities of food eaten outside the three carbohydrate groups (▲◆•) will also add up to enough carbohydrates to raise the blood-sugar level eventually.

6. Your food chart is color-coded and symbolized to make it easier for you to follow. Here are the steps to take:

a. When it is TIME for you to eat a meal or snack, go down the column under the TIME allocated to find out the number of symbols you are allowed for each group.

Example:

Time	4 p.m.
	Snack
FRUIT ▲	1
STARCH-BREAD ◆	1
MILK •	0
PROTEIN ■	1
FAT ●	0
FREE VEGETABLES ✓	0

If your meal plan looks like the above example, then at 4 p.m. you can choose and eat any foods on your chart that are equivalent to symbols: ▲◆■

Here are some examples to help you with meal-planning:

A. 1 small 2" apple
   6 saltine crackers
   1 slice cheese

B. 1/2 oz. box raisins
   1 long graham cracker
   1 T. peanut butter

C. 1/2 small banana
   1/2 ham sandwich (1 slice bread, 1 slice ham, mustard, lettuce, tomatoes)

D. 1/2 c. orange juice
   1 oz. bag Doritos
   1 oz. cheese dip

E. 1 chewy (peanut butter) granola bar
   1/4 c. cottage cheese

7. Remember, this meal plan will change with different stages of your life. For example, when going through a growth spurt, you will need an increase in food intake.

8. Research has suggested that a polyunsaturated fat diet is superior for the WHOLE family. Therefore, it is advisable to use corn or sunflower oils or margarine, to include more lean meats and poultry, to reduce the amount of heavy beef and pork in the meal plan, and to include only skim or low-fat milk products.

9. Your meal plan on ketone/sick days:

a. Ask your dietitian for the "Liquid Exchange List," which is a list of foods more easily tolerated on sick days.

b. Take SMALL, FREQUENT feedings of liquids easily tolerated:

Example: If vomiting   1 tsp. every 10-15 minutes
           If vomiting ceases   1/2 c.-1 c. every 1-2 hours

c. PUSH plenty of FLUIDS for two reasons:
   1. To prevent dehydration.
   2. To flush away ketones.

d. Call your physician if vomiting does not stop and fluids are not being tolerated.

10. Studies show FIBER should be an important part of EVERYONE's meal plan. Some fibers delay carbohydrate absorption; therefore diabetics do not get that sudden shot of sugar in the bloodstream after eating. Check blood sugars to find out how fiber affects your diabetes. (You may need to decrease the amount of insulin you take.) You can gradually increase your fiber intake by substituting fiber-rich foods for foods you already eat. Example: bran cereals, oats, whole wheat bread, beans, brown rice, and most vegetables are good fiber sources.

Copyright © 1984
Paula McMahon, R.D., and Luther B. Travis, M.D.
The University of Texas Medical Branch
Galveston, Texas
All rights reserved

Copyright © 1974, Revised 1977
Jean Claflin, R.D. and Valerie Kohn, M.S

desserts/snacks/special occasions

Snacks & desserts are COMBINATIONS of symbols. These foods contain concentrated sources of carbohydrate (▲◆•), which raise the blood-sugar level. They also contain fat (●), which has A LOT of calories, causing weight gain. Many of these foods are not nutritious; and a larger portion of nutritious foods has to be given up or exchanged for these SMALL amounts of desserts. Therefore, it would be wise to work these foods into your meal plan ONLY on special occasions. So there should be no guilt feelings, if you remember to do the following two things:

1. WORK desserts INTO your meal plan. (Pay close attention to the SMALL amounts allowed.)

2. Eat ONLY on SPECIAL OCCASIONS. (Do not get into the habit of eating these foods daily.)

To all the foods in the shaded area, there are alternatives that may not raise your blood-sugar level quite as high (e.g., sugarless hard candies or mints, dietetic syrup or jelly).

So decide now, what is a special occasion for you, then fill in the three blank squares with your three favorite desserts. If your favorites are not on this chart, ask your dietitian for the exchanges, in order to give you a more flexible meal plan. Be careful to notice the combination of symbols in these particular foods.

Figure 7–1. Front and back illustrations of "Your Daily Diet," an instrument developed and used in our Center for dietary education. Copies of this may be obtained for a nominal charge from American Diabetes Association, Texas Affiliates, Inc.

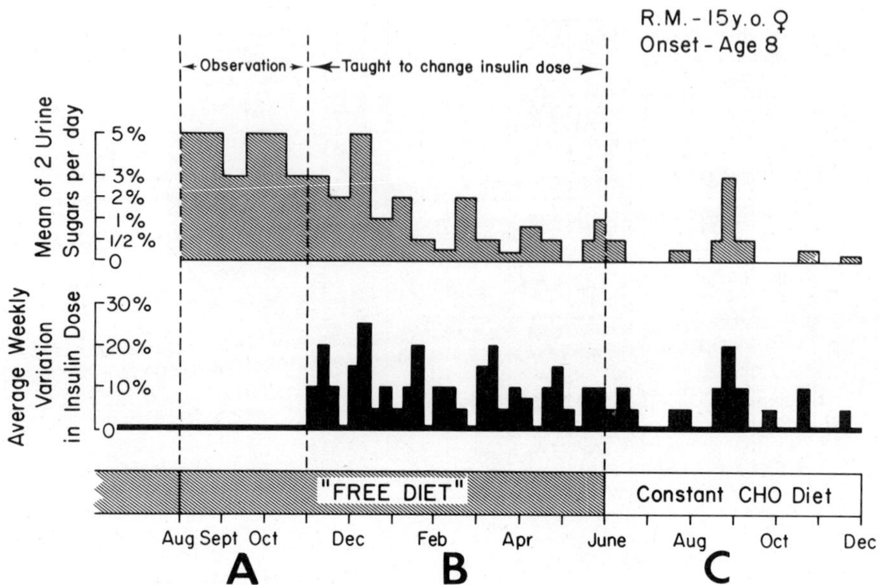

Figure 7–2. This diagram, prepared several years ago, demonstrates the advantage of controlling dietary intake. R. M. first came to us seven years after onset of diabetes. She was on a fixed insulin dosage, urine testing, and a free diet. In period *A*, she continued the usual program but kept accurate urine records, which are recorded. In period *B*, she was taught how to alter insulin dosage based on the degree of glycosuria. Frequent dosage changes were required to bring about a reduction in glycosuria. In period *C*, the diet was changed to a Constant Carbohydrate Diet (see text). In this period, decreased glycosuria was achieved with fewer adjustments in insulin dosage.

many children to deal with and that the entire concept of a free diet delays normal coping by the child with the reality of diabetes.

Weighed and Measured Diets ("Rigid" Diet)

This type of diet is conceptually at the other extreme. Purists require that at each meal, all food components are either weighed or measured and that all concentrated sweets are eliminated. Calories and their specific components (carbohydrates, fats, proteins) are controlled at each meal.

Studies with patients on this type of diet have demonstrated less fluctuation in blood glucose from day to day, coupled with a need to make fewer alterations in insulin dosage. Some families find that this highly structured system is more in accord with their lifestyle than are less rigid diets. Less stress is evoked by the rigidity in this diet than by what might be considered laxity in other dietary programs. Such families should be allowed to use such schemes, with the realization that there is a potential for significant parent-child conflict when peer pressures exceed parental pressures.

The lifestyles of most persons are not con-sistent with the constant attention to food that is imposed by this method. Meal times often become battlegrounds rather than times of family harmony. The undue attention to preciseness often results in wider fluctuations in blood glucose as a result of the stress of the process. Families seem to feel that every morsel (and not one additional) must be consumed, despite the fact that the child's needs and desires may change from day to day. In some children, this conflict leads to periodic overindulgence, while in others, it may lead to occasional anorexia, or to other weird and antisocial behaviors, as demonstrated below:

T. L., a 17-year-old girl with an 11-year history of diabetes, was referred to us for lack of control. History revealed that following a visit to a Midwestern diabetes center five years earlier, the patient's dietary program along with other care aspects had been significantly altered. Dietary consistency was rigidly attempted with complete elimination of "all sugar" and with the measurement of all foods consumed. Mealtimes became hostile for all involved persons. The girl resisted attempts at rigidity in diet, while the parents insisted even more strongly. As a means of family compromise, they adopted a pattern whereby the girl could eat as she desired, but would then selectively regurgitate (at the table) the overeaten food, only then being allowed to consume the "diabetic diet."

Needless to say, this habit had cost her many of her friends, and she had few social invitations. She became more withdrawn and ultimately refused to go to school. Despite all of this attention to diabetes, its control was very poor.

Admittedly, this case is somewhat bizzarre, and this girl and her family may well have had significant psychologic problems even if the dietary area had not become such a major force in her life. But less severe and more common problems do occur when undue attention is focused on any particular aspect of care. In some families, the child reluctantly adheres to the dietary restrictions but becomes noncompliant in other aspects.

Constant Carbohydrate Meal Plan (CCMP)

This is the diet system that has been used in our center for years. It occupies a place somewhere near the middle, between the other two systems. The CCMP, as noted earlier, is a misnomer. Some of its characteristics are noted in Table 7–5.

It is a diet that is designed to give the child some room for freedom of action when confronted with antipodal choices. Suppose that, after completing a hamburger, french fries, and a cola that have been worked into the diet, the teenager is still hungry. Does he merely not eat anything else despite the desires; have some lettuce and pickles; have another hamburger and fries; or merely have another hamburger patty? The believers in the selection of either of the first two choices would obviously be correct from a purely diabetic standpoint, but their understanding of children, particularly teenagers, is suspect. Most teenagers, when confronted with a similar situation, would choose the third option—a hamburger patty, a hamburger bun, the accessories, and the fries—unless they had been taught differently. We believe most of our patients would choose the last option, the hamburger patty alone. The effect of this on blood sugar is quantitatively less than that of starch, and the resultant rise in blood glucose is much slower. Additionally, protein has a satisfying trait that is greater than that of carbohydrate. Thus, our patients are given some flexibility, which we feel overall en-

Table 7–5. CHARACTERISTICS OF CONSTANT CARBOHYDRATE MEAL PLAN*

1. Encourages child's active participation in dietary decisions
2. Uses an expanded exchange system
3. Attempts to keep the exchanges of fruits, starches, and milk constant
4. Eliminates the "forbidden-food" concept
   Allows, but limits, the use of concentrated sweets
5. Acknowledges the contribution of protein to blood glucose concentrations
   But assents to its regulated use
6. Satisfies some of the social and peer-association needs of the child
7. Allows the family to make compensation changes in insulin dosage

*As used by the Children's Diabetes Management Center, University of Texas Medical Branch.

hances adherence and better maintains control.

The CCMP discourages the use of concentrated sugars because of its unstabilizing effect on blood glucose but refuses to participate in "double think." How differently does the body react to 4 ounces of orange juice than to 3 ounces of Coca-Cola? What's the difference between the blood glucose response to two slices of toast with margarine and a 4-ounce glass of apple juice, and that to a peanut butter and jelly sandwich? There is no difference. All represent concentrated sugars, but, whereas the latter products are often "banned," the former items are encouraged. Too soon, children recognize the falseness in these messages, and the chances of working with them as partners are soon lost. Generally, people want what is denied them. We try to counter this by showing people how to use all foods wisely.

At the beginning of the dietary program, it is beneficial for all patients to weigh and measure foods, because most persons have difficulty with approximations until a standard is defined. After a brief period, regular measurements are discontinued, but, for adherence reasons, the families are asked to remeasure periodically—at about three- to six-month intervals.

The CCMP incorporates individuality based on lifestyle. Almost any food can be worked into the meal plan, and the child realizes that an occasional dessert is possible. It allows the child to feel more like those in the peer group. Acceptance of this dietary program by the teenager seems superior to that of other dietary programs.

SPECIFIC ISSUES IN NUTRITIONAL MANAGEMENT

Adherence or Compliance

This subject is addressed at various points in the book, but at this juncture, it is worthwhile to note only that one common explanation for poor control of diabetes is failure of adherence to a dietary program. In a society that is so overtly food conscious and where most social encounters are occasions for gluttony, the child's inability to adhere is not surprising. In North American society, food has psychologic as well as physiologic functions. It is important that the "diet" of the diabetic be viewed in the light of our cultural mores and patterns. To do otherwise forces the child with diabetes to choose between being different and cheating on the diet. The child will usually choose cheating; guilt and self-recriminations often result, and the attendant stress magnifies the problem.

No child can adhere to a diet program all the time. It is neither natural nor normal. Thus, it appears best to recognize this and to work with the child and family, so as to minimize chronic cheating and its consequences. One of our goals is to demonstrate to the child and family that diabetes and its requirements can be integrated into a normal life. Holidays, birthdays, celebrations, slumber parties, and so forth are all part of the normal developmental growth of a child—and food is often a component of each of these events. Consequently, a successful educational program must demonstrate acceptable methods by which the child with diabetes can appear as a normal, healthy participant in these life events.

Methods of addressing and managing nonadherence to diet are dealt with in Chapter 10. Needless to say, a prerequisite is an emphatic understanding of the problems faced by the child with diabetes.

Obesity

One usually thinks of the person with IDDM as being thin or underweight, and such is usually the case at onset. But the problems of abnormal weight gain plague the diabetic as surely as they do the nondiabetic. As with the nondiabetic, genetic and environmental factors appear important in determining propensity to obesity. Obesity-generating eating patterns that were present prior to the child's diagnosis of diabetes are not easily forgotten. Unless the physician and nutritionist work at altering eating patterns of the entire family in such cases, old habits are likely to recur.

There are many environmental and psychosocial factors that may predispose an individual to obesity in the general population, including family eating patterns, inactivity, boredom, depression, and acting-out behaviors. Rarely are there metabolic or hormonal causes for the obesity, and all causes have a common characteristic: the energy consumed exceeds that which is used for normal processes. The same is true for the person with diabetes, but there is another factor to be considered in the diabetic: glucose and insulin, working together, are lipogenic. If the amount of glucose available to the body exceeds that needed for energy metabolism and statural growth, the remainder, in the presence of an appropriate insulin dosage, will be stored as either glycogen or fat. There are two situations in the diabetic when obesity may be the result of management: (1) the chronically, overcontrolled person who is forced to consume extra calories often as a result of too much insulin and its consequence, hypoglycemia; and (2) the young person who is quite conscientious about the blood glucose concentrations but attempts to normalize them by insulin administration alone. The following is an example of the former problem:

E. M. was diagnosed as having diabetes at age 7 years. The parents were both relatively thin individuals. They were well informed about the dangers of prolonged hyperglycemia and both privately pledged to prevent such occurrences. Before the onset of diabetes and after the period of metabolic recovery, the girl's weight was in the 30th percentile for her age and height.

According to her history, over the next three years her diet was rigidly maintained, and she received from two to four insulin injections per day based on both individual and pattern blood glucose values. Her blood glucose was usually maintained between 50 mg/dl to 150 mg/dl, and her glycosylated hemoglobin values were in the high-normal range. She experienced multiple insulin reactions, averaging 10 to 12 per week, the majority being of mild to moderate severity and being easily aborted by food consumption. For most hypoglycemic reactions she consumed either a Coke (6 to 12 ounces), a large glass of orange juice, or some candy. If the hypoglycemic episode was more than 30 minutes from mealtime, she then consumed an "extra" starch exchange.

During the first three years of her diabetes, her weight rose from the 30th percentile for a 7-year-old to greater than the 95th percentile for her age (then 10 years).

Calculations revealed that this girl received, on the average, an extra 1200 to 2000 calories per week (above her dietary needs) as treatment for hypoglycemia. At this rate, she gained almost a pound per month during most of the three years. The problem of excessive weight gain was reversed in this case by reduction in standard insulin dosages.

Obesity often becomes a major problem for the adolescent female and as noted above, sometimes affects the child who is attempting good control. Inactivity in the teenage girl contributes to the problem, and this is compounded by the many social occasions on which food is consumed. Obesity is best treated by a preventive program for, as with the nondiabetic, the success of weight-reduction dietary programs is limited. Appropriate treatment of obesity in the diabetic requires adjustments in dietary intake, insulin administration, and exercise. It is a more complex process than in the nondiabetic.

Occasionally, some "knowledgeable" adolescents discover that they can control weight gain without restriction of food intake. They do this by merely reducing the amount of insulin administered, thereby creating hyperglycemia and glycosuria. Even though this does reduce weight, the resulting hyperglycemia and ketonemia is undesirable and dangerous.

When weight reduction is important to the well-being of a child with IDDM, a detailed program should be developed to address the causes for the obesity as well as its management. The treatment program must be integrated to keep diabetes in balance while weight is lost. Our practice is to first ensure that diabetic control is established with appropriate manipulations in food intake and insulin administration. Carbohydrate intake is stabilized, and as many dietary fats as possible are subtracted from the diet. This reduces caloric intake without significant disruption of the diabetes. If reduction in either carbohydrate or protein consumption is found to be necessary, the reduction is made slowly with appropriate attention to the blood glucose values. An increase in energy expenditure (activity) is encouraged, and its effect is additive.

Dietary Changes With Stages of Diabetes

The stages of diabetes are discussed in Chapter 3. Prior to initiation of insulin therapy, the person is usually in a state of negative balance and has often lost considerable weight. Anorexia may be present. After insulin is started, appetite and food intake increase, and the body becomes anabolic. This period of metabolic recovery may last from two to eight weeks, during which time an enormous number of calories may be consumed. Only after preillness weight has been regained does the patient's appetite diminish and stabilize. The physician and nutritionist must carefully follow the child during this time and make adjustments as necessary.

After the child regains weight and the appetite and nutritional status approach normal, a consistent meal pattern should be established. Periodically, the meal plan should be re-evaluated relative to the child's current needs. This is particularly important during periods of rapid growth.

Fiber

Dietary fiber is that portion of plant food that is not completely hydrolyzed by digestive enzymes of the intestinal tract and that includes cellulose, lignin, hemicellulose, pectins, gums, and mucilages. Foods containing fiber include fruits, grains, legumes, nuts, seeds, and vegetables. Most plant fibers are long chains of complex sugars banded in irregular patterns that prevent them from being fully digested. Some fiber is partially digestible, while other fiber is not digestible at all. The total carbohydrate equivalence of diets reported in most tables includes both fiber that is digestible and that which is not.

The actual importance of fiber in the diet is still debated. Studies suggest that high-fiber diets lower the postmeal glucose surge and ultimately decrease the total amount of insulin needed for control of blood glucose. Current evidence suggests that the presence of fiber decreases gastrointestinal absorption of carbohydrates, and perhaps also of protein and fat. Whether there are other local or systemic effects is not known.

Two potential problems exist concerning

high-fiber diets. The first is the concern that by increasing the fiber amount, the total caloric intake will be reduced. High-fiber foods are low in calories and may occupy the stomach to such an extent that satisfaction is realized prematurely. Growth and nutritional status must be monitored. Dietary fiber may also interfere with the absorption of calcium, iron, copper, magnesium, phosphorus, and zinc, as well as certain of the vitamin groups. Consequently, the mineral metabolism of the diabetic may be impaired.

The advantages of using relatively high-fiber diets appear to outweigh the disadvantages. Most experts suggest that 7 to 10 percent of the carbohydrate content of the diet might reasonably be gotten through high-fiber foods. It appears to be most effective when the total carbohydrate content exceeds 50 percent of the calories and is associated with a low fat intake. Introduction to and use of whole-grain cereals and breads, along with fruits and vegetables, will help the child receive a well-balanced diet with adequate fiber. Adequate portions and fiber content of foods commonly eaten by children are shown in Table 7–6. Patients should be counseled regarding the possible need to reduce insulin doses following the introduction of high-fiber diets.

Sugar Substitutes

Shortly after the diagnosis of diabetes is made, many parents find themselves in the local grocery staring at items marked "dietetic" or "diet." There are dietetic food products including cookies, candy bars, and even eye-catching gift items; elsewhere are found diet soft drinks, canned fruits packed in water, and dietetic ice cream. Shortly thereafter, the child is being overwhelmed with dietetic cookies, peanut butter cups, ice cream, and chocolate wafers. Diabetic control suffers because of the use of these dietetic foods.

Unfortunately, the word "dietetic" is often misinterpreted by the patient, for it means only that one or more ingredients have been replaced with some other ingredient. Sometimes the ingredient removed is sugar, but just as often it is salt. Therefore, it is important that all patients learn to read product labels, not only to find out what ingredient has been replaced but also to find out the nutritional value of the food item and to see how to work it into the meal plan. Some special "dietetic" products are permitted, but none of these costly special foods are necessary. The meal plan for the child with diabetes should be appealing and should appear

Table 7–6. **FIBER CONTENT OF FOODS PER 100 GRAMS**

Food	High Fiber (3 g)	Moderate Fiber (1.5 g)	Low Fiber (0.5 g)	Little Fiber (0.2 g)
Bread			Whole wheat bread and crackers	White, cracked wheat, rye, pumpernickel breads
Cereals	All-Bran (4.8 g/cup) Wheat germ (2.5 g/cup)	40% Bran flakes Puffed wheat Raisin bran	Barley, Cheerios, corn flakes, oatmeal, puffed rice, brown rice, Shredded Wheat, Wheaties	Rice Macaroni Noodles Spaghetti
Vegetables	Green peas (canned)	Green and wax beans, dried beans and peas, broccoli, Brussels sprouts, cauliflower, mustard greens, green peas, okra, pepper, pumpkin, winter squash	Asparagus, beets, cabbage, carrots, celery, corn, cucumber, eggplant, lettuce, mushrooms, onions, sweet potatoes, white potatoes, tomatoes	
Fruits	Fresh blackberries (4.1 g/¾ C) Dried figs (5.6 g/C) Dried dates (2.3 g/½ C)	Apples, berries except blackberries, figs, pear with skins	Applesauce, apricots, bananas, fruit cocktail, cherries, grapefruit, grapes, mangos, melons, oranges, peaches, pears (without skin), pineapples, plums, prunes, raisins	Juices only

"normal" in most respects, and it is unnecessary for preparations to require the purchase of special foods. Special foods may detract from the feeling of normalcy that is sought; additionally, they are expensive. Two dietetic products that might be suitable for the diabetic are gelatins and puddings, since these two products contain fewer calories and are no more costly than the regular items. Two other products that have made life more pleasurable for the diabetic are the "diet" soft drinks and water-packed fruits. The "diet" soft drinks are sweetened with nonnutritive sweeteners that neither affect the blood sugar nor contain many calories (averaging less than 3 calories in 12 ounces). A larger quantity of water-packed fruits can be exchanged for a smaller quantity of fruits packed in syrup.

"Dietetic" or "sugarless" does not necessarily mean that the item does not contain carbohydrates or calories. Sugar substitutes are divided into two categories: nonnutritive and nutritive sweeteners. Nonnutritive sweeteners include cyclamate and saccharin, which have essentially no caloric or nutritive value. They also do not effect the blood glucose level. The nutritive sweeteners are fructose, sorbitol, mannitol, xylitol, and aspartame. These sweeteners must be worked into the meal plan carefully for two reasons: they provide calories (4 calories per gram) and they may raise the blood sugar level at various rates if given in sufficient amounts.

Saccharin

Since 1980, when cyclamate was removed from the market by the FDA, saccharin has been the major noncaloric sweetener purchased in the United States. It may be used in the diabetic meal plan as a free item. This nonnutritive product was discovered over 100 years ago and gained much popularity in World War II when sugar was limited. In 1971, reports raised the question of an association between saccharin intake and cancer. Since that time, conflicting data on this association have been reported. Since 1977, the FDA has sought to ban saccharin, based on the Delaney Amendment, passed in 1958, which states that any food additive found cancerous in animal studies should not be used for human consumption. The FDA attempt has been temporarily blocked by Congress but its future actions remain uncertain.

Fructose

The use of this nutritive sweetener in the meal plan of the diabetic is controversial. Fructose is also known as fruit sugar and is found in many fruits and berries and in honey. It is one and one half times sweeter than sucrose; consequently, a smaller amount is needed.

Most of ingested fructose is absorbed unmetabolized in the jejunum through facilitated diffusion, and its absorption is slower than sucrose, glucose, and maltose. During absorption from the bowel, only 5 to 8 percent is converted to glucose or lactate. Through the fructose-1-phosphate pathway, fructose is rapidly metabolized, mainly by the liver, resulting in a low concentration in the blood and a small urinary loss. The first step of cellular metabolism is insulin independent, but one of the metabolic products of fructose, triose, does require insulin action. Therefore, fructose metabolism is partially insulin dependent.

Studies have shown that, in the patient whose diabetes is controlled, small amounts of fructose do not raise the blood sugar level as high as do complex carbohydrates. An additional advantage of fructose over sucrose is that fructose users have 25 percent fewer dental cavities. In foods, it acts like sucrose and does not leave an unpleasant after-taste.

Sorbitol

Sorbitol has been used since 1929 in commercially prepared foods as a sweetener. These foods are incorporated into the meal plan for the diabetic. Sorbitol is a naturally occurring sugar alcohol found in a variety of vegetables, fruits, and berries. It is produced commercially by the hydrogenation of glucose, but sorbitol is not available for home use. Sorbitol does not promote tooth decay. One disadvantage is that it has only half of the sweetening effect of sucrose. Like fructose, sorbitol contains calories (4 calories per gram). Consumption of a large quantity of this polyol (more than 30 grams per day) will have a laxative effect, as with any of the polyols used as a sugar substitute. Dietetic products contain the same number of calories, regardless of whether sorbitol or sucrose is present.

Sorbitol is slowly absorbed in the gastrointestinal tract and is efficiently taken up in the liver. It is converted to fructose by passive diffusion and is eventually changed to glucose. The initial steps of sorbitol metabolism are insulin independent. If, however, there is insufficient insulin, as in patients with uncontrolled diabetes, the metabolism is dependent on insulin. Studies show that sorbitol has no special advantages over sucrose as a sweetener for the patient with diabetes. The use of moderate amounts of sorbitol is acceptable and may eventually be found to provide some advantages in dietary management of patients who are lean and whose diabetes is controlled.

Xylitol

Xylitol is another polyol similar to sorbitol that is found naturally in many plants. It is commercially produced by the hydrogenation of xylitol found in birch residues and hardwood. One of the characteristics of xylitol is that it is spicy, and like fructose, it is one and one half times sweeter than sucrose. Its spicy taste gives xylitol a palatable sweetness. The amount required to sweeten varies with changes in physical state: xylitol is less sweet when fruit acids are added to it, and it gets sweeter when its temperature is lowered.

Xylitol is the best nutritive sweetener for use in chewing gums, because it causes the fewest dental caries. The calories in xylitol are the same as in sorbitol (4 calories per gram). Xylitol does not seem to increase serum triglyceride levels. When consumed in large doses (30 to 40 grams at a single meal), it causes osmotic diarrhea. After absorption, xylitol is taken up and degraded to trioses in the liver. The initial steps are insulin independent until their final metabolic transformation to glucose.

There is some doubt about the safety of this polyol, based on recent studies of rats fed 2 to 20 percent xylitol in the diet for two years. At present, xylitol has been removed from the market voluntarily and is being evaluated thoroughly by the FDA for possibly causing tumors. When it was on the market it was very expensive (about $3.00 per pound). Most scientists believe the advantages of xylitol are trivial or slight at best when it is substituted for sucrose in the meal plan.

Aspartame

Aspartame (NutraSweet, G. D. Searle and Company) is the newest nutritive sweetener, becoming available in the United States in 1982. It is an amino acid that contains 4 calories per gram. Aspartame is 200 times sweeter than sucrose and has no metallic after-taste. It has been studied by the FDA Bureau of Foods, and the outcome is promising. It is now used in the soft drink industry and has been released for home use.

Despite a few suggestions of toxic side effects, the safety record of aspartame is relatively unblemished. An increasing number of food products contain aspartame and, because it produces no changes in blood glucose, it is the preferred sweetener.

Fats in the Diet

Of the various plasma lipids, cholesterol and triglyceride are the subjects of most concern, because increased serum levels are associated with increased risk of atherosclerosis and coronary disease. People with diabetes are more prone to develop atherosclerotic disease than is the general population. The mechanisms for this are not well understood, but it appears to be unrelated to blood glucose control.

Triglycerides and cholesterol have two sources: they are manufactured in the body (in the liver and intestines) and they are found in foods. Dietary modification in cholesterol, triglyceride, and saturated fat intake along with maintenance of a desirable body weight can decrease the level of plasma lipids. The Food and Nutrition Board and the Council on Foods and Nutrition have recommended this dietary modification and body weight maintenance theory for people with elevated plasma lipids.

The typical American consumes 40 to 45 percent of his or her calories in the form of fat with a polyunsaturated:saturated ratio of 4:1 and a cholesterol content of 500 mg to 1000 mg daily. Saturated fatty acids, found in animal fat, are saturated with hydrogen, causing the firmness of the product. Polyunsaturated fatty acids contain some hydrogen but are not fully saturated; therefore, the molecules are soft or liquid. Vegetable fat contains a large amount of polyunsaturated fats. It has been found that serum cholesterol levels decrease with a polyunsaturated:saturated fat ratio of 2:1 or 1:1. Along with this fat ratio, it is recommended that the total intake of fat be reduced to 30 to 35 percent of the calories consumed and that the intake

Table 7–7. LIQUID EXCHANGE LIST, WITH CARBOHYDRATE CONTENT

Fruit Exchange: 1 fruit exchange = 10 grams CHO*

8 oz or 1 C Gatorade = 1½ fruits + 130 mg sodium + 24 mg potassium
4 oz or ½ C orange juice or grapefruit juice = 1 fruit
⅓ C apple juice or pineapple juice = 1 fruit
2 oz or ¼ C grape juice or prune juice = 1 fruit
4 oz or ½ C Cran-Apple juice or nectars = 2 fruits
4 oz or ½ C Hi-C or Tang = 1½ fruits
1 C presweetened Kool-Aid, lemonade, or punch = 2½ fruits
1 C Sweet'nLow–flavored drink mix = 1 fruit
3 oz regular soft drink = 1 fruit
1 regular twin Popsicle = 2 fruits
2 tsp sugar = 1 fruit
2 regular hard candies = 1 fruit
5 Lifesavers = 1 fruit

Starch Exchange: 1 starch exchange = 15 grams CHO*

½ C cooked cereal = 1 starch
½ C mashed potatoes = 1 starch
1 small baked potato = 1 starch
½ C regular Jello = 1 starch
1 C vegetable or cream soup = 1 starch
½ C vanilla ice cream = 1 starch
1½ C V-8 juice = 1 starch

Milk Exchange: 1 milk exchange = 12 grams CHO*

8 oz or 1 C (½ pt) whole, skimmed, lowfat, or buttermilk = 1 milk
½ C evaporated milk = 1 milk
⅓ C condensed sweetened milk = 1 milk
8 oz milkshake = 1 milk, 1 starch
8 oz malt = 1 milk, 1 starch, 1 fruit
⅓ C ice milk = ½ milk, 1 fruit
½ C regular vanilla pudding = ½ milk, 2 fruits
½ C regular chocolate or butterscotch pudding = ½ milk, 3 fruits
½ C sugar-free custard mix = 1 milk

Free Foods: May be eaten as desired

Diet drinks	Broth
Unsweetened Kool-Aid	Sugar-free gelatin
Unsweetened lemonade	Unsweetened Popsicles (made from any of the first three
Unsweetened tea	above)
Unsweetened coffee	Water

*CHO = Carbohydrate

of cholesterol be restricted to 300 mg or less per day.

Increased levels of triglycerides are a frequent result of hyperglycemia in insulin deficiency in the young patient with diabetes. Triglyceride elevation is less likely in patients whose diabetes is well controlled than in those with poorly controlled diabetes. Therefore, attention to control of the diabetes is the prerequisite in treatment of elevated triglyceride levels. Proper use of insulin and of dietary methods of correcting obesity, with restriction of dietary carbohydrates and fats, is often effective.

No harm is done by encouraging the patient and family to reduce their cholesterol and triglyceride intake. However, there are potential emotional factors involved in commanding an over-restrictive diet. Extreme dietary recommendations for a lower cholesterol and fat intake may become another burden for the diabetic patient and may interfere with normal lifestyle. On the other hand, if a family's history indicates hypercholesterolemia, a fat-controlled meal plan would benefit not only the child with diabetes but also the whole family. Making the diet a family affair helps the child with diabetes feel less different.

DIET AND ILLNESS

Children with diabetes, like children without diabetes, become ill periodically, and this stress places an added burden on their diabetes. The effects of stress on diabetes and its management are discussed in Chapter 11. Suffice it to say here that attention to oral intake is important during such stressful times. Using the liquid exchange list (Table 7–7) will make it easier for the child and family to handle both illness and diabetes simultaneously.

Some of the foods on this list contain concentrated sugars that may be substituted when the ill diabetic patient is unable to consume his or her usual diet. Often illness will cause a loss of appetite. Therefore, the best approach in this situation is to consume small frequent feedings of foods that the patient feels can be tolerated.

Vomiting or diarrhea or both may cause depletion of valuable body minerals and electrolytes. Sodium and potassium are lost and need to be replenished through foods such as Gatorade, ginger ale and other carbonated beverages, tea, and fruit juices. Usually fruit juices are not as well tolerated as the other beverages listed. Fever causes an increase in basal metabolism and consequently in the number of calories used. Therefore, it is desirable to give the child calorie-containing liquids.

DIET AND SPECIAL OCCASIONS

Special occasions, such as birthday parties, slumber parties, dances, and so forth, are common in the day-to-day life of the child. In many social settings, such occasions may appear to happen weekly. The child and parents need guidelines so that the child may participate without compromising the diabetes. There are a number of acceptable methods for handling these occurrences, the best solution usually being one agreed to by the child and parents. Some of the accepted options will be briefly discussed:

1. *Provide Dietetic Foods*
   This is probably the most common method used. The child, parents, or hosts provide dietetic foods and drinks, and the child selects the appropriate ones. With the widespread use of diet soft drinks today, this does not set the child apart.
2. *Exchange from a Meal or Snack*
   Quite often the child has a meal or snack scheduled that would regularly occur close in time to the special occasion. Food exchanges from that meal or snack can be given instead. When this method is combined with the provision of diet softdrinks, the options are plentiful.
3. *Combine Numbers 1 and 2 with Eating a Small Portion*
   A small portion of cake or ice cream, along with the aforementioned options, increases the range of choices open to the diabetic.
4. *Eat What Others Do, But Supplement with Prefood Insulin*
   For the person who understands very well his or her diabetes and its perturbations, this is an acceptable alternative. The patient must have gained some experience earlier so that proper insulin supplementation can be accomplished.

SUMMARY

Dietary management is an important aspect of care. For insulin therapy to be most effective in controlling blood glucose, attention to the dietary intake is necessary. The family, physician, and dietitian must work closely together so that a well-integrated diet plan is developed. Dietary management, like all other aspects of care, is a dynamic process and must be continually evaluated and appropriately altered.

8

Exercise

By tradition, exercise has been one of the key elements of management programs for persons with insulin-dependent diabetes. Early studies demonstrated that exercise produced an augmentation of the effect of insulin on blood glucose lowering, and exercise thus became one of the cardinal features of attempts at achieving carbohydrate control. Despite sharing this lofty perch with insulin and diet, exercise programs have, in general, not been incorporated into most management programs with the same vigor; partly because evidence supporting a beneficial, long-term effect has been difficult to document. The recent heightened interest in exercise programs has been prompted in part by a national enthusiasm for physical fitness but also by an accumulation of data concerning dynamics of exercise programs. Physiologic studies in both nondiabetic and diabetic individuals have now documented some short-term benefits and have suggested potential long-term rewards. In dealing with patients with IDDM, clinicians have noted that individual responses to standard exercise programs are variable, occurring because of differences in type of diabetes and because of differing levels of carbohydrate control at the time of observations.

CARBOHYDRATE METABOLISM DURING EXERCISE

Nondiabetic

To understand some of the perturbations of carbohydrate metabolism that occur dur-

ing exercise in the patient with insulin-dependent diabetes, it is perhaps best to start with a brief review of the physiologic alterations that occur with exercise in the nondiabetic individual. The metabolic state in the nondiabetic during rest is depicted graphically in Figure 8–1. Extracellular glucose is the primary energy source for the liver, the adipocyte, resting muscle, and all non-insulin-dependent tissues. Extracellular glucose that is not used in the energy phase of the metabolic cycle is stored as glycogen (liver and muscle) or as fat. Insulin is necessary for glucose entry into insulin-dependent tissues as it binds with specific receptors at the cell membrane. Resting muscle is also able to use free fatty acids to meet some of its basal energy demands.

Figure 8–2 represents some of the more important and complex changes that normally occur when exercise commences. One of the first and most important consequences of exercise is the relative inhibition of pancreatic insulin secretion. This inhibition is mediated by neural mechanisms and by early elaboration of catecholamines, primarily epinephrine. The small amount of insulin that remains is insufficient to prevent glycogenolysis and lipolysis but does facilitate glucose use by the exercising muscle. Much of the early energy requirements are met by the elaboration of free fatty acids from fat stores. Glycogenolysis is further enhanced by increased secretion of glucagon and growth hormone, while cortisol stimulates gluconeogenesis. Through these interactive processes,

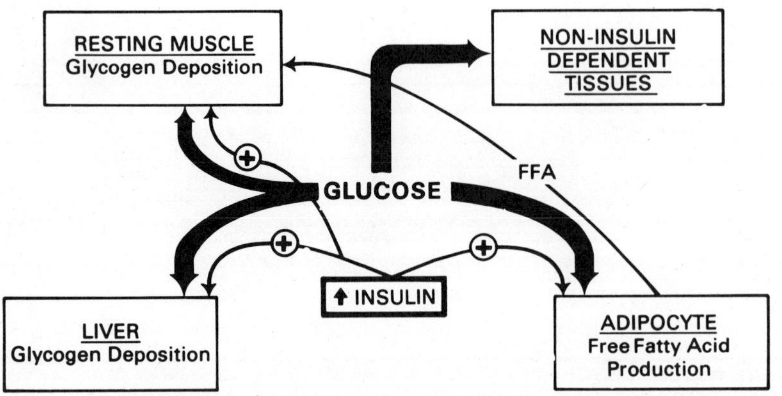

METABOLIC STATE—RESTING NORMAL

Figure 8–1. This figure is similar in some respects to one seen earlier in Chapter 6. Here, in the context of exercise, it is merely intended to demonstrate the positive effects of insulin in (1) preventing glucose production by the liver, (2) facilitating glucose entry into muscle cells, and (3) promoting free fatty acid (FFA) production. Plasma glucose remains "normal."

the extracellular concentrations of glucose are held relatively constant as demands of exercising muscle and non-insulin-dependent tissues are proportionally met by the increased glucose production. Afterward, during the recovery phase following exercise, the process is reversed and glycogen is resynthesized.

Diabetic

A single major difference occurs during exercise in the insulin-dependent diabetic, and this difference leads to important overall responses by the body (Fig. 8–3). In IDDM, the insulin is usually being partially, if not completely, delivered into the extracellular space from a depot subcutaneous site. As exercise commences, there are neural and adrenal medullary responses similar to those of the nondiabetic, but insulin delivery from the depot is not interrupted. In point of fact, delivery of insulin from the depot site may even be enhanced because of the increased blood flow accompanying exercise. Consequently, the liver does not effectively accelerate glucose production in the face of ex-

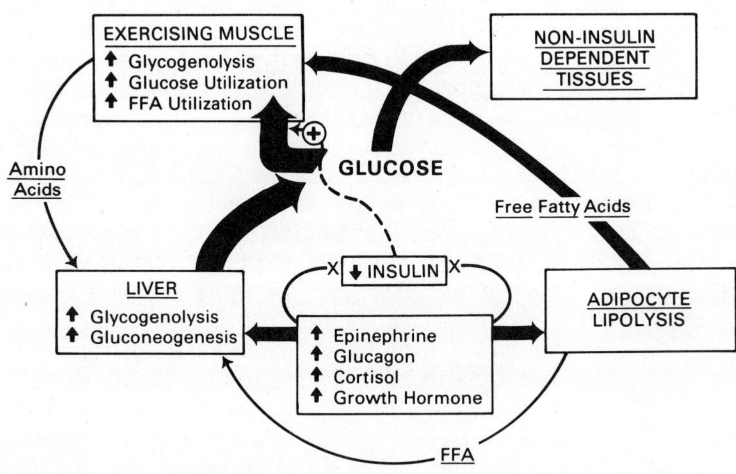

METABOLIC STATE—EXERCISING NORMAL

Figure 8–2. When exercise commences in the nondiabetic, there is an increase in secretion of hyperglycemic hormones (that is, epinephrine, norepinephrine, glucagon, cortisol, and growth hormone). These produce hyperglycemia by (1) inhibition of insulin secretion and (2) stimulation of glycogenolysis and gluconeogenesis. Additionally, most of these hormones are lipolytic, and there is a rise in free fatty acids (FFA), and subsequently in ketone bodies. Glucose is made more readily available for use by exercising muscle.

Figure 8–3. In the diabetic, the same hyperglycemic factors are operational, *except* insulin delivery from the subcutaneous depot is not blocked. If free insulin levels are high, the liver may not be able to increase its glucose production. In some instances, the adipocyte will not be able to increase delivery of free fatty acids (FFA). As the exercising muscle uses more glucose, the blood level may fall to hypoglycemic levels. If sufficient energy is not available from either source, early fatigue occurs. As might be expected, the underinsulinized person gets an accelerated release of both FAA and glucose, potentially leading to hyperglycemia and ketosis.

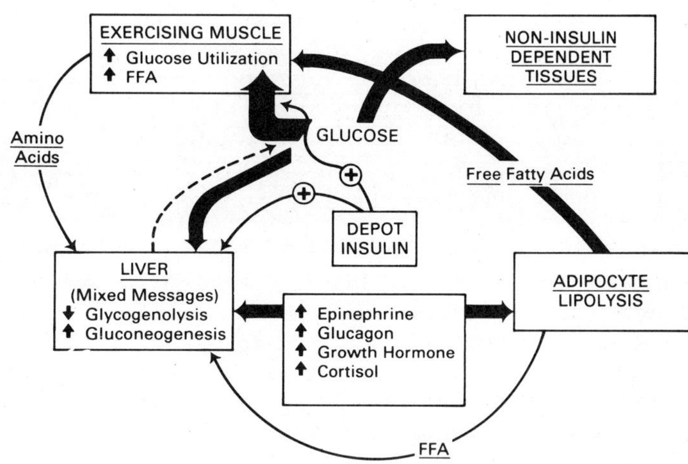

METABOLIC STATE—EXERCISING DIABETIC

aggerated needs. Glycogen deposition may be occurring simultaneously with blunted glycogenolysis. Thus, plasma glucose levels commonly fall in response to exercise, and symptomatic hypoglycemia may result.

In the well-insulinized diabetic, the magnitude of hypoglycemia is dependent on several factors, the most important of which appear to be (1) the relative rate of insulin absorption from the depot site, (2) the time interval from the last meal, and (3) the composition of the meal. Consequently, if the exercise period coincides with the peak absorption of depot insulin (usually 6 to 10 hours after injection), plasma-free insulin concentration is likely to be higher and the potential for postexercise hypoglycemia greater. Likewise, prolonged activity of the extremity in which depot insulin has been administered is more likely to cause earlier absorption and peaking of blood insulin levels. Thus, someone who has administered his or her depot insulin in the thigh is more likely to exhibit rapid insulin absorption while jogging than is someone who has given the injection in arm, buttocks, or abdomen. Whereas a reduction in blood glucose concentration is expected in the well-maintained and adequately insulinized patient, this effect may be different in the person whose diabetes is poorly controlled or who is ketotic. Studies have demonstrated that in these patients both plasma glucose and ketones rise, further hindering attempts at glucose control and increasing the potential for symptomatic ketosis.

EXERCISE FOR THE YOUNG PERSON WITH DIABETES: IS IT DESIRABLE?

In general, there are multiple advantages to an exercise program for the patient with IDDM. Table 8–1 demonstrates a few of the documented benefits, some which are common to all persons and some which are unique to the diabetic. In the well-controlled diabetic, there is often a reduction in the amount of insulin required to achieve a comparable level of glucose control. Studies have demonstrated that the ultimate effect of

Table 8–1. ADVANTAGES OF EXERCISE PROGRAM FOR IDDM PATIENTS

In the patient with controlled diabetes, exercise:
Decreases insulin requirement
Decreases peak blood glucose levels following meals
Increases number and affinity of insulin receptors
Reduces ketonemia
Aids in control of weight (helps prevent obesity)
Improves conditioning and work capacity
Improves cardiovascular stability
Reduces hyperlipidemia
Improves self-image and self-esteem

physical training on glucose control is not only immediate but lasts well beyond the period of activity. There is a suggestion that exercise three to four days per week may be adequate to maintain this effect. Additionally, if the exercise is conducted shortly following meals, the peak level of blood glucose is decreased, thereby preventing rapid shifts. The antiobesity effect of exercise is also important in the person with diabetes. Not only does the person benefit from the caloric expenditure engendered by the activity, but also there is now convincing evidence that conditioning has an anorectic reward over time. Based on studies in the nondiabetic, there seems to be validity to the widely held belief that hyperlipidemia and cardiovascular stability are improved.

The positive effects on self-image and self-esteem noted in a number of studies are of particular importance to the young person with diabetes. Because of the very nature of this disease, there are a number of negative factors that influence the patient's sense of identity and self-worth. Physical conditioning seems to have a tranquilizing effect on the psyche of the adolescent and gives another outlet for some of the stresses that so markedly influence diabetic control.

Potential Problem Areas

Although the advantages of an exercise program far outweigh any disadvantages, it would be folly to conclude that the latter are of no consequence. Potential problems must be identified and a program developed to prevent or circumvent as many as possible. A close working relationship must be established among the physician (diabetes management team), the diabetic and his or her family, and athletic instructors (coaches and so on). When such is done, there are few problems that cannot be handled by a thoughtful educational and management program.

The two most notable problems encountered are exercise-induced hypoglycemia and exercise-exaggerated hyperglycemia and ketosis. Attention must also be directed toward a third possibility: that some of the older teenagers and young adults may have degenerative complications (for example, retinopathy, hypertension, neuropathy, and nephropathy). Consideration of the potential consequences of exercise in these persons must be weighed. Because of the possibility of degenerative complications, it is essential that any person whose duration of diabetes exceeds 10 years have a complete physical assessment before a vigorous athletic program is begun. Periodic reassessments should also be mandated.

Hypoglycemia

As noted earlier, the drop in blood glucose concentration that occurs during exercise in the well-insulinized patient is primarily related to decreased hepatic glucose production in the face of exaggerated muscle use. Deprived of its primary fuel substrate, the muscle responds with decreased work performance, manifested primarily as early fatigue. Non-insulin-dependent tissues are also deprived. The nervous system is primarily affected because of the essential role of glucose in its functioning. Early symptoms of decreased availability of glucose to the central nervous system are confusion, disorientation, alterations in personality, and, if not corrected, unconsciousness, and convulsions or coma or both.

As a result of the fall in blood glucose, and often before there is evidence of "brain symptoms," neural and hormonal systems are brought into play in a counter-regulatory response. Epinephrine, norepinephrine, glucagon, growth hormone, and cortisol are elaborated with resultant release of hepatic and muscle glucose. These neural and hormonal responses produce ancillary signs and symptoms: shakiness, tremors, rapid heart rate, constriction of peripheral blood vessels (pallor and "cold" skin temperature), and increased sweating. As is evident, these are some of the same clinical signs associated with vigorous exercise or anxiety or both, and it may be difficult for the patient or clinician to discern the true etiology.

Prevention of Significant Hypoglycemia

This is a cardinal feature of good diabetic management. The first aspect of prevention involves the patient's knowledge of his or her own diabetes and its specific nuances. The diabetic should be aware of his or her body's own responses to exercise and be cognizant of the factors involved that might either precipitate or prevent hypoglycemia. Addition-

Table 8–2. **PREVENTION OF SIGNIFICANT EXERCISE-RELATED HYPOGLYCEMIA**

Knowledge
  1. Of the specific interactions of insulin, food, and exercise
  2. Of the symptoms and signs of patient's own hypoglycemia

Attitudes
  1. Willingness to make some alterations in management
  2. Willingness to act on early symptoms and signs
  3. Willingness to involve a friend

Insulin
  1. Alterations in overall schedules
     Fewer problems with 2 or more injections per day
  2. Alterations in site of injection
  3. Specific decisions on type of insulin and time of injection

Food
  1. Take complex carbohydrates *before* activities
  2. Have simple carbohydrates available during activities

ally, the diabetic should also be able to distinguish the early symptoms of hypoglycemia and be prepared to prevent further falls in blood glucose.

Certain precautionary actions can generally reduce the likelihood of significant hypoglycemia. Table 8–2 outlines some of the most important aspects. As noted earlier, it is vital for the person with diabetes to have a full understanding of the interaction of insulin, food, and exercise. It is likewise important to be aware of specific clinical symptoms and signs that result from rapid drops in blood glucose. However, knowledge is not enough, for the diabetic must be willing to make alterations in overall management and to take action on the early symptoms and signs. If the early symptoms include confusion, the consequences of inaction may not be appreciated. Having a friend nearby who is attuned to the prodrome of hypoglycemia ("buddy system") is well worthwhile.

Hypoglycemia is more likely to occur during exercise if the peak of insulin action approximately coincides with the exercise time. Since NPH and Lente insulins generally reach their peak actions between 6 and 10 hours after injection, hypoglycemia is most likely at this time. If insulin is given before breakfast, then one might anticipate problems with exercising between 3:00 and 5:00 PM. If management has consisted of a single morning dosage of insulin, the afternoon peak will be higher and the potential for hypoglycemia increased. Consequently, a two shot per day program, by lowering the peak,

is associated with a reduced incidence of exercise-induced hypoglycemia.

Crystalline or Regular insulin exerts its maximum hypoglycemic effect two to four hours after administration. Consequently, if a dose of Regular insulin is routinely administered before the evening meal, hypoglycemia might be anticipated during exercise that occurs between supper and bedtime. Occasionally, such hypoglycemia may be delayed into the early morning sleeping hours. In such instances, consideration should be given to modifying the dose of evening Regular insulin when vigorous exercise is planned. Obviously, the insulin should be given in a site away from the most vigorously exercised part of the body.

Extra food intake is the most effective method of preventing exercise-induced hypoglycemia. To be maximally effective, the type or quantity of food should be geared to the nature or extent of the exercise. Additionally, timing of the food intake in relation to the exercise program is important. For the highly motivated teenager who desires to perform well while maintaining good diabetic control, it is advantageous to perform blood glucose testing before and after sample exercise periods in order to determine the amount of food intake needed to prevent hypoglycemia.

The food must be given prior to the exercise, and it should provide a carbohydrate source primarily in the form of starches. Simple sugars are absorbed too rapidly to provide any significant sustaining action. For most moderate exercise periods of about 30 minutes' duration, approximately 15 grams of carbohydrate (1 starch exchange) is sufficient. Programs with higher energy expenditure, such as soccer or basketball, may require more carbohydrate intake; while others may require less.

Some diabetics have attempted to prevent hypoglycemia by purposely lessening or decreasing overall control of their diabetes. This is accomplished by either reduction in the routine amounts of insulin or by unregulated increase in the usual dietary carbohydrate. This practice is to be discouraged for several reasons. First, it may place the young person at greater risk for hyperglycemia and ketosis and will definitely lower his or her eventual work capacity. More important, however, is the fact that during periods of underinsulinization, glycogen stores are being progressively depleted. Consequently,

Table 8–3. **SYMPTOMATIC HYPOGLYCEMIA**

Mild
  Weakness, tiredness
  Shakiness, tremors, anxiety
  Increased hunger
Moderate (Above Symptoms, Plus)
  Altered consciousness (sleepy, lethargic)
  Change in personality (inappropriate behaviors)
  Increased pulse rate
  Pale, cold skin
  Feels either hot or cold
  Inappropriate sweating
Severe (Above Symptoms, Plus)
  Unconsciousness (coma)
  Convulsions

in the event of hypoglycemia, the body may be unable to raise blood glucose spontaneously, which increases the risk of developing more severe hypoglycemia.

Treatment of Symptomatic Hypoglycemia

Mild symptomatic hypoglycemia is common during exercise in the well-controlled diabetic. As noted earlier, hypoglycemia of this degree can be frequently prevented by appropriate handling of insulin and food intake. Mild hypoglycemia is generally recognized readily by the person with diabetes and is easily avoided by stopping the exercise and ingesting a small amount of quick-acting carbohydrate (a simple sugar). Most children and young adults will handle these mild episodes themselves without others knowing. In most instances, exercise may be resumed within 10 to 15 minutes.

More serious episodes of hypoglycemia often require attention from those around the diabetic (coaches, friends, and so on). Table 8–3 lists some of the symptoms and signs commonly exhibited. A change of personality is common, and the person's behavior may suddenly become inappropriate to the situation. The diabetic may be sufficiently confused so as not to personally recognize the symptoms. Generally, there will be some combination of the following symptoms and signs: altered consciousness (sleepiness, lethargy, hyperactivity), skin pallor or coldness, inappropriate sweating, tachycardia. Such symptoms and signs usually respond, within minutes, to rest and the administration of about 10 to 20 grams of carbohydrate (given in the form of two to four sugar cubes or three to six ounces of a regular soft drink). After the person has responded, administra-

tion of an additional starch exchange and another 10 to 15 minutes of rest is appropriate, after which return to activity is usually safe.

If the child becomes unresponsive (unconscious, semicoma, or coma) or has a convulsion, the attendant should respond quickly and appropriately. If the diabetic is able to swallow, small sips of a regular soft drink should be given. Alternately, a tube or dispenser of a commercial concentrated sugar may be squeezed into the side of the person's mouth. If this brings no response within 5 to 10 minutes, administration of 1 mg (1 cc) of intramuscular glucagon is indicated. This should be supplied for the athletic personnel or school nurse, with directions for its use being given by physician and parents. Such therapy should always be initiated before the child is transported to a hospital or sent home. Injectable glucagon is safe, and even if given when not needed, no actual harm will occur. On the other hand, failure to initiate proper therapy in such a situation may lead to serious brain injury. Table 8–4 provides a graduated program for management of hypoglycemia.

Hyperglycemia and Ketosis

As noted earlier, the person whose diabetes is out of control (poorly insulinized) may have a response to exercise manifested by further increases in blood levels of glucose and ketoacids. On occasion, symptomatic diabetic

Table 8–4. **TREATMENT OF SYMPTOMATIC HYPOGLYCEMIA**

Mild
  Usually treated by individual
  1 or 2 fruit exchanges (2 to 4 sugar cubes, 3 to 6 oz
    Coke)
  Rest for 15 minutes after symptoms leave
  1 starch exchange before restarting activity (e.g., 2
    peanut butter or cheese crackers)
Moderate
  Diabetic may need help in management
  Same as for "mild"
  May need to repeat "mild" treatment
Severe
  Diabetic will need help in management
  Sips of regular soft drink, if swallowing
  Tube or dispenser of concentrated sugar
    Squeeze entire container into side of mouth
    Assist in swallowing
  Glucagon: 1 cc (1 mg) given by injection (at site)
    Should be supplied by physician/parent
  Secure help from one competent in care
  Transport if does not respond immediately

ketoacidosis may be precipitated. Thus, it is essential that the diabetic who wishes to be actively engaged in athletic programs have his or her disease in balance. The desire to perform athletically can be a strong motivator for establishing and maintaining diabetic control. Parents must be helped to understand that exercise is not a replacement for insulin in lowering blood glucose levels.

Dehydration

Persons with diabetes have a higher potential need for water than do nondiabetics. This is caused by hyperglycemia with attendant glycosuria and its associated increase in obligatory urine water. All diabetics are susceptible to dehydration, but the underinsulinized person with persistent hyperglycemia is most at risk. Thus, free access to water should be allowed and the diabetic person should be encouraged to drink whenever thirsty. Diabetic patients in poor overall control may show evidence of excessive loss of extracellular electrolytes, particularly sodium. This is rarely a problem in a person with well-controlled diabetes.

Degenerative Complications

Significant complications rarely occur until after a diabetes duration of 10 to 15 years. There is convincing evidence that the degree of control of carbohydrate metabolism is a contributing factor to the development of such complications as neuropathy, hypertension, retinopathy, and nephropathy.

Neuropathy of a sensory nature may present problems for the athlete. Occasionally the person has painful sensations, particularly of the lower extremities, which may interfere with activities. More frequently, there is either hypothesia or anesthesia of the feet. Such diminished sensation leads to the potential for unrecognized trauma and repeated or prolonged tissue injury. Neuropathy, more than vascular insufficiency, leads to significant foot problems. Attention should be given to proper footwear and foot care, and intensive treatment should be instituted for either injury or infection, however insignificant these appear.

Hypertension at rest is more frequent in the young diabetic than in the population at large. In addition, the untrained person with diabetes may experience a greater rise in both systolic and diastolic blood pressure following exercise than do nondiabetic peers. On the other hand, aerobic conditioning seems to lower the blood pressure in a fashion similar to that of the nondiabetic. However, isometric exercises (for example, weight lifting) may cause an inappropriately high blood pressure response in the diabetic. If the person also has retinopathy, the potential for problems is real. A thorough physical examination, with blood pressure taken before and after exercise, is desirable at regular intervals during conditioning. With a proper rate of conditioning, the harmful effects on blood pressure diminish.

Retinopathy of the severe type generally occurs only after 15 years' duration of diabetes but may be seen occasionally after a duration of 10 years. In the presence of acute problems (that is, proliferative retinopathy, neovascularization, vitreous hemorrhage, retinal detachment, and so forth) or immediately following photocoagulation, rigorous exercise appears contraindicated. This is particularly true when the exercise is accompanied by a rise in blood pressure. More modest degrees of background retinopathy are not contraindications to an exercise program.

Nephropathy of clinical significance is unusual before 15 to 20 years' duration of diabetes. On the other hand, fixed proteinuria may begin somewhere between 10 and 15 years' duration, and exercise-induced proteinuria may be seen after five years. There is no evidence that exercise or athletic conditioning is associated with worsening of the renal lesion.

SELECTION OF ATHLETIC ACTIVITIES

Although there are few, if any, athletic or exercise activities in which the young person with diabetes cannot engage, there are some activities that are preferred. In general, the selection of an activity should take into account such factors as the capability of the individual to pursue that activity throughout life and the advantages of its aerobic conditioning. Thus, the selection of an activity that can be enjoyed singly or that requires no more than one other person is preferred. Examples might be jogging, swimming, aerobic dancing, tennis, and racketball. Such em-

Table 8–5. **GUIDELINES FOR HIGH-PERFORMANCE ATHLETICS**

Secure eligibility statement from physician
  (diabetologist) (should ensure compatible
  insulin/food/exercise program)
Have coach/trainer and team physician made aware of
  essentials of diabetes and potential problems
Instruct coach/trainer and team physician on
  recognition of hypoglycemia
Instruct coach/trainer and team physician on treatment
  of hypoglycemia; including the administration of
  glucagon
Encourage "buddy system"

---

phasis on individual activities is not intended to exclude team sports, but these should be thought of as extras rather than as the primary activity. Some of the more hazardous sports, such as scuba diving, hang gliding, mountain climbing, and so forth, are not generally recommended and should be pursued only if there is a close "buddy system." As mentioned earlier, strengthening or toning (anaerobic) exercises such as weight lifting are not recommended as the diabetic's sole form of exercise.

The Diabetic and Competitive Athletics

Most young persons with diabetes can participate competitively, and there are many examples within professional ranks to document this statement. Compared with nondiabetic peers, the young person with diabetes does have more problems to overcome, some of which have been noted earlier. Another problem, not previously mentioned, is a tendency for parents to be overprotective toward children who have grown up with diabetes. It is somewhat difficult to break this handicap, but the family should be encouraged to allow the young person some latitude to participate in competitive athletics.

Table 8–5 identifies some guidelines for coaches or team physicians (or both) who encounter young persons who wish to engage in high-activity, competitive athletics. A com-

plete physical examination by a physician, preferably a diabetologist, should be obtained. The eligibility statement should ensure a compatible program involving insulin, food, and exercise. The team coach or trainer, as well as the team doctor, should have an overview of diabetes and be aware of potential problems. The coach or trainer should be able to recognize hypoglycemia and be prepared to handle it. This person must be able to administer intramuscular glucagon should the need arise. It is not sufficient to merely have the team physician aware of these factors, for team physicians are rarely present during practice sessions, and episodes of hypoglycemia are even more common at these times than during an actual game.

ACTIVITIES FOR THE UNINTERESTED, NONATHLETIC DIABETIC

As indicated earlier, an exercise program has certain desirable features related to diabetic control. Many families are not oriented toward regular programs of exercise, and it is difficult to motivate their offspring toward such goals. Certain techniques, long applied to other aspects of care, may be used in motivating these children also. First and foremost, the entire family must become participants; thus, an activity that is concordant with family lifestyle should be elected. Regular periods of walking are often overlooked as a reasonable activity as one tends to forget that the calories used in walking one mile are almost identical to those used in jogging or running that same distance.

An educational program should outline the advantages of regular exercise. The diabetic should be encouraged to set goals, keep records, and periodically review progress toward achieving those goals. A periodic assessment of actual performance (that is, improvement in work capacity) is a strong motivator for continuing activity programs.

9

Psychologic and Family Factors

Insulin-dependent diabetes mellitus (IDDM) presents a formidable challenge not only to the individuals who are afflicted (children and adolescents) but also to those in their immediate environment (their parents, siblings, teachers, health care providers, and friends). These young persons with diabetes must maintain a delicate balance among daily insulin requirements, exercise, and diet just to survive and function normally. To maintain this balance, they are taught to test blood or urine glucose levels several times a day, administer one or more injections of insulin daily, adhere to some restrictive dietary requirements, and pay attention to exercise and activity. Attempts at maintaining a metabolic balance are paralleled by the need for a psychologic balance in relation to the illness and its sometimes inordinate demands. Despite careful adherence to the diabetic regimen, the child with IDDM may experience periods of loss of metabolic control, owing primarily to the capricious nature of the illness. Additionally, children with IDDM are often taught that if they are consistently responsible in performance of their diabetes-related functions (for example, monitoring glucose levels, keeping records, administering insulin, adhering to diet, and so forth), they can live reasonably normal lives, participating in activities similar to those of their peers. The fallacy of this premise is soon recognized as the child realizes that there is nothing "reasonably normal" about administering multiple shots a day, constantly monitoring body systems, and following a controlled diet. This ultimately fosters anger and resentment and delays effective coping in many children.

The diabetic regimen exposes the child during the most intimate of functions (for example, urine testing) as well as during the most public and social of functions (for example, administering injections, meal times). The network of persons collaborating to assist the child in health care functions is wide and varied, including physicians, nurses, dietitians, exercise physiologists, teachers, parents, and siblings. Because of the pervasive nature of IDDM, it is reasonable to assume that the maintenance of metabolic control will involve a complex interaction of physical, psychologic, familial, social, and environmental variables.

This chapter examines the historic basis of this assumption and the current empirical foundation from which to assess the role of psychologic and familial factors in treatment. Past literature has focused primarily on the incidence of behavioral, emotional, and family problems of children and adolescents with IDDM. This chapter, on the other hand, will emphasize the interaction of characteristics of the illness and those developmental tasks of childhood that affect the normal psychologic and physical growth of such children.

The relationship between psychologic and family factors and the effects of the disease on the achievement of developmental tasks are further emphasized in order to enhance effective treatment of these children. This chapter will also attempt to maintain a "delicate balance" between the consideration of physical factors and the consideration of psychosocial factors. The child in good metabolic control who is withdrawn, depressed, and socially isolated or who is aggressive, hostile, and resentful is not a healthy child. Nor is the child who is functioning well socially (at home, at school, and with peers), while demonstrating consistently high blood glucose concentrations, a healthy child. In this chapter, we will further delineate those psychologic and familial factors that have implications in treatment and appear important in fostering optimal emotional and physical health of children and adolescents with IDDM.

HISTORIC PERSPECTIVE

The importance of the role of psychologic factors in diabetes has long been recognized. In the 17th century, Thomas Willis attributed the cause of diabetes to "prolonged sorrow." In the 1930s, Menninger reported on the association between the mental states (particularly anxiety and depression) and the physical states of diabetic psychotic patients. Initial attempts to define the relationship between physiologic and emotional states peaked in the 1950s, when authors focused on a search for the "diabetic personality," a search for correlations between personality traits and a predisposition to diabetes. Simultaneously, and along similar lines, attempts were made to relate a specific neurotic, nuclear conflict to the development of diabetes. The basic care conflict of the diabetic person was hypothesized to be one between the desire to care for others and the wish to be cared for. Intuitively intriguing as they may be, the "diabetic personality" and care conflict theories are not supported by empirical evidence. In a critical review of the diabetes literature from 1940 to 1980, Dunn and Turtle (1981) state, "there is still no evidence for a 'diabetic personality' that is uniquely and directly associated with the disease itself, distinct from that associated with any other chronic illness."

The investigation of psychologic factors in the search for the "diabetic personality" declined; however, there remained a number of investigators who contended that the incidence of emotional and behavioral problems was higher in persons with diabetes than in those without the disease. Two new lines of research became prominent, one focusing on the influence of psychologic factors on the *onset* of diabetes and the other focusing on the influence of psychologic factors on the *course* of the diabetes. For a complete review of this literature, the reader is referred to Johnson (1980). Aspects of this literature will be noted in later sections of this chapter. From a historic viewpoint, it is important to note that the questions involved are extremely complex and that the methodology used to address them has often been overly simplistic. Investigators have approached the problem from a unidirectional viewpoint, studying the effects of psychologic factors on the onset or course of diabetes or studying the impact of diabetes on the psychologic adjustment or physical health of the child. These narrow points of focus on the relationship between an individual and his or her disease are not sufficient to adequately account for findings relative to either the ability to cope with diabetes or the degree of metabolic control. The child functions not within a vacuum but rather within a network of social environments, the most influential of which is the family.

Although the focus of research changed from the individual child to the family, investigations continued to be of a unidirectional nature, assessing the impact of the family on the diabetic child or the impact of the diabetic child on the family. From a theoretical point of view, it seems most profitable to conceptualize the diabetic child as one part of an ongoing family system. The diabetic child is affected by patterns of family functioning, reflected in parental attitudes and behaviors; and has an impact on the family in areas of communication, marital integration, parental self-esteem, and so forth. Both child and family functioning are affected by the particular characteristics of the illness experience itself: age of onset, duration, and degree of control. Although there is currently a great deal of theorizing about the relationship between family functioning and the diabetic child's physical and psychologic health, there are few empirical tests of the hypothesized associations. Minuchin and his collaborators (1978) have attempted to do so; however, the lack of appropriate control groups, the small number of families studied, and the lack of specificity in the definition of family typologies make results difficult to interpret.

The process of examining the roles of psychologic and family factors in diabetes has become increasingly refined. With the recognition of the importance of treating the child within the context of his or her family, investigators have begun to address two common questions: How is family functioning affected by the presence of a child with diabetes? How is the child's ability to cope with diabetes affected by family factors? The answers to these questions are integrated by a family systems model that focuses on the reciprocity and interdependence of parts in a social context.

In the historic models, scant attention has been paid to the interactional effects of stage of childhood development, psychologic and family factors, and the illness itself. The small number of children with specific chronic illnesses has resulted in a pooling of age groups for investigation. Because children view their world differently at various ages and stages of development, their coping mechanisms vary accordingly. Additionally, the interaction of the child's illness with specific developmental tasks of the child's age group may profoundly affect the intervention methods available to enhance child and family coping abilities. For example, identity, independence, body integrity, privacy, and a desire to be similar to peers are all major concerns of adolescence. Each is a factor that is affected by the daily health regimen of the teenager with diabetes. The way in which particular characteristics of this illness interact with particular age-related developmental tasks warrants further investigation and discussion.

EFFECTS ON DEVELOPMENTAL TASKS

Through naturalistic observation, empirical study, and societal consensus, a series of childhood and adolescent stages has been delineated to correspond to the physical, emotional, and cognitive tasks required of children within particular age ranges. These tasks describe the characteristic behaviors expected of children within these age ranges and thus become our yardstick for the assessment of healthy growth and development

and for the anticipatory guidance thereof. The developmental tasks of life are those things children must learn if they are to be judged, and to judge themselves, as reasonably happy and successful individuals. Task accomplishment constitutes healthy and satisfactory growth in our society.

Description of the tasks within stages draws heavily from the works of developmental theorists in specific content areas: general development (Havighurst), personal-social development (Erikson), cognitive development (Piaget), moral development (Kohlberg), and development of children's understanding of health and illness (Bibace and Walsh). Maturation and experience interact at each stage to enable the child to address and achieve particular tasks and then to progress to more advanced levels. Processes or events—physical, psychologic, and environmental—that interfere with either maturation or experience will disrupt the normal sequence of attainment of these developmental tasks. Chronic illness is one such disruption. Chronic illness modifies both the maturational processes and the experiences of the child, which in turn affect the achievement of developmental tasks, often making them more difficult to achieve or attainable only at a slower rate.

In using the developmental task model as a conceptual framework on which to base discussions and investigations of the treatment implications of psychologic and family factors in diabetes, several points about the model need emphasis. First, it must be recognized that developmental tasks arise from several interdependent sources. One set of developmental tasks, including crawling and walking, is tied mainly to physical maturation. This physical maturation is often the necessary precursor to the teaching of appropriate social attitudes, values, and behaviors, such as those of bladder and bowel training. A second set of tasks, such as learning to read and to obey societal regulations, arises primarily from sociocultural pressures. A third set (for example, the choice of and preparation for an occupation) is linked to the personal values and aspirations of the individual. Thus, *physical maturation, sociocultural pressures,* and *individual characteristics* are three dimensions that will influence not only the delineation of age-related developmental tasks but also the individual's attainment of these tasks, socialization, and adaptation to the environment. A chronic condition such as diabetes will affect all three sources of developmental tasks.

Second, the inter-relationship among the three dimensions (physical maturation, sociocultural pressures, and individual characteristics) must be emphasized. All three function in multiple reciprocal relationships within an ecologic framework that includes the individual's race, socioeconomic class, religion, and family constellation.

Third, the progressive, unfolding nature of the developmental task model must be noted. Although timing is an important aspect of the evaluation of task accomplishment, the sequencing of task accomplishment is more important. The achievement of developmental tasks at each stage is dependent on the successful accomplishment of tasks at previous stages.

The child with diabetes is faced with the delicate balance not only of physical maturation, sociocultural pressures, and individual characteristics within the normal developmental progression but also of exercise, diet, and insulin in the maintenance of psychologic and physical health. The role of psychologic and family factors in assisting the child to achieve these delicate balances within each developmental stage is the subject of the following discussion and of hypotheses for future research and clinical intervention.

Infancy and Toddlerhood

Infants spend their first year and a half in a dependency relationship with adults. During this time, they face some of life's greatest challenges. They must physiologically adapt to life outside the womb. Because cognition develops through sensorimotor mechanisms, the development of the physical skills of eye-hand coordination, sensory discrimination, and motor skills is important to learning. Infants must perceptually attain object performance, adapt to eating solid foods, and achieve emotional stability. In terms of personal-social development, infants must establish trust in others to fill their basic needs, develop emotional ties to others, experience and master the first stage of stranger anxiety, and begin to develop a sense of intentionality of their own acts. Infants' needs during the early part of this period include nurturing, as well as touch and other sensory stimulation; during the latter part, the freedom to move independently and explore becomes important.

The beginning of the ability to symbolize thought processes in language marks the end of infancy and the beginning of toddlerhood. Cognitively, the toddler begins to use imagery and memory and learns through conditioning and rote learning. Cognitive, language, and moral development are all egocentric, which defines the term "my stage" for this period of development. Toddlers are pleased with themselves and with all the new things they imagine and do. As they increase their self-reliance, toddlers must work hard to overcome a constantly ambivalent situation; they want independence but are still dependent on adults. Toddlers master skills in walking, talking, and controlling body eliminations. On the personal-social level, they depend on approval and want autonomy; these desires are often incompatible, because some newly acquired skills provoke the anger of caretakers. During this stage of great exploration, toddlers assert themselves and must learn to adjust to socialization demands. When toddlers overassert, they may become terrified and need comfort and security. Although during this period they begin social play, toddlers absorb the emotions around them, relate poorly to peers, and have difficulty sharing possessions. They face such tasks as developing autonomy and testing limits.

The hallmark of infancy and toddlerhood is the egocentric inability to differentiate between self and world. Concepts of sickness and health may be beginning to develop, but children's responses are most often in terms of a "place" where it hurts. Children's attempts at responding to health- and illness-related questions will often involve expression of a personal or irrelevant experience.

Effects of Diabetes

It can be hypothesized that the effects of diabetes on the attainment of developmental tasks in infancy and toddlerhood are most pronounced in the area of development of trust and autonomy. Infants and toddlers who must be hospitalized for initial stabilization of their diabetes will experience disruption of home routines, separation from parents, painful medical procedures, and interaction with numerous strangers. The development of trust in infancy depends on early experiences of having needs met in an appropriate and timely manner: when the infant is hungry, he or she is fed; when "gassy," he or she is burped; when wet, he or she is changed. Consistency in need fulfillment contributes to the infant's sense that the world is a safe place, but such consistency is often difficult to achieve in a hospital environment.

The infant is only beginning to develop a concept of object performance, including the knowledge that when parents leave, they will return. The toddler, who has attained object performance, still has no time concept, however; five minutes may seem like five hours, or five days, or forever. Fears of separation from parents may increase the child's anxiety (stress) and cause additional complications in the attainment of metabolic control. Since toddlers cannot differentiate fantasy from reality nor thought from behavior, they may very well attribute their illness to punishment for thinking bad thoughts or for behaving poorly. Toddlers also often appear to retaliate in anger at parents who in the past have been able to ameliorate the pain from cuts and scratches but who seem powerless to protect the child from scary and sometimes painful hospital procedures.

Once the diabetic toddler returns home, the parent may initially restrict the child's activities in fear of hypoglycemia reactions. The developmental necessity of exploring and practicing newly acquired motor skills thus may be hampered. Parents may also find that previously attained developmental tasks such as bowel and bladder control and talking in sentences may be temporarily lost.

Psychologic and Family Factors

There are no studies on the role psychologic or family factors play in the ability of infants and toddlers to cope with diabetes. The incidence of diabetes during these developmental stages is low, and studies have relied on assessment methods (interviews, drawings, and questionnaires) appropriate only for older children. Since children who have had diabetes for longer durations have been found to cope less well than those who have had the illness for shorter durations, this is a fruitful area for future investigation. There are also no data on how the diagnosis of diabetes affects the development of the early parent-child relationship or on how intervention at this stage could enhance optimal child development in the attainment of stage-related tasks.

Treatment Implications

Consistency is most helpful for infants and toddlers who experience hospitalization during the initial stages of diagnosis and stabilization. Parents should be encouraged to bring familiar items from home to the hospital and to remain with the young child during the hospitalization.

During the period of initial diagnosis, both toddler and parents may experience overwhelming emotions. Toddlers have little control over the emotions they so readily pick up from environmental cues. Therefore, they need and will use adult models. Adults can help the child by providing words or actions to imitate, by empathizing with the child, and by enabling the expression of these feelings in shared talk or play.

High levels of anxiety in the young child can be decreased by preparing the child for even the smallest of procedures and separations, with facts repeated over and over again. Any sense of panic experienced by toddlers can be lessened by helping them to re-establish a sense of control. This can be done by offering them simple environmental choices, such as choosing between juice and milk or between the green shirt or the blue shirt.

Just as the toddler will need a balance among the factors of exercise, diet, and insulin, he or she will also need the continued balance between "love" and "limits." Parents of children with physical problems often continue to treat their children as "vulnerable," the effects of which are evident in restriction of age-appropriate activities, overindulgence, and in consistent limit-setting. Parents' confidence in their ability to parent may be shaken by the shock of realizing that they will now be parenting a child who initially appears so "sick."

Parental support, perhaps in the form of exchanging feelings, concerns, and knowledge with other parents of diabetic children, and an increased knowledge of child development are two interventions vital to this stage of development of infants and toddlers with diabetes. A third intervention for the health care provider to consider is assisting the parents in the implementation of child management techniques that will help them discipline their child. The "terrible threes," which often began as "terrible twos" is a normal (albeit frustrating for parents) period in children's lives as they struggle with the attainment of autonomy. When the struggle focuses on mealtimes and eating, however, the behaviors may have serious effects on the health of the diabetic child.

For the young child, the parents can be encouraged to make a picture chart that they can use to reinforce positively those behaviors they want to see performed by the toddler. Parents may obtain a piece of white poster paper and a grease pencil. They may glue on the poster four large pictures representing behaviors they wish the child to perform: for example, a plate with food (eating breakfast), a toothbrush (brushing teeth), a toilet (going to the bathroom), and a syringe and insulin bottle (taking shots). The paper may then be covered with clear contact paper. Whenever the child performs a desired behavior, the parent smiles, lavishly praises the child, and takes the child over to the chart, where he or she can mark a big X over the appropriate picture with the grease pencil. The children love the praise and the motor activity involved, are proud to see their accomplishments, and quickly set forth to "do another picture" on the chart. The chart is designed for the ease of the parents, who can wipe off the grease pencil marks with a tissue and reuse the chart the next day.

Two effective methods of helping parents increase toddlers' sense of control over their diabetes and to decrease their fears are play and role modeling. Parents can encourage the child to play with dolls and health care equipment, such as toy syringes. In playing "doctor," the child pretends to assume control over the medical regimen and often "plays out" feelings of fear, loss of control, anger, or pain. Parents can help the child continue the play by showing the positive consequences of the child's performing healthful behaviors (the child may then play with a favorite toy, the child feels good, and so forth).

The use of a role model is a powerful teaching technique. The more similar the model is to the child (age, sex, ethnicity) and the more clearly the model is rewarded for the performance of healthful behaviors, the more the diabetic child will imitate the model. Arranging a session in which the young child can watch another child perform the behaviors of the diabetic regimen is therefore beneficial to all involved.

Early Childhood

The preschooler continues to develop the skills of independence and exploration. Games such as "king of the mountain" and fantasy roles such as Superman and Wonderwoman reflect the child's newly developing sense of "I can do it." Physical tasks of early childhood involve the refinement of both general body control and fine muscle control. Intellectually, children in early childhood are learning through exploration, manipulation, and play. Stage-related tasks involve developing and refining concepts of social and physical reality, learning about sex differences, and developing an accurate body concept.

The norms of society-at-large begin increasingly to affect the social and personal tasks to be accomplished in early childhood. The child must learn about cultural rules and expectations, about sex roles, and about right and wrong. As magical thinking is resolved and as children become more reality oriented, egocentrism gives way to a desire to please parents and significant others. Being a "good boy" or "good girl" becomes an important focus of both thought and action. The discovery of rules, order, and relationships and the growing ability to compare may often result in a constant barrage of "it's not fair" statements. The emotional relationships developed within the family are now generalized to relatives, peers, and other adults. At this stage, children become more affectionate and can imitate but cannot empathize. They still have great difficulty with the concept that others have feelings different from their own at the moment. Also typical of emotional development at this stage are frequent nightmares and phobias and the fear of body part loss.

The early school-age child must develop his or her sense of initiative and curiosity simultaneously with the task of development of increased impulse control. Adults in the child's environment fill stage-related needs by setting and maintaining clear limits, providing protections, and fostering a developing sense of competence, control, and power.

In accord with the preoperational style of thought of children in early childhood, children center on a concrete, single aspect of their own experience to define illness. Bibace and Walsh divide early childhood into two stages that reflect children's understanding of health and illness. In the first of these, "phenomenism," the child defines illness in terms of a single external symptom. This symptom is most often a sight or sound that the child has at one time associated with the illness. The cause of the illness is attributed to a source that is often spatially remote and inappropriate. A young child cannot comprehend the cause link between an illness and its source and cannot articulate the link in terms other than co-occurrence or magic.

How did you get sick? "Out in the sun and I went to the doctor." How did the sun make you sick? "The sun . . . " How did you get better? "I went home."

In the later stage of preoperational conceptualization of health and illness, a stage termed "contagion" by Bibace and Walsh, children describe illness in terms of a single environmental occurrence that is often a physical activity and is often restricted inappropriately to one body part. The source of the illness is seen as someone or something close to but not touching the child or an activity or event that occurs prior to but not simultaneous with the occurrence of the illness itself. Similarly, cure is thought to consist of a person or object in the child's immediate environment or an event or activity occurring subsequent to the illness. The child still centers on a single, concrete aspect of the illness and cannot articulate a connection between the source or cure of the illness and the illness itself, but the single concrete aspect and the source are now invoked from a class of events both spatially closer to the child and more appropriate to the domain of the illness.

Why do you have diabetes? "From drinking too much water before bed." How did drinking too much water before bed make you have diabetes? "Too much water before bed makes you sick."

Effects of Diabetes

Children in the stage of preoperational thought (early childhood) and those in the stage of concrete operational thought (middle childhood) perceive their world in different ways and can also be expected to experience their diabetes differently. Unfortunately, investigations of the effects of diabetes and the role of psychologic and family factors in diabetes have not progressed along developmental lines. Study samples usually range from early childhood through early adolescence, with numerous samples extending through late adolescence. The following discussion will therefore be addressed to the developmental tasks of middle childhood.

Middle Childhood

School-age children are more cooperative and reasonable than preschool-aged children; their industry and ambition are reflected in an orientation toward learning and skill acquisition. Cognitively, they are in the stage Piaget labels "concrete operations," in which they attain the ability to use logical operations, such as conservation and reversibility, for thinking and other problem solving.

A chief task at this stage is the mastery of the "three R's" in school, the "learning to learn" through reading and other informative activities, and the amassing of basic facts in the sciences and humanities. Children also learn through hobbies, especially those in which they collect and classify, and through recreational activities. Children in middle childhood have learned to distinguish fact from fantasy and are developing realistic concepts of birth, death, and religion.

During middle childhood, children gradually change their orientation from one of pleasing specific persons to one of upholding rules and laws. They are now able to generalize from specific situations to the general rules of behavior. These changes help children to develop conscience, frustration tolerance, and self-regulation of behavior.

In the personal-social realm, the tasks of the child in middle childhood become more complex and varied. Children in this stage must relate to a widening group of teachers and other unfamiliar adults, achieve independence within the family, meet the expectations of their peers, and cope with sex role expectations and myriad other external pressures. The school age child needs opportunities to make choices and for physical release and activities, peer support, and team socialization.

The major developmental shift of the concrete operational period is the ability of the child to differentiate between self and world, to distinguish between what are internal and external events, and to generalize from the specific case to the general situation. The child's major focus is still on concrete external events and objects—the "what is" as opposed to the "what will be"—but now the child can manipulate these events and objects in terms of operations such as classifying, categorizing, adding, subtracting, multiplying, and dividing.

The concrete operational stage is also divided into two periods that reflect the child's growing understanding of health and illness. The earliest of these periods is termed *contamination*. During this substage the child does not differentiate between mind and body. "Bad" behavior as well as contact with germs or dirt can cause illness. The child now defines illness in terms of multiple symptoms and will refer to external body functions. While the source of an illness is still perceived as external, the child can articulate a causal link between the source (bad behavior, dirt, germs) and its effect on the body (illness). Both illness and its cure are transmitted through physical contact. Avoidance of contact with the source of illness, either by preventing the body from touching the contaminated source or by not engaging in the contaminated "bad" activity, is the initial way children assume some control over the cause and cure of illness.

What is chicken pox? "They're bumps and red spots." How do children get them? "From touching chickens." What makes chicken pox better? "Rubbing the stuff from the doctor on 'em."

During the latter period of middle childhood, the child begins a stage called *internalization*, in which illness is globally described as being within the body. The child focuses on the *way* in which illness is internalized and not on the internal functioning of the body. The child can articulate the process by which the source and the cure are internalized. A direct relationship is seen between an external contaminant or an unhealthy body state (such as "fat," "old," or high blood pressure) and internal organs. At this stage, the child is also becoming aware of the body's own healing powers and can recognize his or her ability to prevent illness through proper care.

It is important to note here that the child's focus is on the process of internalization of cause or cure of illness and not on the internal physiology of body parts. Children cannot articulate how internal organs function and, when they attempt to do so, usually resort to concrete analogies (such as "the heart is a pump").

How do children get diabetes? "From eating too much sugar." How does that give you diabetes?

"It goes into your blood." And? "It gives you diabetes, I guess."

Effects of Diabetes

Children in the early and middle childhood stages must be given the opportunity to explore their environment and to gain an increasing sense of independence within the family. In the family with a diabetic child, these tasks often demand attention of focus on achieving an appropriate balance between child responsibilities and parent responsibilities. During these stages, parents assume the major responsibility for the child's performance of health behaviors, and therefore independence within the family may be difficult for the child to achieve.

It is important for children to develop a sense of initiative and industry during these years, a sense that "I can do" in relation to controlling the physical processes of their own bodies, developing a sense of emotional self-control and the ability to tolerate frustration, and learning about the world around them. This sense of "I can do" must be fostered within the framework of successful control of diabetes as well. It can be hypothesized that children challenged with the aspect of a positive achievement in attaining control will do better than children who are confronted solely with the "I can't do" aspects of their diabetes. Because of the particular emphasis on learning and categorizing facts and figures, this is an optimal time to teach factual data about diabetes (for example, techniques of injection, of HBGM, and of recording; physiologic parameters such as insulin, food, and exercise). The educator must recognize, however, that the ability to understand conceptually the application of this knowledge in a day-to-day setting will not be attained until early adolescence.

In addition to the effect of diabetes on tasks of exploration, initiative, industry, and learning, one can expect the illness to interact with those tasks relative to self-perception, both in a physical and psychologic sense. A common fear of early childhood is the loss of a body part, and the young child may have fearful misconceptions about the purpose of injections or what's happening inside that has produced diabetes, or the meaning of periodic "blood-letting" (either in the physician's office or during HBGM). The developing sense of body control may be jeopardized by inexplicable feelings of loss of control during hypoglycemia.

Children in early and middle childhood have social and developmental tasks to accomplish as well. Important at these stages, especially in middle childhood, is peer support and the ability to participate in team endeavors. Any condition that engenders a feeling of being "different" from friends will interfere with the development of peer relationships. Enhancement of peer relationships is often best accomplished during this stage by the opportunity to participate in clubs and sports, activities that may necessitate additional attention to the balance between exercise, diet, and insulin.

From a developmental point of view, these childhood years are a crucial time for the development of self-esteem, the ability to see the positive products of one's endeavors. Children who are not allowed to exert their growing independence, who are restricted from opportunities to interact with their peers, and who do not experience success in the control of their diabetes may be at risk in the development of a positive sense of self.

Psychologic and Family Factors

In an extensive review of 16 empirical studies, Johnson (1980) noted that there are few psychologic traits or problems consistently associated with diabetes. When objective tests of self-esteem were used, she found children with diabetes to demonstrate adequate self-perceptions. Additionally, the studies reviewed demonstrated little evidence that high anxiety is a common characteristic of children with diabetes. The majority of studies also found no evidence for heightened aggression or hostility among children with diabetes, and the two studies that did find such evidence can be criticized for having methodologic problems. Only peer relations and social problems are reported with any consistency. Since any chronic illness requires some social readjustment, these results may not be specific to diabetes. Some children appear more successful in this readjustment than others.

Although most authors find minimal psychologic disturbance in their samples of children with diabetes, there is general agreement that those children who do exhibit problems in emotional adjustment have greater problems with diabetes control. A high prevalence of psychologic disturbance has also been reported in families of children with poor diabetes control. From Johnson's analysis, the most common family patterns that appear to negatively affect the diabetic process are (1) overanxious patterns, (2) overindulgent patterns, (3) overcontrolling patterns, (4) patterns of resentment and rejection, and (5) uninterest and neglect.

Treatment Implications

It appears that medical practice has sufficiently conveyed to children with diabetes a sense of self-worth and a sense of their ability to live with their illness. Assessments of self-esteem, anxiety, resentment, and hostility are not significantly different from those of the nondiabetic. Children with diabetes do appear to have difficulty, however, with peer and social relationships, but the inter-relation of these problems is unclear. Do these children maintain their internal psychologic health at the expense of peer and social relationships, or are nondiabetic peers unaccepting of those who are "different" by virtue of their diabetes? Until this differentiation is made, intervention on the part of parents, teachers, and health providers must take a two-pronged approach. The child could profit from the teaching of social skills concerning the relationships and diabetes. Modeling, role playing, and social reinforcement have been shown to be effective in teaching social skills to both adults and children in a variety of situations. The child needs to know how to respond to information-seeking, embarrassing questions, and teasing from peers. "Is it catchy?" "Yecch, needles," "Diabetics can't eat sugar," and "How come you get to eat a snack in class?" are among the more common comments and inquiries that children with diabetes respond to by either withdrawal or hostility.

Children need to learn and practice the "exact words" to use when confronted with such questions. Talking generally about what the children can do in such situations is not sufficient to get them to use their skills when the situation of need arises. An effective method of teaching these skills is for the health provider to have the child call a teacher, grandparent, aunt, or other supportive adult from the office to tell the adult about his or her diabetes. The health provider can help the child address relevant points such as the word "diabetes," what it means, how to stay healthy with diabetes, that diabetes is not contagious, that the child can still do most of the things other children do, why snacks are required, and so forth. This session will get the child over the first hurdle of "What do I say?" and "What words do I use?" The session can also be referred to in the future ("Remember what you told Aunt Barbara") to point out to the child that he or she does have the skills to address these questions when asked by peers.

In this context, peers and adults do not need a medical textbook explanation of the illness, its regimen, or its consequences. The health provider can help the child with simple, specific, and honest words that are appropriate to his or her level of understanding. A young child with diabetes could say, "I have diabetes—that means my body doesn't use sugar the same way yours does. That's why I take shots and watch what I eat." Or "You get a shot when you are sick and it helps your body do what it's supposed to do to fight being sick and stay healthy. I have diabetes and my body doesn't do what it's supposed to do to turn my food to energy. I take shots to help my body do that and stay healthy." Or "You've got blond hair, I've got brown hair. Is that catchy? I've got diabetes, you don't. It's not catchy either."

Another part of the intervention approach is a focus on educating healthy children about diabetes. Teaching normal differences between people presents a formidable challenge when the variable of similarity has been shown to be the most powerful factor in whether people like each other or not. While "opposites attract" may be convenient to describe the odd couple, the norm is more apt to be "birds of a feather flock together." So too with childhood relationships. Children like children who are most similar to them. Normal differences must therefore be taught to children within a context of similarity: "Johnny has diabetes. He can eat everything you can eat, in balanced portions." Or "You took a flu shot to prevent you from getting sick. Julie takes her shots to prevent her from getting sick. She just has to take hers every day."

Still another intervention approach is that involving maintenance of self-esteem, enhancement of appropriate parent-child relationships, and fostering of increased child responsibility for health behaviors. Despite the large number of studies showing the efficacy of using social learning techniques to enhance the parent-child relationship and to

foster child compliance to a wide range of behaviors, these methods are rarely used in enhancing child adherence to the diabetic regimen. In one study, Schafer, Glasgow, and McCaul (1982) used self-monitoring, goal setting, and behavioral contracting procedures to increase the regimen compliance of three nonadherent diabetic adolescents. Adherence increased and was maintained at the desired level for two of the three subjects; the third, whose family was experiencing a variety of severe problems, did not show reliable improvement. With the use of behavioral techniques such as contingent reinforcement and behavioral charting, parents can incorporate health behaviors into a systematic framework that encourages their children to be responsible for a wide range of general behaviors as well. As with the parents of infants and toddlers, a concerted effort to focus on the teaching of child development knowledge and child management techniques is necessary. Often, perhaps out of fear, anxiety, guilt, or resentment, parenting becomes focused solely on the child's diabetes. It is often encouraging for parents to learn that there is no physiologic association between their daughter's dirty room and her diabetes!

The charts used with these older children become more sophisticated. The purpose of the chart is to positively reinforce, or reward, the child for the performance of clearly defined behaviors. If a child's action is followed by a reward, the action is more likely to recur than if it were not rewarded. Rewards can be social (such as verbal phrases, smiles, a pat on the back, an extra privilege) or material (such as a special gift or an increased allowance). Charts help parents avoid the overuse of criticism and "nagging," both of which increase the attention paid to the behaviors and serve as a reward, leading to recurrence of the undesired behavior.

Charts have been used effectively for well over a decade to help parents increase the frequency of their children's positive behaviors, such as getting up on time in the morning, doing homework, getting along well with a sibling, and cleaning their rooms. These same techniques can be used to increase the frequency of health behaviors in the diabetic child. Parents are encouraged to put between four and six items on the chart. All items should be behaviors that the parents desire from their child and not behaviors that are undesirable; in other words, all items should be phrased positively. The items must be written with sufficient clarity that both child and parent can easily, and without argument, determine whether the behavior is important or not. The items listed should provide the child with as much information as possible about how the reward might be earned. For example, "Have a clean room in the morning" tells the child little, for what does a "clean room" entail? Does it mean one shoe under the bed, two shoes under the bed? "All toys in the closet and off the floor at 5:00 at night" gives the child a much clearer message. Whether or not this has been achieved is easily determined by counting any toys on the floor and by looking at the clock.

In choosing the four to six items for the chart, the parent should list two or three that the child is doing already. In this way, the child will receive reinforcement on the very first day, and this reward will increase the probability that other behaviors on the chart will be performed in the future. Starting with a "morning chart" is often a good idea because morning behaviors are usually more easily specified. If the morning is successful, the remainder of the day is likely to go better. Specific morning behaviors might include (1) gets up at 6:30 with a single call, (2) tests blood (or urine) glucose, (3) eats breakfast, (4) brushes teeth, (5) makes bed, and (6) catches bus at 7:45.

Each behavior item on the chart must have its own reward; it is not a two-out-of-three or four-out-of-six system. Rewards should be decided on by the child and parent and should be congruent with the family's values and lifestyles. Simple as it may sound, rewards are only valuable if they are rewarding, and the child alone can determine the rewarding value. For young children, stars put on the chart are often sufficient reward. When combined with verbal praise, a star identifies for the child the precise behavior for which a reward was given. Each behavior could also earn material rewards, such as five minutes extra TV time before bed or five minutes to play alone with Mom or Dad without other siblings around. For older children who understand the concept of an exchange system, each behavior could be worth a number of points that the child could earn toward a specifically designated privilege. However, such rewards are valuable only if they are spent, and it is most effective to reward the child as soon after the performance of the behavior as possible. The younger child should be able to collect the rewards earned at the end of the day, because waiting until the end of the week is too long a time period. Older children can profit from a weekly system.

Families in which disengagement and enmeshment are well balanced, in which environment is delimited by appropriate rules and procedures, and in which the parents are in general agreement about their perceptions of the family have been shown to have children who are in good metabolic control. It can be hypothesized that rules set positively, with rewards for compliance, will enhance adherence to diabetic regimens and give the child a positive sense of self-esteem in his or her accomplishments. Restrictive rules with consequences for noncompliance are apt to only increase child rebellion. Such "rules about rules" further emphasizes the delicate balance parents must maintain to promote both the physical and psychologic health of their children with diabetes.

Adolescence

Adolescents are in a stage of contrast and ambivalence; they are neither children nor adults. Puberty adds new stresses to life; emotional and physical changes are often perceived as a loss of one's former self. Quick mood changes accentuate this seemingly irresponsible, irrational, and inconsistent time of life. In adolescence, there is an attempt to master many of the developmental tasks of childhood at a new and more mature level.

In adolescence there is reduced dependency on the presence of objects and on imagery for thinking. The teenager moves into the initial stages of a cognitive period termed *formal operations* with an enhanced ability to comprehend purely abstract or symbolic content. This ability in turn enables the adolescent to master philosophy, higher mathematics, and theoretical aspects of the sciences and humanities. Learning takes on an additional focus: the ability to apply knowledge needed for adaptation in general and for one's occupation in particular.

The personal-social tasks of adolescents become more complex and rooted in a delicate interplay between social norms and mores and the developing individual value system. Youthful idealism is often starkly pitted against realism as the adolescent begins to develop a more sophisticated moral code that can distinguish between such concepts as morality and legality, rules and justice. Teenagers find themselves questioning old values and either reaffirming them or finding new ones.

Much is demanded in the teenager's preparation for adulthood. Adolescents must make sense out of the world, set realistic goals and limits, learn that rules are not the same for all individuals, and learn to balance their own individual rights and the rights of others. This stage culminates most successfully with the achieving of gradual independence from adults; achieving intimate personal relationships; and ultimately choosing a mate, vocation, and life philosophy.

In adolescence, the teenager is no longer bound to reality but can now hypothesize and think abstractly about possibilities. This new cognitive flexibility is reflected in more mature and complex conceptualizations of health and illness.

In the *physiologic* stage of understanding health and illness, the young adolescent describes and explains illness in terms of internal body organs and functions. Although these children are aware that illness may be triggered by an external event and can describe how multiple external causes affect internal body parts, they are most interested in describing internal functions. There is also an increased recognition that personal actions can contribute to health and illness outcomes. Characteristic of formal operational thought, the child's conceptualizations of health and illness depart cautiously from concrete reality. The adolescent can now describe illness in terms of multiple causes and symptoms, can describe functions and structures that are neither external nor visible, and can make hypotheses about the relationship between the body and the environment.

What is a hypoglycemia reaction? "It's like when you forget to eat and then there's too much insulin in the blood." What happens during a reaction? "Not enough sugar gets to the brain. The brain doesn't run right without enough sugar. You can't think right and get confused, dizzy, and shaky."

The most mature conceptualization of health and illness occurs in the *psychophysiologic* stage of the older adolescent. Illness is still defined in terms of internal physiologic structures and functions, but now psychologic factors are included among the causes and symptoms. The malfunctioning of internal organs is used to explain the immediate cause of illness, and psychologic events are perceived among the less-immediate causes. Likewise, among multiple cures is the relief of sources of psychologic pressure. Although children in the psychophysiologic stage can articulate how the mind affects the body, they do not seem able to describe ways in which the mind or psychologic events are controllable.

What is ketoacidosis? "It's sort of like the opposite of hypoglycemia. It's when you have too much sugar and not enough insulin in your blood." What causes ketoacidosis? "Ketoacidosis is caused by a lot of different things—poor control, not enough insulin, being under stress, getting an infection." What do you mean by being under stress? "You know, like worried or nervous about tests at school." How does stress cause ketoacidosis? "When you're real nervous and anxious, your body releases some chemicals that cause more sugar to go into the blood and you don't have enough insulin to burn that sugar." What can you do to prevent it? "Well, you can make sure you're drinking enough liquids, and you can increase the amount of insulin you take if you think that's necessary."

Effects of Diabetes

Among the developmental tasks of adolescence are (1) adjustment to and acceptance of emotional and physical changes of puberty, (2) solidification of a sense of body integrity and identity, (3) gradual attainment of independence from adults, (4) re-examination of personal values, (5) learning of mature ways to cope with peer pressures, (6) development of intimate personal relationships, and (7) choice of future educational and vocational directions. At no other stage does diabetes so negatively interact with the achievement of these developmental tasks. During adolescence, life-altering implications of diabetes become most salient and demanding—precisely at the time when the person is least motivated to heed them.

Concerns about being different assume renewed importance during adolescence. The teenager who adamantly demands to be treated as an individual within the family is also the one who worries about the most minute details of personal style with a concern that they might not conform to the scrutiny of peers. Prior to the adolescent years, the parents assume much of the responsibility for diabetic health behaviors, and part of the child's medical education may have focused on the "normal" lifestyle that could be attainable with appropriate attention to insulin, diet, monitoring, and exercise. With the arrival of adolescence and the assumption of diabetes self-care, the teenager is confronted with realization of the abnormal or atypical nature of life with diabetes. Differences from peers are accentuated, at least in the teenager's mind. The early adolescent concept of an idealized body image is disrupted daily as the teenager further mars an imperfect body with needles and stylets. Many adolescents are angered by the necessity of a second or third insulin shot in the evening, a ritual that forces the adolescent to acknowledge having diabetes at some other time than morning. Only if the adolescent senses some improvement in immediate health is he or she happy with the extra attention devoted to diabetes care. Teen preoccupation with modesty and growing sexuality is also often subverted into anger and resentment by the connection between the genitals and urine testing and by parental involvement in the testing. This is one factor in the general acceptance of HBGM as an alternative to urine testing. The gradual assumption of independence by the adolescent, often turbulent under the best of conditions, is further complicated by even the most well-meaning of parental watchfulness, concern, or intrusion into the health care regimen. Altering various therapies and rejecting diet, urine or blood glucose testing, and even insulin reflect the attitude of experimentation, rebellion, and independence that is a necessary part of adolescents' development as they work toward a definition of their own identity. However, when this attitude finds expression in the rejection of the therapeutic program, consequences are serious and potentially fatal.

During adolescence, the reward system for effectively adhering to the diabetic regimen also changes. When parents held the major responsibility for child compliance, rewards for adherence may have been in the form of star charts, additional allowance money, verbal praise, or extra privileges. By the time the adolescent assumes full responsibility for his or her health care, parents and health providers often assume that the performance of health behaviors will be internally rewarding. Unfortunately for the health of the teenager, the immediate reward of acceptance by a peer group or a one-night fling at a party far outweigh the values for performance of health behaviors, which are seen as restric-

tive. It is well known that the long-term consequences of aberrant health behaviors are not sufficient to promote adherence to any medical regimen. Teenagers who see the daily evidence of their "bad" behavior in terms of poor results of blood or urine tests face a potential attitude of what Seligman (1975) termed "learned helplessness," through repeated failures at a time when a stable, strong identity and positive self-esteem depend on seeing productive results of one's own actions. Regaining metabolic control may not provide any immediate reward in terms of "feeling better." Adolescents often describe the experience in terms of driving an automobile with poor shock absorbers. The car is in poor shape, but since the driver has learned to compensate for the bumps and pits in the road, the car feels comfortable to the driver. But, because the car is unsafe, new shocks are applied. Now the car is "healthy" but feels uncomfortable to the driver. When the adolescent regains metabolic control, he or she is now more healthy, but the functioning feels uncomfortable and "different." This difference in feeling may be very disconcerting to the person and may last as long as a week or more. Teenagers, who are not known for their ability to delay gratification, often will not wait out these changes in physical feelings and will resort to less-restrictive regimens that promote high blood sugars.

The particular health regimen required for good diabetic care and the public nature of the associated health care behaviors interact with some of the most vital tasks that an adolescent must attain in the progression of healthy psychologic and physical development: independence, body image, identity, sexuality, responsibility, and self-esteem. How well adolescents with diabetes cope with these potentially negative effects is illustrated in current research on psychologic and family factors.

Psychologic and Family Factors

Many of the findings related to the role of psychologic and family factors in diabetes have been discussed in previous sections that reported results of studies that focused predominantly on school-aged children but that also included small samples of adolescents. Those investigators who studied samples consisting mainly of adolescents are faced with the complex problem of accurately identifying the factors contributing to a rise in the incidence of children in poor metabolic control during adolescence. While this can be partially attributed to some of the hormonal changes occurring during this developmental period, it would appear also to be attributed to the increase of normal life stresses that occurs during adolescence. Severe and prolonged stress is associated with the production of the various stress hormones with associated metabolic consequences, such as an increase in free fatty acids and in blood glucose levels. Controlled studies on the effects of stress on diabetes consistently report a rise in free fatty acids, with a more variable response in blood glucose levels. Such results and ample anecdotal experience support the concept that diabetic stability is significantly and directly influenced by the stresses of life.

In general, most adolescents with diabetes seem to handle these increased stresses reasonably well. As with those trends noted in samples of younger children, the personality patterns of adolescents are similar to those of healthy control subjects. Sullivan (1978) found no significant differences between the self-esteem of diabetic and nondiabetic teenage girls. Although the group of girls with diabetes were found to be more depressed than were their nondiabetic peers, Sullivan suggested that this was attributable to a depression instrument that assessed physiologic symptoms rather than the purely psychologic symptoms of depression.

Positive attitudes toward diabetes are also positively correlated with many other adjustment factors, such as peer relationships, family relationships, and school adjustment. In fact, a majority of studies report the healthy attitudes of adolescents toward their illness. Teenagers report seeing themselves in the same light as other teens in many important areas of personal freedom and responsibility in their daily lives, and they exhibit a realistic view of their own control. One group of adolescents studied by Partridge and colleagues (1972) felt they had been asked to take responsibility for their health care at an appropriate age and reported assuming other responsibilities, such as managing money, at the same age as nondiabetic peers. Adolescents report telling their friends about their diabetes, developing occupational goals sooner than their nondiabetic peers, and planning to marry and have children. Although encouragement of such positive attitudes is certainly warranted, it must also be

noted that adolescents may also be denying some of the hard realities of their illness; they often believe that diabetes will not affect their future plans or cause health complications, nor would they trade their diabetes for a less life-threatening condition such as obesity or acne. These are part of the invincible feelings of many adolescents.

Most of the current evidence thus supports a picture of psychologically healthy diabetic adolescents; however, some exceptions have been noted in comparison to healthy peers: feelings of seriously damaged body images, lower levels of ego development, and less self-image complexity. Some of the reported problems may be attributed to the large number of misconceptions that teenagers have about diabetes. Bibace and Walsh note that children do not begin to conceptualize health, illness, and cure in physiologic or psychophysiologic terms until the advent of formal operations and abstract thought in adolescence. Much of the intensive medical education of the child, however, occurs during the school-age years. There are no studies that investigate the effects of a diabetic education program based on the cognitive-developmental stages of children's thought. Parents and health professionals may overestimate the adolescent's conceptual understanding of diabetes; written examination on knowledge and facts may not adequately assess skill in day-to-day disease management. Knowledge alone has been shown insufficient to predict good diabetes control; knowledge plus positive attitudes about diabetes may be the key to adequate diabetes management.

Adequate diabetes management in adolescence, as in previous stages of development, appears related to family factors. Poor family adjustment is associated with poor diabetes control, and findings have been discussed in other sections of this chapter. It is worth reemphasizing the lack of empirical tests of the relationship between parental or family patterns and the child's diabetic condition. Psychologic and family factors may affect the adolescent directly through stress-associated metabolic derangements or indirectly through effects on adherence to treatment regimens.

Treatment Implications

Stress, disturbed family patterns, and potential effects on self-esteem appear to be the major psychologic and family-related complications of diabetes in the adolescent. Several particular intervention approaches are implied.

The first involves an expanded educational program aimed at correcting any misconceptions held by the adolescent about the illness, introducing more complex concepts of physiologic functioning and the role of psychologic factors in health, and addressing psychosocial issues that are relevant to the developmental tasks of adolescence. Now that the adolescent is focused on thoughts about the future, issues related to sexuality, genetics, and vocational considerations become important.

Although the ability to conceive and bear healthy children is an important concern of adolescents, the health provider must also address their more immediate concerns of sexual performance and sexual gratification. Sexual performance is most commonly addressed in the discussion of the vascular or neuropathic effects of diabetes and the risk of impotence in young men. The complications of diabetes may, however, affect the sexual gratification of both young men and young women and must be addressed when adolescent diabetics question their ability to fully experience sexuality.

Another aspect is the encouragement of realistic, direct discussions between the parent and teenager and between the health professional and teenager: discussions that empathize with the adolescent, acknowledge feelings of difference, encourage appropriate experimentation with regulation of the therapy program, and encourage discussions of concerns with other adolescents with diabetes.

A third aspect of intervention involves the maintenance of a positive reinforcement system for the performance of health behaviors. As mentioned earlier, once the adolescent assumes full responsibility for the health care regimen, parents and health professionals all too readily assume that the performance of these behaviors will be internally rewarding; but that is not often the case. Parents, worried about the degree to which their teenagers are assuming full responsibility for health care, are often apt to pay only negative attention to the regimen. This attention comes in the form of embarrassing behavior check-ups and in the form of nagging, neither of which is a positive reinforcement that will promote continued beneficial health behaviors.

The loosening and final cutting of apron-strings is a difficult enough task for parents and adolescents, even when uncomplicated by diabetes. Sincerely concerned and caring parents often sadly and perhaps guiltily feel that one thing, diabetes, has already "happened" to their child and are fearful that another negative occurrence may happen. What may be merely a series of school-related problems for other teenagers often produces serious health ramifications for the adolescent with diabetes. The period of adolescence is quite like a chess game between parent and child, a game that the parent *must* gradually lose. If, however, the parent loses "too quickly" (that is, allows the teenager to assume responsibilities with which he or she is not yet ready to cope), the adolescent becomes overwhelmed and cannot make beneficial, effective decisions. If, on the other hand, the parent loses the game "too slowly," the adolescent emerges into adulthood ill equipped to make his or her own decisions about what is now an independent life. Unfortunately, there is a wide range between "too fast" and "too slow," and the timing that contributes to the optimal growth of maturity in the adolescent has not been determined.

Parents can be counseled to have faith in the decisions their adolescents are making. Their chief role during this period is to help their teenager to see the positive and negative consequences, both long-term and short-term, of their reactions in a nonevaluative, open, honest discussion. As difficult as it is for parents to realize, the final decision concerning a specific course of action will most probably be made by the adolescent. Parents can be helped to choose their house rules carefully at this time; rules such as "Be in by 11:00" and "You have to test your blood (or urine) sugar four times a day" are ineffective if there are no enforceable consequences. The number of enforceable consequences decreases as the child grows older. Constant threats of "what will happen" only undermine the adolescent's view of the parent as an accurate describer of the world.

It is during this time that the health provider can guide the adolescent to the realization that it is the teenager who owns the diabetes and that it is he or she who will experience the major positive and negative consequences of the illness. If parents assume the responsibilities of and the feelings concomitant to the illness, there is no reason for the adolescent to do so. During adolescence, the health provider can help remove diabetes from the parent-child independence-dependence arena by solidifying his or her relationship with the teenager. The teenager can be encouraged to schedule his or her own appointment and discuss methods of attaining progressively more independence. The health provider must be cautioned not to assume a parent-surrogate role and not to serve as merely another battleground for the assertion of adolescent autonomy.

When parents and their adolescents find themselves in a pattern of negative interaction that increases stress levels and in turn makes the diabetes more difficult to control, family therapy is often indicated. Successful treatment of adolescents with "brittle" diabetes through family therapy that addresses unproductive patterns of communication has been reported by Minuchin and his colleagues (1978).

Relaxation techniques and biofeedback have also been used to ameliorate stress and control diabetic symptoms. Reports of these techniques have noted reduced insulin requirements and improved glucose tolerance. Relaxation techniques would appear to be an especially useful intervention for teenagers: they address the increased stress reported to occur in adolescence. Additionally, the interventions teach methods of self-control that enhance the autonomy and independence of the teenager, fostering the attainment of important stage-related tasks.

CONCLUSION

The developmental task model provides an effective framework from which to assess the ramifications of diabetes on the psychologic and physical development of the child and to plan effective intervention. It also provides a basis from which to form hypotheses and investigate the psychologic and familial implications of diabetes on its onset, course, and treatment.

Except for those occurring in adolescence, the effects of diabetes on the accomplishment of developmental tasks at progressive stages have been studied. The small number of children with specific chronic illnesses has resulted in the pooling of age groups for investigation. Because children perceive their world differently at various ages and stages of development, coping mechanisms will also vary over time. Additionally, the interaction of the illness with the specific developmental tasks of an age group may profoundly affect the methods available to enhance the role of the family.

Unfortunately, statements about the role of psychologic and family factors in intervention in diabetes will remain suspect until more faith can be placed in the adequacy of currently used research designs and the reliability and validity of measurement techniques. Many studies have been retrospective "fishing expeditions," with multiple measures and inadequate control and comparison groups. Small subject samples and lack of representation from all socioeconomic backgrounds limit generalization of findings. Many studies have relied solely on clinical observations or anecdotal information. Results of investigations using more objective, empirically based measures, on the other hand, often report contradictory findings as different measures are used by different investigators to assess the same construct.

Such methodological considerations must be overcome in our search for the answer to the question, "What intervention is most appropriate at what point in development?" Intergroup comparisons of homogeneous samples of children with diabetes are probably more productive than are continued studies of diabetic versus normal subjects. Prospective longitudinal variables are effective methods of investigating the effect of the relationship. Increasing attention to the use of psychosocial measures that relate directly to the specific behaviors of the diabetic regimen should also increase the ability to predict future behaviors. Global measures of psychologic and family functioning have shown some relationship to the psychologic functioning of diabetic children but little association with their metabolic status.

The importance of psychologic and family variables is based on the rationale that if such variables can be identified, then they can be modified to enhance coping abilities and metabolic control. As relevant psychosocial variables are identified, they must be manipulated in prospective clinical trial studies. Likewise, only well-controlled experimental investigations of various educational or psychotherapeutic interventions—studies that use randomized control-group or single-subject designs—will yield cause-and-effect information regarding efficacy of intervention. Only caution and careful attention to methodologic concerns will enhance application of knowledge about the treatment implications of psychologic and family factors in diabetes.

10

Education

Education of the child with diabetes and his or her family is carried out in an effort to enable the clinician eventually to turn many aspects of day-to-day care over to a partner who is knowledgeable and competent. Why this is important and how it is best accomplished are primary issues explored in this chapter. The clinician needs to know whether the educational program is working effectively, and some of the methods for assessing this aspect are also covered.

Education of the person with diabetes in certain aspects of self-care has always been identified as a necessary component of management. Diabetes is a participatory illness. Insulin must be measured and injected correctly, food intake must be monitored appropriately, and exercise must be undertaken carefully to prevent potential imbalances. Additionally, the person with diabetes must recognize the early symptoms and signs that suggest problems and be able to handle these appropriately.

Traditionally, the educational program was conducted almost exclusively by the physician, with occasional support from either a nurse or dietitian. Then, as now, the competent, dedicated, and conscientious physician is usually successful in dealing with an intelligent, emotionally intact, and well-motivated child and family. However, when any of these characteristics are missing—whether in the physician, child, or family—the likelihood of successful diabetic management decreases.

During the last two decades, several unrelated factors have made it difficult for the physician to be as successful as in the past: recent advances in diabetes requiring more knowledge and more time, imposed on the physician, and disruption in the traditional family structure. There has been an explosion of new knowledge in the area of diabetes, with increasing evidence supporting the value of tight control in circumventing complications. To achieve tight control, the family of the child with diabetes generally requires more intense supervision and more consistent availability of the health professional. The relatively low frequency of IDDM in the child and the increased demands on the physician's time in other areas have had a negative effect on perceived competency, both in the physician's mind and in the opinions of the public. Add to this the fact that the stability of the American family has weakened. Fewer families appear to have the supportive characteristics so necessary for the optimum care of diabetes. Also, health professionals in the nonmedical fields often have expertise not acquired in the traditional medical training programs. It is easy to see why fewer and fewer physicians feel inclined to undertake an educational program alone.

WHY EDUCATE?

Obviously, to live effectively with a chronic illness, the child and parents require skills and knowledge in many aspects of care. They need life-sustaining and health-maintaining information. Parents need to learn facts and skills for the safe and appropriate care of their child at home. Later, as responsibility for care is shifted to the child, the need to re-educate is apparent. Hence, teaching, as a means of imparting knowledge, helps the person with diabetes to integrate this knowledge into his or her life.

Education attempts to satisfy an intellectual curiosity, a need or desire to know. The educator becomes a resource for the child and family, a source of information to help satisfy this curiosity. This thirst for information is particularly apparent in the young child. A four-year-old girl handling an insulin syringe and giving a doll its shots may appear to the casual observer as though she were playing, although this child is actually exploring and learning.

A major reason that patients and families need to learn is to enable them to make informed choices and intelligent decisions. It is becoming increasingly apparent that patients and parents want and expect this role in management of their health needs. They want to be involved in health care decisions that affect them and their lives. For them to be active participants, the child and parent need information that is timely, germane, and that can be understood and processed intellectually.

There are, of course, other reasons to educate and inform children and their families. A number of authors have postulated that education promotes better patient adherence to treatment plans, more efficient use of the health care provider, and possible reduction in costs of hospitalization and medical care. Another benefit, in our legal-conscious society, is that the person who is knowledgeable and who participates as a partner in overall care and decision making is not as likely to pursue litigation.

McWeeny in 1980 addressed the rights of all individuals concerning education about their health. She lists patient education rights as (1) the right to accurate information, (2) the right to be taught as a unique individual, (3) the right to learn what the patient wants to learn, (4) the right to accept or reject patient teaching, and (5) the right to expect quality education. Others have also looked at patient rights. Regulating agencies and third-party payers have identified the patient's need and right to knowledge. In 1972, the American Hospital Association issued its "Patient's Bill of Rights." This document addresses, among other topics, the health care consumer's right to information regarding diagnosis, informed consent, professional relationships, hospital rules, and human research. In its 1974 White Paper, Blue Cross cited studies to support the cost effectiveness of patient education and strongly encouraged state plans to "assist health care institutions to establish and operate patient education programs and to support them through existing payment mechanisms."

The overall reasons to conduct an educational program are to provide children and families with the resources to live in the healthiest state possible and to assist them in adapting to their illness in a positive manner. Each professional health contact that is made with the child with diabetes and his or her parents is a potential teaching and learning situation. Since several persons may be involved, it is imperative that the philosophy be consistent and the data accurate. Although the style of teaching will be personal and unique for each individual, the content should be directed toward similar outcomes. In most instances, it is best for a single person to coordinate all the information.

PATIENT EDUCATION: THE GROUNDWORK

Quality patient education is based on the caregiver's philosophy of overall heath care for children and their parents, knowledge of teaching and learning principles, and specific communication skills. The patient educator's philosophy of care includes knowledge about human health-seeking behaviors. In addition, the educator holds beliefs about children's understanding of health, about the role family members play in child care, and about the value of education. The patient educator also must identify his or her own role in the provision of health education: Should that role be in a traditional teacher-learner situation? Or should the patient educator serve as a facilitator and a resource of knowledge? The effective patient educator must build a conceptual framework or theoretical foundation for patient education. Such a system includes knowledge of children's cognitive development, theories of learning, and theories about behavior change and motivation. Only after this is accomplished can the educator begin to consider the specifics of diabetes.

Cognitive Development

The patient educator teaching children and parents about diabetes mellitus must have a working appreciation of how children and adults learn. The child's cognitive development follows a predictable course. Infants learn about their world as they begin to trust their caregivers. Their psychomotor activity and senses allow them to gather information. Toddlers have mobility and are beginning a language and evolving independence. These children live in an egocentric, concrete world. Changes in their environment or routine are upsetting to them and not well understood.

Teaching children at these ages focuses on allowing their control within the parameters of their care needs. For example, toddlers are not developmentally ready to understand the reasons for insulin injections. They do, however, learn how to respond to them. Parents who give the shots skillfully and without delays and who provide love and reassurance afterward are teaching these children that injections are an accepted part of their lives.

Preschool children learn about their world by doing. They are imitators, explorers, and experimenters. They live in the present, and their ideas remain somewhat vague and unstable. Fantasy and imagination provide explanations to their questions. Play is their medium for learning. Surprisingly, even preschoolers can fairly accurately imitate injection technique in doll-play situations.

School-age children enter the phase of cognitive development described by Piaget (1952) as concrete operations. These children use groupings, classifications, and numbers to order their world. There is the beginning of use of logical reasoning. The child can appreciate cause-effect relationships.

Teenagers learn through formal operations—a system of logical thought, abstract reasoning, and flexible problem solving. Cognitively, teenagers learn the same way adults learn, but adults actually have certain basic differences. Adults bring their own level of psychosocial development to the learning situation. Adult learners are influenced by their role in society, in work, and in the family. For example, the father who in the past has had little to do with child care may hesitate to learn the day-to-day care of his diabetic child. Adult learning is further affected by a reservoir of past experiences and knowledge.

Domains of Education

How children and adults learn is important for the educator. What they learn is equally important. Although the relationships are not entirely clear, educational psychologists have identified three major domains of education: cognitive, psychomotor, and affective.

The *cognitive* domain includes knowledge of facts, theories, and generalizations and a level of understanding, interpretation, and application. Sophisticated functioning in this domain includes analyzing, synthesizing new structures, and evaluating or judging values. For example, it is necessary for a child to know that he must take insulin every day (fact). It is desirable that he be able to predict the consequences of forgetting or missing his shots (analysis). It is helpful if the child or family or both can formulate a plan of action in the event that shots are missed (synthesis). Some children and families will only be able to learn facts, whereas others are able to analyze and evaluate their actions. The diabetes educator assists the child and parent not only in learning facts but also in applying this knowledge and evaluating the outcome of its application.

The *psychomotor domain* includes sensory perception, physical and emotional readiness for action, and guided responses. The child learning to test urine must first identify the testing materials and then be willing to handle the urine. Initially, each step of urine testing will require careful thought. After repeated supervised and guided practice, the child achieves a level of complex motor movements without having to think about each successive step. The same is true for measuring blood glucose or for administering insulin. To perform a motor skill, the learner must possess a functioning neuromuscular system and be able to create a mental image of each step in the skill. Hence, teaching psychomotor skills to a child under 5 or 6 years of age can be both frustrating and futile. The diabetes educator uses techniques of shaping, modeling, fading, and chaining to teach motor behaviors (Table 10–1).

The *affective domain* of education includes the child's and parent's value systems and philosophy of life. How learners feel about themselves and about their abilities will affect how well they learn and use that knowledge. Educators traditionally have focused on the cognitive and psychomotor aspects of diabetes education. However, the learner's atti-

Table 10–1. **TEACHING PSYCHOMOTOR SKILLS**

	Technique	Application
Shaping	Building on small aspects of behavior to attain more complex skills	Reading the syringe scale before learning to put insulin in the syringe.
Modeling	Teacher demonstration to show the learner what to do	Teacher demonstrates use of blood-testing materials on self.
Fading	A gradual withdrawal of teacher participation	Teacher holds syringe while child pushes in plunger. Eventually child self-injects.
Chaining	Teaching a series of behaviors from the *last* step to the first	Teaching injection technique first, then measuring and mixing insulins.

tudes toward their care, their health needs, the teacher, and the teaching/learning situation affect the outcome of education. In fact, attitudes may have a greater impact than knowledge on long-term behaviors and compliance. Although learners will bring past opinions and feelings with them, they will be exposed to other values in their diabetes education. The educator can promote attitude formation by providing positive role models and satisfying learning experiences. Positive self-care attitudes are further fostered when the educator has high credibility. The diabetes educator is seen as credible when he or she is seen as both knowledgeable and trustworthy.

Change Theory and Motivation

People learn when they have a need or desire to learn. Their motivation to gather information, in this case, results from a sense of imbalance or dissonance. The "health belief model" addresses the human health-seeking behaviors. In describing this model, Rosenstock (1960) found that persons will take health action if they believe that (1) they are susceptible to the disease in question; (2) the disease would have deleterious effects on their life should it be contracted; (3) they are aware of certain actions that, if taken, may reduce their susceptibility or the severity of the disease; and (4) the threat of taking action is not as great as the threat of the disease itself.

Parents of newly diagnosed diabetic children respond in the same way. The child typically has symptoms for a few days or weeks. Finally, the parent decides that "It is more than the flu." In bringing the child into the physician's office, the parent is seeking information to explain the child's health. The parent has been motivated to seek help. By definition, motivation is a state of tension resulting from unsatisfied needs. To return to a state of equilibrium and ease, the individual moves to change or to maintain certain behaviors. Researchers are studying change and motivations as means of predicting and promoting patient compliance to treatment programs.

There are a few things that are already known about motivation and learning, however. The patient who is motivated to learn does so. Motivation is seen in the child and parent who interpret diabetes education as a means of restoring equilibrium. Motivation may be enhanced by the learning process. Motivation to learn is promoted when content is relevant, when skills are used actively, and when learners feel that they are successful in learning and applying their knowledge.

Basic Principles of Learning

In addition to the fact that motivation affects learning, the educator must be aware of other teaching and learning principles:

1. *Learning is enhanced by a moderate level of anxiety or tension.* This tension produces a need to learn. If anxiety is too high, however, the person becomes more involved with managing the fear or the stress. High stress uses energy, leaving little attention for learning. Such a situation often exists in parents when they hear their child's diagnosis. Fears, guilt, and anxiety, as well as lack of physical rest, all make their learning difficult.
2. *Learning is more effective if the learner participates.* Choosing goals with the instructor makes learners partners in their education. Children especially profit from active involvement in their learning. Learning is further enhanced when children can immediately apply their knowledge.
3. *Learning is facilitated by building on previous knowledge.* Relating new material

and information to already familiar knowledge enhances learning. Analogies and stories help children to learn new concepts.

4. *Most learning occurs from concrete to abstract.* Just as the child's cognitive development moves from concrete to formal operations, the learning of new material proceeds in such a direction. The parent must understand when insulin action occurs (concrete) before he or she can safely change insulin doses (abstract).

5. *Learning is enhanced when teaching style fits learner's style.* Some children and parents learn best when moving from general concepts to specific ideas. Others learn best in just the reverse order. Most families are extremely concerned about how diabetes will affect them personally. For these families, specifics of care are more important initially. Assessment of learning style is important if the diabetes educator is able to individualize the instruction.

6. *Learning is promoted when the environment is conducive.* A nonthreatening, trusting, and supportive external environment facilitates trial-and-error learning. It allows the child or parent to try new skills in a safe way and in a manner that supports their sense of self-esteem. Behavior that is rewarded is more likely to be maintained and to recur. Rewards in the teaching and learning processes may be extrinsic, such as praise or tangible items. Rewards may also be intrinsic, such as the sense of accomplishment from answering questions correctly or from injecting insulin painlessly.

The conceptual framework for diabetes education is derived from theories of cognitive development, from teaching and learning principles, and from theories on change and motivation. These concepts provide a background for planning, implementing, and evaluating diabetes education.

Teaching is communication. As such, its effects (documentation) must also be communicated. Documentation of patient education is necessary to meet legal and accreditation requirements and to ensure continuity of care. Legally, the recording of teacher activities and learner achievement documents the professional's attempt to meet health care needs and patient's rights. Documentation is a requirement of the Joint Commission on Accreditation of Hospitals' Standards. Probably more important is the role documentation plays in communication. Sharing educational objectives and progress promotes consistent and comprehensive care. Documenting educational plans, progress, and evaluation can be time-consuming. The use of patient education forms and checklists assists the educator in reducing the amount of time in documentation. Unfortunately, the education forms in diabetes are varied and often incomplete. Sample forms used in the Children's Diabetes Management Center in Galveston, Texas, are included in the appendix of this book.

PATIENT EDUCATION: ASSESSING THE LEARNER

If one believes that the child or parent is motivated to learn because of a need, then it seems reasonable to assess aspects of that need. What the learner brings to the learning encounter (past experiences, beliefs, and knowledge) will affect the success of the present learning situation. To individualize diabetes education, the educator establishes a data base of information about the child and family. This assessment covers cognitive-emotional and sociophysiologic readiness. The initial assessment helps the educator to identify areas of incorrect or absent knowledge and begins involvement of the child and parent in care.

The interview is one method for data collection. The health professional's manner of interview and interpersonal skills should communicate to the family a sense of caring and trustworthiness. Information about present cognitive and psychomotor functions is often better obtained with questionnaires and observations of skills. Attitudes also may be gleaned from careful interview and simple questionnaires.

Cognitive-Emotional Readiness

Cognitive Development

Children's cognitive level of functioning will most assuredly affect their ability to learn concepts and skills. The educator gathers data regarding age, school functioning, and previous learning experiences. Asking children what they like in school, what their school grades are, and what they like to read provides additional information about cognitive abilities. Observing young children in a learning situation provides further data. Can they differentiate colors (as in urine testing)? What do they know about their bodies? What do they know about diabetes?

Assessing the parents' cognitive level includes an evaluation of diabetes knowledge and history of previous learning experiences. Talking with children and parents together provides information about their language, use of diabetes terminology, and style of communication.

Coping Skills

How well the child and parent learn may depend on how effectively they are adapting to the diagnosis of diabetes. If a parent is fearful for the child's immediate health and is overwhelmed by the new demands, energy will be directed toward reducing these tensions. Little emotional energy will be left to meet the demands of education. Until adaptive coping is reached, the educator will need to use special approaches to the teaching and learning situation (Table 10–2). A teenager who is actively denying the disease sees little need in learning about diabetes; consequently, traditional approaches to education may not be effective in this case.

Attitudes

Children and parents will bring to the learning situation their past experiences with education, educators, and health professionals. They will have preconceived ideas and beliefs about illness in general and about diabetes in particular. The child will often share the parents' attitudes in these issues. If the learner values education and basically trusts the health care system and its professionals, then information is more readily accepted. If, as in some ethnic cultures, the learner distrusts professionals and feels little personal control over the future, then the information will be received with skepticism.

Assessing this area of learner readiness involves asking such questions as: How did you feel about first hearing your child's diagnosis? How are things now? What seems to be the worst thing about having diabetes? How will diabetes affect you and your family? Assessment of nonverbal behaviors is equally

important: How comfortable is the child in discussing diabetes and its care? Does the parent seem anxious, confused, or uninterested?

Motivation

Assessment of attitudes, cognitive development, and coping styles aids the diabetes educator to make predictions about the learner's motivation. It is often helpful to determine the learner's source of motivation or locus of control. Internal motivation tends to enhance the learning experience. Whether the learner asks questions, and the types and content of the questions, are clues to the learner's motivation.

Sociophysiologic Readiness

Health Status

How well the child feels will determine how intently he or she can focus on educational goals. Attempting to educate the acutely ill child is futile. The time is better spent in supporting the child and family and in meeting their emotional and physical needs.

The diabetes educator must further assess the child's sensory and neuromuscular system. Reading may be difficult for the child recovering from DKA and its associated temporary visual alterations. Will the parent or child have difficulty reading the syringe markings? Does either child or parent have problems with dexterity or eye-hand coordination?

Cultural Background

Health beliefs, folklore, religious beliefs, and ethnic background may have an impact on the learner's readiness. Persons from cultures that basically distrust strangers, resist changes, hold fatalistic views, and are present-time oriented will be confused and reticent when placed in a typical health education system that values change, self-directed care, and delayed gratification.

Not only education but also how the child's family interprets and implements other aspects of his or her diabetes care will be affected. The family that has little orientation to time and schedules will have difficulty adapting to a routine of injections and con-

Table 10–2. **PSYCHOSOCIAL ADAPTATION AND PATIENT TEACHING**

Stage of Adaptation	Patient's Beliefs/Behaviors	Reducing the Barrier to Learning
Disbelief (denial)	Patient's thoughts: "There's nothing wrong with me." "It can't be happening to me!" Patient's actions: Disregards activity or diet restrictions. Ignores nurse's attempts to teach about self-care measures to be done after discharge.	Provide careful orientation to hospital surrounding and unit policies affecting the patient. Teach with a present-tense focus. Provide careful explanation of each procedure while it is being done. Assure patient that he or she is safe. Teach family members about what is happening to the patient. Concentrate on a one-to-one relationship for teaching.
Developing awareness	Patient's thoughts: "Why is God punishing me?" "If only I had been more careful (not eaten so much, smoked so much, and so on), maybe I wouldn't be sick. Patient's actions. Places blame for illness on self and/or others. Strikes out at others to relieve own pent-up hostilities.	Listen carefully to what the patient is saying. Continue to teach with a present-tense focus. Understand that hostility needs venting and that it is not personally directed at the caregiver. Avoid arguing with the patient.
Reorganization	Patient's thoughts: "I wonder how my loved ones feel about me now? "I'm beginning to see how my life is changing." Patient's actions: Avoids bringing up subject of illness or life changes with family members. Asks more questions about his condition.	Ask the patient how he or she feels about having this disease. Build communication between patient and family, especially in terms of working together toward problem solution. Provide increased reassurance for patient's family members. Begin to teach some material the patient will need to know in the future. Maintain one-to-one teacher-learner interactions.
Resolution	Patient's thoughts: "I see how my life has changed." "I recognize that other people with this same condition are functioning well." Patient's actions: Seeks out other patients with same condition. May be more likely to openly express emotions (especially crying).	Encourage expression of feelings. Allow patient to cry. Begin to use group instructional setting. Have a recovered patient visit this patient.
Identity change	Patient's thoughts: "I have changed, and life is going to be different from now on." "There are limitations on my life because I have a disease." Patient's actions: Actively seeks out information about his or her own disease (in the library, for example). Seeks level of greater independence.	Concentrate teaching content on the future, but also continue to teach about what is happening at present. Allow the patient to become as independent as possible.
Successful adaptation	Patient's thoughts: "I resign myself to this change for the rest of my life." "I wonder which is more important, quality or quantity of life?" Patient's actions: Chooses which of physician's orders he or she is going to follow.	Refer the patient to an agency that can continue the teaching-learning interaction after discharge from the hospital. Allow patient to discuss alternatives of following or not following doctor's orders (as well as consequences of each alternative). Maintain open communication by avoiding judgments.

Reprinted with permission from Bille D: "Barriers to the teaching-learning process," in Bille D, ed.: *Practical Approaches to Patient Teaching*. Boston: Little, Brown, 1981.

stant mealtimes. The family that is present oriented may not make follow-up visits but seek help only in crisis situations. Families that are expected to follow the health beliefs of grandparents and other elders may have difficulty implementing contemporary health practices. The child or family who believes that God and religious faith will cure diabetes will have special needs related to education. If the family believes that medical professionals are omnipotent and are to be obeyed unconditionally, the child and parents may be reluctant to share fully in decision making in diabetes care.

The diabetes educator should not only assess the child's cultural beliefs but should also determine which extended family members are the most significant to the beliefs of the child and parents.

Resources

Learner readiness depends in part on the child's and parents' access to family, friends, and funds. The family history should determine not only which family members have diabetes but also the type of diabetes and its treatment. How much has the learner heard about diabetes from family members? How available and supportive are the parents?

Economic status may dictate certain aspects of diabetes management, such as methods of monitoring, menu planning, and follow-up care. Families concerned about the financial impact of diabetes will need to receive some reassurance and to acquire some problem-solving skills, often before further interventions such as education can be initiated.

Barriers to Readiness

The child and parent exhibit a readiness to learn when they are attentive, inquisitive, and interested. Their success in the learning situation will depend on many intrinsic and extrinsic factors.

Barriers to the learner's readiness include such *intrinsic* factors as feelings of fear or guilt, poor cognitive abilities, and a lack of interest in learning. How the family perceives diabetes as an illness may affect its learner readiness. For example, parents who perceive no problems in handling the diabetes, who see little danger, or who lack appreciation for the potential seriousness of diabetes may not take education seriously.

An *extrinsic* barrier to readiness that is often overlooked is the effect of ill health (such as DKA) on the child's ability to attend to education. Education sessions are frequently begun while the hospitalized child is still feeling unwell. It may be that diabetes education is better accomplished in segments. Initial education, shortly after diagnosis, should focus on survival skills (see section on "Implementing the Teaching Plan" at the conclusion of this chapter). Further education, within the first few weeks after diagnosis, should cover additional self-care issues, such as managing ketones, sick days, and changing insulin dose.

Table 10–3. ASSESSMENT OF LEARNER READINESS

Cognitive-Emotional Readiness
DEVELOPMENTAL LEVEL:
__________ Level of education (grade in school)
__________ Reading ability
__________ Learning strategies/how child learns
PREVIOUS DIABETES EDUCATION:
__________ Level of diabetes knowledge
__________ Family history of diabetes
__________ Previous experience with diabetes
__________ Previous experience with chronic illness
COPING SKILLS:
__________ Fears, concerns
__________ Previous coping patterns
__________ Ability to relax
ATTITUDES:
__________ General health beliefs
__________ Feelings about education and teachers
__________ Immediate concerns about diabetes
Sociophysiologic Readiness
HEALTH STATUS:
__________ Intact sensory systems
__________ Neuromuscular status
__________ Anxiety level
CULTURAL BACKGROUND:
__________ Ethnic background
__________ Time orientation
__________ Religious beliefs
__________ Significant others
RESOURCES:
__________ Extended family
__________ Family assessment
__________ Economic status
MOTIVATION:
__________ Response to education plan
__________ Interest
__________ Aspects of the child or parent that will serve as motivators
__________ Participation and involvement in care
Potential Barriers to Readiness
Attitudes
Perceptions of diabetes
Availability of family during the child's education
Language differences

More extensive education and, in fact, re-education should be planned at points throughout the child's life.

Documentation

Assessment tools are widely used to document learner readiness. Such tools should include the information outlined in Table 10–3.

Creating the Teaching and Learning Environment

Educating children and parents includes not only assessing their readiness but also creating an environment conducive to learner success. The diabetes educator prepares the physical surroundings, establishes an interpersonal environment, and readies himself or herself for teaching.

Physical Surroundings

An environment that enhances education is quiet, well-lighted and comfortable, with minimal distractions and limited interruptions. Such surroundings are usually unavailable on hospital floors. In this situation, the diabetes educator may have to use some creativity in securing a conducive environment. As much as possible, the educator should modify the child's environment. If teaching must be done on the nursing unit, drawing the curtain and requesting colleagues not to interrupt classes may help decrease distractions.

Interpersonal Environment

When parents are asked, years later, what they remember most about hearing their child's diagnosis, they typically recall *how* they were told and not so much *what* they were told. Children and parents accept information more readily from the health professional when that information is given in a caring, sensitive manner by a person who is trusted and liked. To teach effectively, the diabetes educator must be able to employ certain communication skills and techniques.

Parents learn to trust the health professional when they feel that their needs are being met. Active listening, positive responses, and reflection of feelings are methods that promote rapport. The willingness to listen communicates understanding and support. Praising positive behaviors promotes the parents' sense of worth and ability. Parents need the assurance that their actions and decisions are appropriate and helpful to their child's well-being.

Communicating with children requires special techniques. Young children are often fearful of strangers and are particularly wary of strangers in white coats. However, even the young child should be made to feel included in the care, so the educator should spend time with and talk to the child. Children should be addressed at their own eye level. Other methods of establishing a trusting relationship with the child include using simple language and allowing the child time to react and respond to queries. Consideration of what interests the child and an unhurried discussion of the child's interests, hobbies, school, family, and pets is sure to succeed. Play is a particularly effective vehicle for communicating with young children.

Qualities of the Teacher

The diabetes educator's role is to assess learner needs, stimulate interest, and facilitate learning. The teacher first and foremost must be knowledgeable about diabetes, and his or her knowledge must be current and accurate. Studies reported by Etzwiler demonstrate the general lack of diabetes knowledge found among persons who might be expected to teach about diabetes.

Learning is facilitated when the diabetes educator also has a clear philosophy of care and education. Positive attitudes and acceptance of learners' individual differences are equally important. The educator must be knowledgeable in a variety of educational methods to meet the individual and developmental needs of children. Educational techniques useful with adults are usually inappropriate for the young child. Many times, routine discussions are more effective than scheduled classroom lectures. The educator must, further, be sensitive to the timing of the educational sessions. Short sessions with limited objectives are most effective.

The teacher should be comfortable with using words that are clear, concise, and familiar to the family. Often, however, it is not what the educator says but how it is said that is most penetrating. A caring attitude and a sharing of goals and plans with the family is necessary. The diabetes educator must know when he or she does not know something and must be willing to admit this to the child and parent. Vague or incorrect replies confuse the child and parent and may lead to loss of trust.

The diabetes educator must have a commitment to his or her professional continuing education. Continuous literature review, professional conferences attendance, and even review of current lay literature on diabetes all help the educator to maintain a grasp on current, accurate knowledge. Working as a member of a team is also of benefit because sharing and an interchange of ideas will promote professional growth.

PLANNING THE TEACHING PROGRAM

After a careful assessment of learner needs and of available teaching resources, the diabetes educator is ready to plan the educational program. Such planning requires that the educator establish goals and objectives and determine priorities. It is sufficient to say that the goals, objectives, and priorities for education must be the same as the health care goals and objectives. These have been covered in Chapter 4 and will not be repeated here. The child and parents should be included in this process to the degree that they are willing and able.

Objectives

Learner objectives are often useful to the diabetes educator as a "road map." If well written, objectives serve to clarify content and to identify the learner's responsibility in the educational process. Objectives guide the educator and identify acceptable levels of learner performance. They are also important evaluative tools. The *Curriculum for Youth Education* (1983), available from the American Diabetes Association (ADA) (New York), was prepared by one of us (LBT) and provides a reasonable starting place. Lesson plans adapted from this curriculum and used in our center are included in the appendix.

Objectives should be clear, realistic, measurable, and understandable to the child or parent. Simple, clear objectives each identify only one learner behavior. Realistic objectives are those that take into account aspects of the learner's needs. For example, it would be unrealistic to plan for a learner with limited reading ability to "read chapter on insulin before tomorrow." Objectives must be measurable in order to be useful as evaluation mechanisms. Objectives that require the learner "to know," "to think about," or "to learn about" are generally unclear and not readily subject to assessment of learning. Measurable objectives demand the learner's active participation. Statements such as "to describe," "to state," "to demonstrate," and "to identify" describe observable learner activities.

Content

Some children and parents will be unable to absorb or learn all the information typically presented in a diabetes education program. Learning problems, language differences, and poor motivation all contribute to the parents' or child's difficulty in learning the basics of diabetes care. For these families, it is more important to concentrate efforts on "survival information and skills." Suggested survival information has been identified in the appendices.

The child's motor development and cognitive developmental level will determine which skills and knowledge are realistic. Diabetes care skills seem to be attained progressively and are reached at fairly predictable developmental levels (*Curriculum for Youth Education*, ADA). Table 10–4 lists skills that are appropriate for different ages of children. Even the very young child should have a responsibility for some aspects of self-care.

Sequencing of Learning

In planning the teaching program, the diabetes educator must consider the order or sequence of instruction. This sequencing is determined by (1) what the child or parent wants to know and (2) the logical order for presenting the information.

By starting the discussion with what the child or parent wants to know, the child's and parents' interest and motivation are stimulated. Often, the first information educators want to provide relates to the physiology of diabetes, and certainly this would seem a reasonable starting place. However, most children and parents are more concerned initially with injections, diet, and monitoring. Meeting their learning needs first will enhance their attention to other information later.

Sequencing education by presenting information in a logical manner is equally important. For example, the learner needs a basic understanding of food use in the body before he or she can appreciate the role of ketones in energy metabolism. Throughout the educational program, the educator must frequently assess the learner's grasp of basic information before adding more complex knowledge.

Teaching Methods and Materials

Children and adults learn best when the presentation is varied, interesting, relevant, and in some respects entertaining. They

Table 10–4. **TASK ACCOMPLISHMENTS**

	Diet	Insulin	Testing
4–5 years old	Helps pick foods	Gathers supplies; helps pick injection sites; pinches up skin; wipes skin	Gathers supplies; collects urine; watches parent do testing; observes color test results on records
6–7 years old	Can tell if food has no sugar, some sugar, or lots of sugar	Pushes plunger in after parent gives shot	Performs urine tests; records results; may need reminding, will need supervision
8–9 years old	Selects foods based on exchanges	Gives own shots (at least one/day)	Does own blood tests
10–13 years old	Knows diet plan	Rotates sites; measures insulin dose	Looks for patterns in test results
14 + years old	Plans meals and snacks	Mixes 2 insulins in one syringe	Suggests insulin changes based on test patterns

learn best when many of the senses are involved (Fig. 10–1). For example, the lecture method, although a valuable teaching tool, has an impact for the most part only on the sense of hearing. When a lecture is combined with pictures or with simulated practice, the learner must involve multiple senses. Assessing how a child or parent learns will aid the educator in using approaches that will improve that learning. Many children and some adults learn best through doing, touching, or seeing, rather than through hearing. For these people, a short lecture combined with a great deal of hands-on learning experience is beneficial. Other people need to hear explanations and think through the actions before doing. For these learners, discussion with adequate question time are the methods of choice.

The *lecture* is a technique known to all

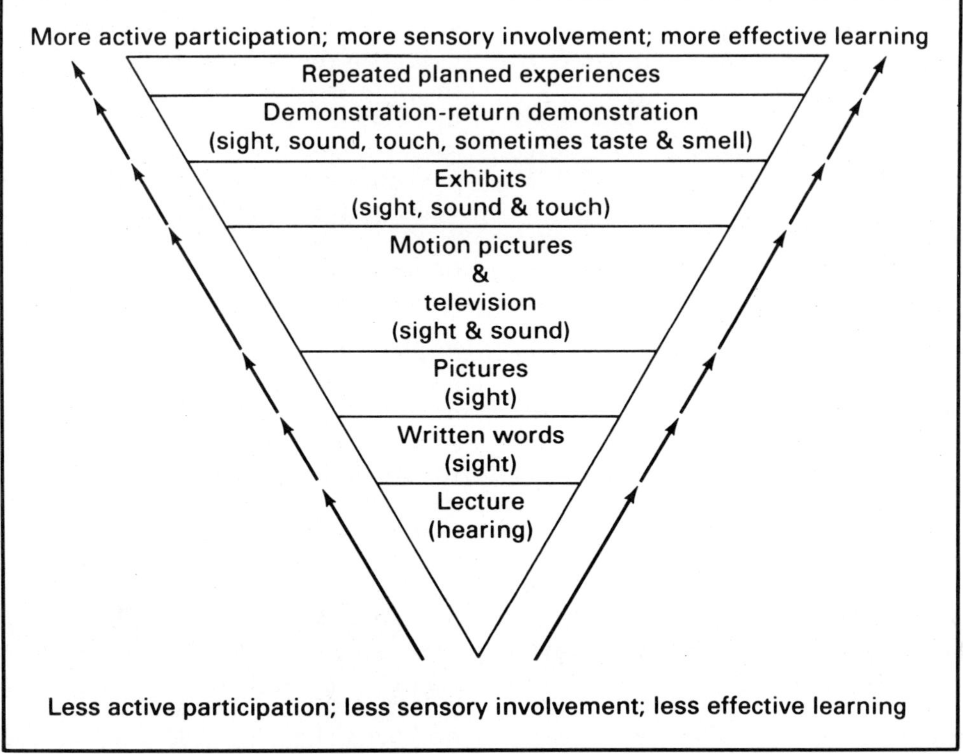

Figure 10–1. Learner is more apt to acquire information as active participation increases and as more senses are involved. (From Bille DA: "The teaching-learning process," in Bille DA, ed.: *Practical Approaches to Patient Teaching.* Copyright © 1981 by Little, Brown and Company, Inc. Reprinted by permission.)

students. It is a method that can impart a great deal of information in a relatively short time. Lecturing is most often performed in the presence of large groups. Major disadvantages to this technique include (1) lack of learner involvement, (2) difficulty in individualizing education, and (3) ineffectiveness with children.

The *discussion* is useful in small-group situations. With this technique, the lecture includes learner participation. The educator should be skilled in guiding the discussion so that it is truly educational.

Role playing, or *simulation,* is a technique that involves the learner to a large degree. The learner must perform activities specific to an assumed role. In diabetes education, role playing is a useful tool to form attitudes, help with problem solving, and evaluate the child's or parents' understanding. Some situations lend themselves well to teaching by role play: what to tell friends about diabetes, what to do during a reaction, how to handle well-meaning friends and relatives, what to do at a party. Simulation involves practicing or rehearsing in a trial situation. Problem-solving issues are effectively taught using this technique (for example, coping with hypoglycemia, ketones, changing dose, and behavior management). Some of these simulations can be done with programmed instruction or individual study. Simulation experiences followed by group discussion not only teach ways to handle the problem but also reinforce the benefits of group support.

Games, puppets, and play are techniques effective with children. Homemade games such as "diabetes bingo" or "diet flashcards" are both entertaining and educational. This supportive method allows the child to structure his or her play environment in a safe way, and it is an assessment tool as well. How young children view their world and their diabetes is sometimes apparent in their play. By providing diabetes-related materials for play, the educator may learn further about the child's misconceptions or inaccurate information.

Quizzes or tests are generally threatening to children and parents alike. However, they are valuable teaching tools when used in a positive way. Again, a quiz followed by group discussion tends to reinforce learning. As a teaching method, quizzes help the educator to determine learner needs.

Using *peers as educators* is a method that is increasing in popularity, as we learn more

Table 10–5. **TOPICS FOR GROUP SHARING**

Feelings about initial diagnosis
Dealing with family/friends
Handling social situations (parties, school, dating)
What is easy or hard about diabetes
What things are worried about
What a newly diagnosed child and family should know
One word to describe diabetes

about peer influence and motivation. It is particularly useful if the educator finds that the group of learners contains individuals with different levels of skills and knowledge. The effectiveness of this method is noted at summer camps. Children learn self-care skills readily from their cabinmates. Parent and teen support groups are examples of using peers as educators. Support groups are especially useful in facilitating attitude formation. Topics to use for encouraging group discussion are listed in Table 10–5.

Self-instruction is valuable for the learner who is self-motivated and who is able to retain information from reading. Most young children are unable or unwilling to use this method. Reading assignments and homework are forms of self-study and may be effective with school-aged children and teenagers. The educator must have previously evaluated all material to ensure that it is written at the level of the child or family and that the material is concordant with other instruction. Programmed instruction may be used with adult learners.

Audiovisual media are used increasingly in education to complement other methods of teaching. Media may be as simple or as elaborate as the teaching program can afford. Regardless of the type, audiovisual material should be carefully evaluated by the educator (Table 10–6). The educator may be lulled into thinking that "more is better" and may distribute packets of information from many sources. All media used should be assessed for applicability, readability, sensory involvement, and type of audience, a brief discussion of which follows.

Applicability. Do the media present accurate, clear information? Is the content consistent with the program's philosophy, objectives, and information? Is the content too simple, too complex, or incomplete?

Readability. Printed material should be evaluated for its ease in understanding. There are a number of readability scales or assessment tools. The SMOG readability formula and Fry's readability graph (Redman,

Table 10–6. **COMPARISON OF AUDIOVISUAL MEDIA**

Media	Advantages	Disadvantages
Visual		
Books/Pamphlets	Inexpensive Readily available Child may keep copies	Requires reading ability
Posters/Flip-charts	Inexpensive Easy to make Good for visual handicaps	Small groups or individual instruction only Bulky Sometimes cluttered with information
Transparencies	Portable Colorful Reusable May be used in large groups	Needs projector
Photographs/Slides/ Photobooks	Portable Colorful Easy to develop May use for self study	Processing time required Skilled preparation required Needs projector
Audio		
Audiotapes	Portable Inexpensive	Requires script Limited use If used alone, may be boring for a child
Audiovisual		
Filmstrips	Least expensive of this group Colorful Widely available commercially	Need special projector Need wall or screen Cannot update visual easily
Slide/Tapes	Easy to update Use with individual or groups	Requires tape editing and slide-sound synchronization
Videotapes	Best for depicting action More realistic Becoming more available commercially	Need videoplayer Costly Need production staff Requires editing Not easily updated
Films	Finer quality than videotape Realistic Available commercially	Most expensive production

1980) are two easily applied tools. Both require counting polysyllabic words in selected sentences. The more frequently polysyllabic words are used, the higher the grade level of the reader must be to comprehend the content.

Sensory Involvement. Are the media technically sound? Is written information legible? Is the format pleasing or distracting, colorful or plain? What senses are involved in using the material? Is there learner involvement or interaction with the media?

Type of Audience. For what audience are the media most appropriate? Does the format complement the content? Can the media be used for both parents and children?

Selecting media is a necessary skill for the diabetes educator. Educational materials on diabetes are more accessible today than ever before. The National Diabetes Information Clearinghouse provides lists of media categorized by special interest or need (Spanish language literature, educational materials for youth, and so on). Pharmaceutical services usually provide patient educational materials without charge (see Appendix). Print media (books, pamphlets, pictures) are versatile, portable, and generally economic. Handouts (homemade or otherwise) should be specific to the needs of the child or parents or both. Nonprint media (films, slide programs, videotapes, computer instruction) are generally expensive, both with initial purchase or production, and later with revision. Nonprint media should be selected carefully with a concern for its applicability in the future as well as in the present.

Any media should be used as a supplement to a complete, personal educational program. Audiovisual materials do not take the place of the instructor. When used properly, audiovisual materials can facilitate learning and enhance the value of the time that the learner spends with the instructor.

Media and Children

At the Children's Diabetes Management Center in Galveston, a variety of educational tools are used to teach children and families. Table 10–7 outlines some of the techniques and media found useful at different ages. The basic text used by children and families is *An Instructional Aid on Insulin Dependent Diabetes Mellitus* (Travis, 1985). This text serves the purpose of unifying the basic philosophic aims of the team. All other materials are modified to maintain this uniformity. In addition to commercially available films, the team uses many "home-grown" materials. Children and parents receive pamphlets and handouts that specifically relate to each of the major educational topics. Some handouts have corresponding worksheets for use in self-study or group discussion.

At our center, posters decorate the classroom (Fig. 10–2), which is located away from the hospital ward setting and has the character of a private consultation room. Some of the posters were created by summer campers for their "Diabetes Fair" and represent a form of peer education. Other posters, developed by professional educators, are interactive in nature. These include charts or graphs that are covered with a plastic film, such as a clear Con-Tact paper (Rubbermaid) or clear acetate. This process allows the child to write on the poster with temporary markers, making the poster reusable.

An effective teaching tool for the young child is a colorful felt board with large cardboard pieces (Fig. 10–3). Each piece has sandpaper or Velcro on the back. Topics such as physiology, hypoglycemia, and ketones are readily described by moving the pieces around the "bloodstream" and "cells." Young children particularly benefit from the visual (colors) and the tactile (moving pieces) sensations.

Discovery learning, a term used by child educators, is a technique easily implemented with children. For example, pictures from a pharmaceutic service's brochure illustrating the mixing of insulin may be cut out and pasted on cards. Each card is numbered on the back, so that when placed in order, the pictures will depict the steps in the procedure.

Educational materials should be available to the families whenever such materials are actually needed. For example, experience has shown that when parents need to use glucagon in the management of severe hypoglycemia, they are usually anxious and "all thumbs." They often forget the necessary steps in its preparation. Parents are therefore taught the necessary skills during class and are then instructed to tape a 1 cc syringe and a small card of instructions to the box of glucagon (Fig. 10–4). In an emergency, the card serves as a quick reminder of the steps that should be taken.

In addition to providing films and child-focused materials about diabetes, the educators in the Children's Diabetes Management Center use films and handouts on general health care. Booklets and coloring books on exercise, dental health, nutrition, and teenage issues are available from specialty organizations and health agencies. All of these are readily worked into the child's educa-

Table 10–7. **TEACHING TECHNIQUES WITH DIFFERENT AGES**

Cognitive Developmental Level	Patterns of Learning	Diabetes Teaching Strategy
Sensorimotor, Birth–2 yr	Exploration	Parent education
	Use of senses	Relaxation strategies with parent
	Developing trust	Play
Preconceptual, 3–5 yr	Use of hunches	Feltboard
	Magical thinking	Movies
	Short attention span	Pretend games
		Puppets
		Drawings
		Therapeutic play
Concrete operations, 6–11 yr	Very little abstract thought	Competitive games
	Uses rules	Rules
	Present oriented	Worksheets
	Beginning logic	Films
Formal operations, 12 yr–Adult	Abstract thinking	Debates
	Interest in details	Challenging games
	Can form theories	Group discussion
	Can think of "possible" as well as actual	Problem solving

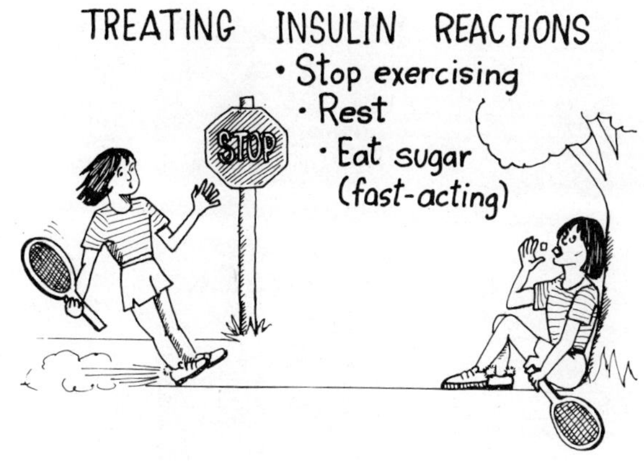

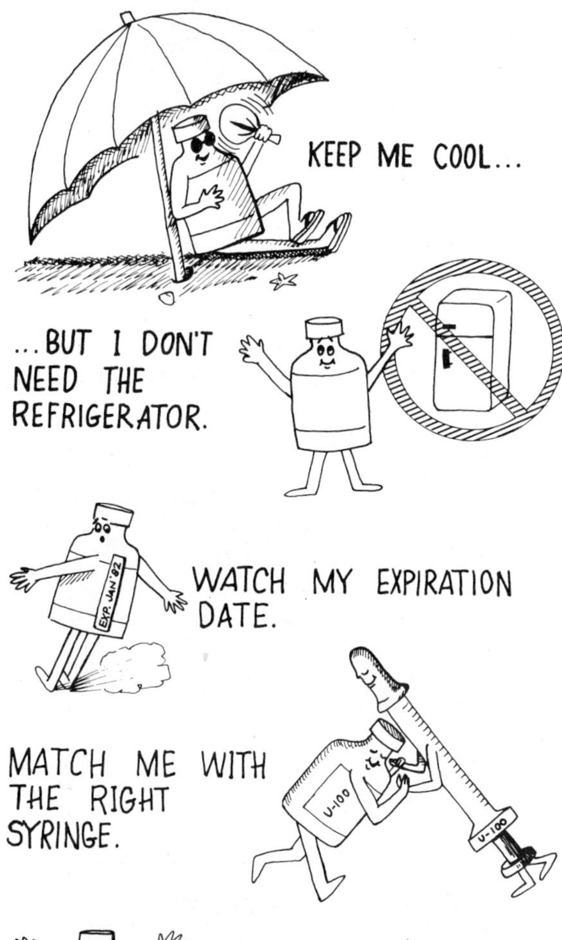

Figure 10–2. Posters offer a colorful way of teaching the child.

tional program. Addressing general health issues reminds the family that diabetes is only a part of the child's overall health needs.

IMPLEMENTING THE TEACHING PLAN

As one may discern from foregoing discussions, providing diabetes education is much more than teaching "off the cuff." Assessing the child's readiness to learn, getting to know the family's needs, and planning the education are necessary preliminaries to actually teaching the content.

Teaching Sessions

The amount of information given to a newly diagnosed child can be overwhelming. Classes should be arranged to provide one topic or skill at a time. The learner's attention span and interest should help determine class length and frequency. Often three or four 20-minute sessions are more effective than a single two-hour marathon session. The following guidelines outline the proper way to conduct the teaching sessions:

1. *Introduce yourself and the topic.* After introducing himself or herself to the learner, the educator should briefly outline the agenda for the session. This introduction allows the learner to organize his or her own thoughts and to focus attention on the task at hand.
2. *Present the content in a logical sequence.* Relate the current topic to previous knowledge. Building on existing knowledge throughout reinforces learning and will further aid the learner in fitting the new information into the overall picture.
3. *Have all materials ready and working.* The educator should have sufficient handouts for all participants. Checking audiovisual equipment for its workability prior to classes not only saves time but also prevents needless distractions.
4. *Summarize and review.* At key intervals throughout the lesson, information should be summarized. This is particularly important when a great deal of new information has been introduced. For example, when explaining hypoglycemia, a summary statement should be

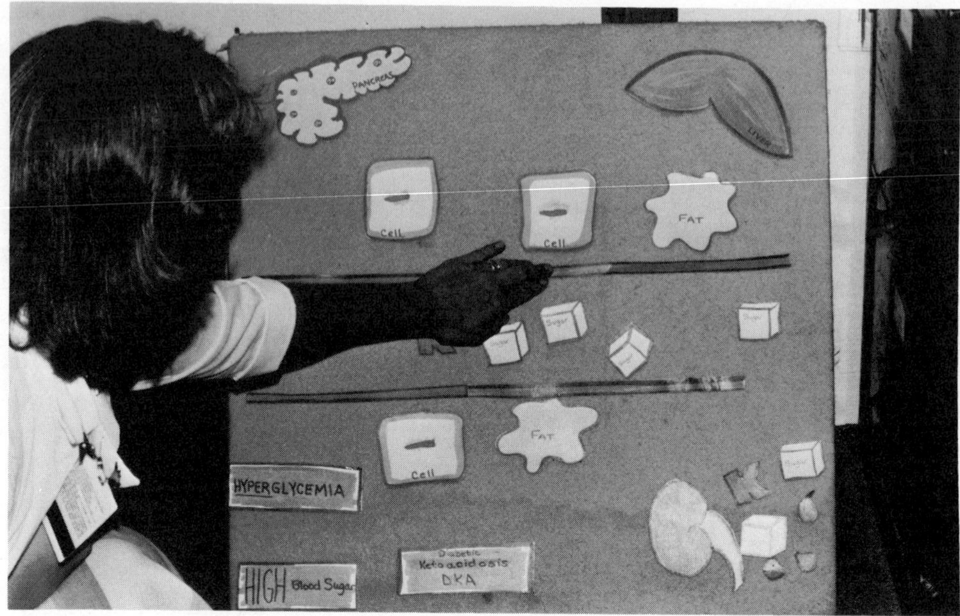

Figure 10–3. The use of felt boards presents the child with an opportunity to experience interactive learning.

made after teaching about causes, symptoms, and treatment of mild reactions and then again after teaching about severe reactions.

5. *Interact with the learner.* The educator strengthens the development of trust when he or she reinforces the learner's correct responses and recognizes the learner with nonverbal cues. The educator should use questions and problem-solving techniques with the learner, to evaluate understanding. Especially with a child, the educator must observe for waning or lost attention. Making eye contact and recognizing and responding to nonverbal cues are important.

6. *Use interactive time effectively.* Educational research has indicated that most instructors inappropriately allow less than one second for the learner to respond to a question. For the interactive time to be most effective, the learner needs an adequate amount of time to hear the question, to think through the question, to formulate a response, and to answer the instructor. Research has suggested that the educator allow a three- to five-second pause after posing each question.

7. *Reinforce learning as it occurs.* If the child makes errors in a skill, such as urine testing, the educator must help to correct the error. However, the educator should also comment positively on the parts of the skill done correctly. For example: "You are holding the dropper just right. Let's try again to get the correct number of drops." Such a response tells the child that his or her successes are being recognized.

Documenting Education

The educator should record the diabetes educational teaching sessions clearly, concisely, and completely. Documentation should include what was taught and, in some cases, what technique was used. Checklists are helpful but must occasionally be supplemented with a narrative description.

EVALUATING DIABETES EDUCATION

In any educational program, evaluation of learning is essential. Evaluation serves to (1)

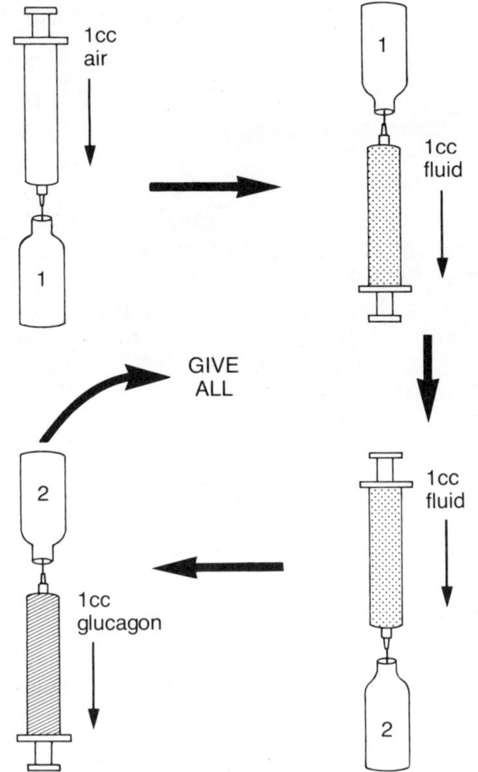

Figure 10–4. A learning-reminding tool developed to aid the parent in remembering how to give glucagon. This card is taped to the box of glucagon.

reinforce education, (2) identify needed changes in behavior, and (3) determine the effectiveness of education. The educator therefore should be evaluating both the learner and the program. Evaluation should be an ongoing process, proceeding throughout the educational program.

Evaluating the Learner

In evaluating the learner, the educator assesses the knowledge level, the competence in self-care skills, the attitudes, and the health status. On a day-to-day (short-term) basis, the educator assesses the child's or parents' participation. Does the learner ask questions? Is the learner assuming aspects of self-care as they are learned? Is the learner alert, responsive, interactive?

Evaluating long-term effects of the educational program is more difficult: How frequently is the child having diabetes-related problems? Is the child adhering to the treatment plan? Is the child hospitalized or ill frequently as a result of diabetes? Is school missed more often than normal? Are the goals of diabetes management being achieved.

If the child is not doing well, he or she may or may not need further education. The diabetes educator performs a vital function for the team by analyzing the cause of the poor performance. It must be recalled that behaviors are facilitated by knowledge but that attitudes or motivation are even more important in affecting appropriate behavior. A correct assessment of the cause of the therapeutic failure allows more appropriate intervention.

During the education process, the educator uses tests, discussion, question-and-answer sessions, and observation to evaluate the learner. An effective evaluation tool is the "what if" situation. To use this tool, the educator creates a problem situation and explores possible solutions with the child and parent. Examples of problem-solving questions are included in the content outlines (Appendix B). Written tests are often used by diabetes educators. Evaluating learner achievement through quizzes is useful, but the educator must carefully select tests that are valid and reliable.

As mentioned earlier, the educator must document the learner's achievements during the education process. Often, this documentation may be summarized in a discharge note or checklist. It should include statements about whether or not the child or parent has met the learning objectives. The documentation should also include a listing of future educational goals.

Evaluating the Educational Program

The program of education must also be evaluated. Program evaluation includes analyzing the effectiveness of the instructor and the usefulness of the methods and materials. Program evaluation also includes an analysis of costs and benefits. Satisfaction questionnaires, chart audits, and budget reviews are tools for evaluating education programs.

In evaluating the educational program, the educator compares program performance with predetermined standards: Does the program meet the needs of its consumers? Is it cost effective? Does it result in improved health (that is, better control)?

CONTINUING EDUCATION

Revising an educational program is a preliminary to meeting further educational needs. Learning to live with diabetes is an ongoing challenge for the child and family. As the child enters new developmental stages, cognitive abilities change. Indeed, the child approaching adolescence should receive comprehensive re-education in diabetes care. Although complete re-education is not necessary for everyone, periodic continuing education or reviews are important. Continuing education serves to (1) review skills and knowledge, (2) provide new concepts and self-care techniques, and (3) renew motivation.

The diabetes educator should plan with each learner for his or her individual continuing education. Follow-up visits with the diabetes team are vehicles for education, and each contact (visit, telephone contact, and so forth) with the child and family should be used as a time for teaching and learning. Crisis times may also be opportune times for further education; such times often serve as motivators. Another means of continuing education is diabetes summer camp. Here, the camper with diabetes draws on peer support, daily supervised repetition of skills, and opportunities for knowledge application. The child and family are encouraged also to subscribe to organizational literature from health agencies and pharmaceutical firms. Periodically, this literature is discussed with members of the team.

TEACHING STRATEGIES FOR SPECIAL NEEDS

The Learner with Limited Reading Ability

Educating the child or parent who does not read poses a particular challenge to the educator, since much of the available material is printed. In such cases, the educator must assess the learner's background and learning style with care and sensitivity. Classes may need to be shortened. Teaching materials must be primarily of the nonprinted variety, such as movies, slide programs, or videotapes. Drawings, feltboard, and photographs are appropriate media for such learners. Evaluating the illiterate learner may be accomplished through the use of oral quizzes, return demonstrations (mimicking), and observation.

The Uninterested Learner

The diabetes educator will often find a child or parent who seems uninterested in the education or uninvolved in the care. A careful assessment of learner readiness should be made. The educator may need to determine appropriate interventions necessary to promote motivation before the educational program is resumed. It may be necessary to use outside support systems for the child with an uninterested or denying parent. Such support may be found in school nurse, school counselors, public health nurses, or extended family members. The child who is not interested in learning is particularly difficult to educate. In fact, such children generally need to acquire immediate survival information and skills initially, followed by comprehensive education when they become ready to learn.

The Very Anxious Learner

Although a moderate level of anxiety enhances learning, high-anxiety levels may immobilize a parent or child. Learners who are anxious may also lack confidence in their skills and judgments and experience a loss of control.

In these cases, frequent supportive contact with good use of therapeutic communication is more effective, initially, than are classes on diabetes care. Allowing the anxious child or parent to explore new feelings and concerns is a necessary prelude to education. The learner who is anxious requires such support and reassurance. This support may need to extend well beyond the educational intervention. Initiating the family into self-care skills in a reassuring manner affords the parent or child a means of controlling some aspect of care.

The Young Child and Needle Fears

Injections and fingersticks, basic requirements in diabetes care, are very frightening to some children. The young child, particularly the preschooler, has a poor sense of body integrity and misconceptions about

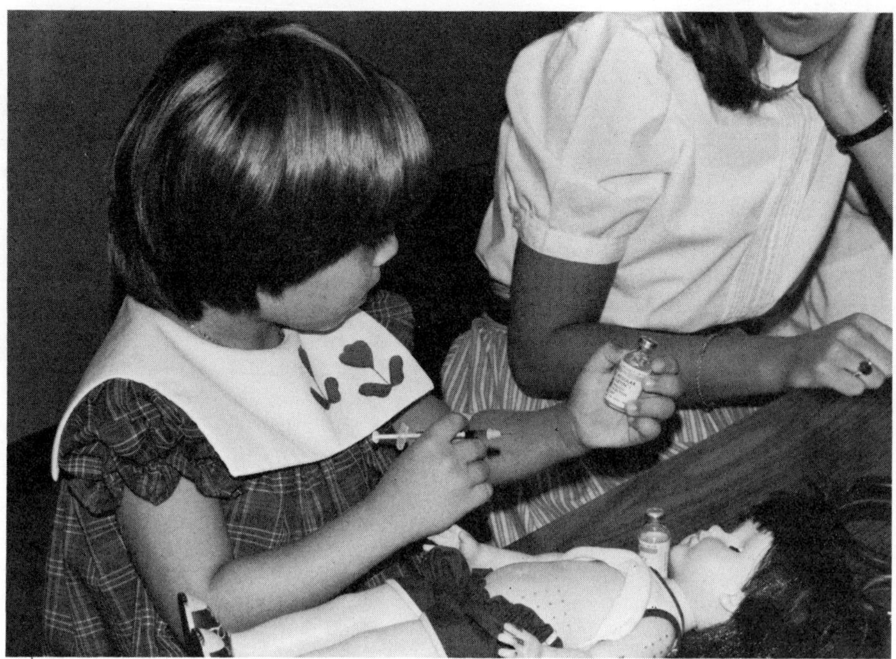

Figure 10–5. Overcoming a young child's fear of needles.

body function. Consequently, children in this age group view shots and blood tests as invasions that hurt and that may result in loss of precious body fluids. Preschoolers truly believe that once a portion of the blood supply is lost, it will never be replenished.

In addition, the child does not make the connection between the minor discomforts of diabetes care and good health. These children simply know that Mom or Dad inflict pain on them daily. They easily associate this pain with punishment and are confused that their loving parents would willingly allow this pain every day. Some children have specific fears, nurtured by their fantasies. Such fears include being afraid that the needle will break off or that their fingers will never stop bleeding.

Working with young children who have these needle fears requires a careful plan to progressively help the child to accept injections and fingersticks. First, the educator must ensure a positive successful environment. Assume the child will do well. It helps to find and praise some existing strengths in the child. For example, does he or she hold still for injections, does he or she help with any steps of the procedure? Next, offer the child opportunities for therapeutic play.

Dolls, stuffed toys, syringes, and supervised play help these children to manipulate and control their environment as they communicate their feelings and fears (Fig. 10–5).

For the older child who fears and dislikes injections, the educator may use such techniques as relaxation and imagery. Focused breathing and deep muscle relaxation are helpful techniques for the anxious child and teenager. Children who report frequent painful injections should be thoroughly evaluated in their procedural skills. Often a minor change in how the child gives his or her insulin will alleviate painful shots.

Parents dislike the thought of giving their child injections, and most parents will be very reluctant and anxious during the initial days of insulin therapy. Often, their fears are based on their own past history of injections (for example, immunizations, antibiotic injections, and so forth). They feel guilty that they must inflict such pain on their child. There is no better way to help parents assuage their guilt than to encourage them to give themselves or each other a simulated shot. Invariably, the parent will be pleasantly surprised that the educator was right: "It doesn't hurt that much." If the child wishes, he or she should observe the parents trying shots. The child then knows that at least the parents know what it feels like.

SUMMARY

Educating the child and parent about diabetes is necessary for adequate self-care. This chapter has explored the theoretical bases for learning and teaching. Suggested techniques and media for educating children have been presented. Fitting the educational plan to the learner's needs and developmental level has been discussed.

Finally, the need to evaluate the learner and the teaching program has been presented. Diabetes education is a process of assessing, planning, evaluating, and revising. The diabetes educator functions as a guide and resource throughout the education process.

A well-planned comprehensive program prepares children and parents for competently handling diabetes—for being in charge of their lives.

Stress, Hyperglycemia, and Ketosis

11

Stress, in the context of this chapter, is defined as a state of pressure or tension placed on an individual by external forces, either physical or psychologic. This is not meant to exclude those tensions that seem to be derived from internal forces but merely to suggest that the initial stimulus is most often external. Physical forces that produce stress include such things as illness, infection, injury or trauma, burns, surgery, disorders of hydration or metabolic balance, and hypothermia. Psychologic stress-producing factors are the anxiety-producing life issues with which all persons must live, including pressures related to performance standards (for example, school, work, athletics), to peers, to sexual identity and orientation, to economic concerns, and to interpersonal problems. It is important to note that most physical factors have a psychic component.

The body's response to a stressor is one of adaptation. The adaptive responses are both physical and psychologic. The psychologic adaptation, covered in Chapter 9, is adjustment, or coping. The physiologic response, extensively studied by Selye and others, is predominantly a neuroendocrine reaction and may have profound effects on the metabolic stability of the person with diabetes mellitus, particularly those with IDDM. It is this physiologic component with which we will be primarily concerned in this chapter.

PHYSIOLOGIC RESPONSE TO STRESS

The physiologic response to any stress is predominantly a coordinated reaction of the central nervous system and various endocrine organs. Figure 11–1 graphically describes how this response affects metabolic balance in the person with diabetes. Obviously, this does not cover the many other varied responses of the cardiovascular system, some of which are purely neurogenic and others neuroendocrine. Here we will consider primarily the responses that supply fuel (glucose, ketones) for energy metabolism.

Central Nervous System (CNS)

Much remains unknown about the precise mechanisms whereby the central nervous system controls energy metabolism, either in the fasting state or in response to the increased demands during stress. It is sufficient to say

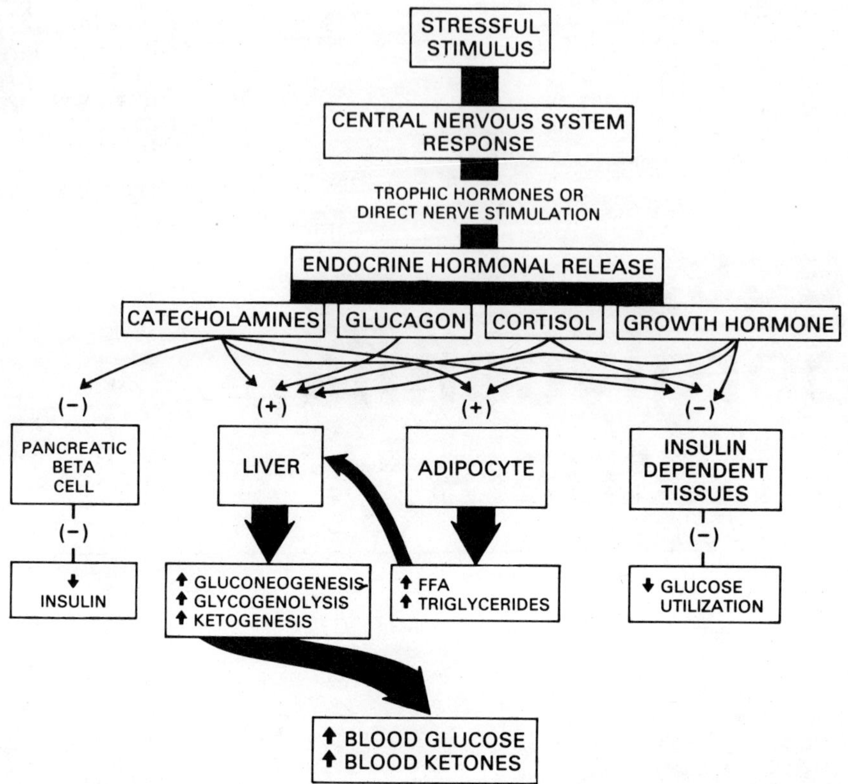

Figure 11–1. The physiologic adaptation to stress is a neuroendocrine response in which the end result is an increase in blood glucose and ketone bodies.

that stress hyperglycemia is a phenomenon that is almost totally regulated by the CNS. Owing to the absolute dependence of the brain on glucose for its energy needs, there are redundant neuroendocrine systems that are operative.

The CNS receives its information regarding stressful stimuli from sensory receptors, and specific neuropeptides are released, similar in most respects to those released under the stimulus of hypoglycemia. The median eminence of the hypothalamus is felt to be the most likely of several proposed sites for this regulatory function. In this area, there is no blood-brain barrier, and there are receptors for small peptides. Additionally, stimulation of this area in experimental animals results in an elevated blood glucose associated with increased levels of blood glucagon and decreased levels of insulin. Cortical signals may be transmitted from the forebrain to the midbrain by a number of fiber tracts. If CNS uptake of glucose is decreased by any of several methods, there is increased release of epinephrine, glucagon, adrenocorticotropic hormone (ACTH), and growth hormone,

with a concomitant decrease in insulin secretion. This results in hepatic glycogenolysis and gluconeogenesis and a mobilization of free fatty acids.

Stress Hormones

The stress hormones are sometimes referred to as counter-regulatory hormones, because they have actions that are counter to those of insulin and that are secreted in response to hypoglycemia. Although neither term adequately describes their overall role in enhancing energy substrate availability, that of *stress hormones* seems to be the better of the two. The stress hormones are catecholamines (epinephrine, norepinephrine, dopamine), glucagon, cortisol, and growth hormone.

Their primary collective action is to activate catabolic enzymes so as to provide the body with the necessary substrates required to maintain metabolic balance. Individually, each can mobilize both carbohydrate and lipid stores, but their collective action is greater than the sum of their individual actions.

Catecholamines

These hormones are synthesized and secreted by sympathetic nerve endings and have the primary role of neurotransmitters. Epinephrine and norepinephrine are alpha- and beta-adrenergic agonists. Whereas hypoglycemia stimulates mostly the release of epinephrine, other stress situations are predominantly associated with norepinephrine release. Secretory response is almost immediate, but the half-life in circulation is short (less than a minute). With respect to fuel metabolism, the catecholamines (1) block insulin secretion (perhaps of minimal significance in the insulin-dependent diabetic), (2) stimulate glycogenolysis, (3) decrease peripheral use of glucose by insulin-sensitive tissues, and (4) activate lipase with subsequent hydrolysis of stored triglycerides to nonesterified fatty acids and glycerol. The overall effect of catecholamine secretion in both normal and diabetic states is hyperglycemia and increased serum concentrations of free fatty acids.

Glucagon

The precise stimulus for glucagon secretion during stress is unknown, but concentrations in the portal vein have been reported to more than triple during certain nonhypoglycemic stress conditions. The effects of glucagon secretion are immediate and include (1) enhancement of hepatic ketogenesis, (2) stimulation of glycogenolysis, and (3) stimulation of gluconeogenesis.

Cortisol

The secretion of cortisol is in response to ACTH, which in turn is released in response to corticotropin-releasing hormone from the hypothalamus. Cortisol secretion is usually delayed by 30 to 60 minutes following stressful stimuli and is then bound to cortisol-binding globulin, thus increasing its physiologic and biologic half-life. In stress, the plasma cortisol concentration may increase 10-fold, and the resultant elevations may last from several days to weeks. Cortisol (1) stimulates ketogenesis, (2) stimulates gluconeogenesis, and (3) blocks peripheral glucose use. Plasma alanine concentration is also increased, which in turn, further stimulates glucagon release.

Growth Hormone

The secretion of the growth hormone from the pituitary is regulated by releasing factors from the hypothalamus. Its biologic half-life is short, and its primary actions are (1) to promote lipolysis and (2) to stimulate ketogenesis. Additionally, there is some evidence that secretion of the growth hormone decreases peripheral glucose use and augments the glycogenolytic and gluconeogenic actions of other hormones.

Although all persons have similar neuroendocrine responses to stress, the magnitude of the response differs dramatically from one person to the next. Some people appear to have only a moderate outpouring of catecholamines in response to a standardized stress stimulus, whereas other people have a significantly greater initial release of norepinephrine and epinephrine. Other studies have suggested a similar individual variability in cortisol and growth hormone secretions. In any group of patients with diabetes, the same variations exist, and some studies have suggested that the hyper-responder is seen more often among this group than in the population at large. Certainly, if studies include only the hyperlabile or "brittle" diabetic, investigators are more likely to obtain this result than they would in a random population survey of all persons with IDDM.

In response to stress, there is a rapid outpouring of these glucoregulatory hormones. Figure 11–2, taken from the work of Schade and Eaton (1983), demonstrates response curves of the stress hormones to pyrogen-induced fever in six persons with IDDM who were being continuously infused with insulin. This figure clearly demonstrates that the rise in stress hormones occurred before the rise in temperature but after a shaking chill. Further studies by these same authors (Fig. 11–3) demonstrate the subsequent elevations of free fatty acids, ketones, and glucose. It is striking that plasma concentrations of three of the hormones (catecholamines, cortisol, and growth hormone) were still elevated eight hours after the single pyrogen challenge.

In the nondiabetic, the rises in glucose and free fatty acids are modulated by a subsequent rise in plasma insulin activity. In the person with IDDM who is purely dependent

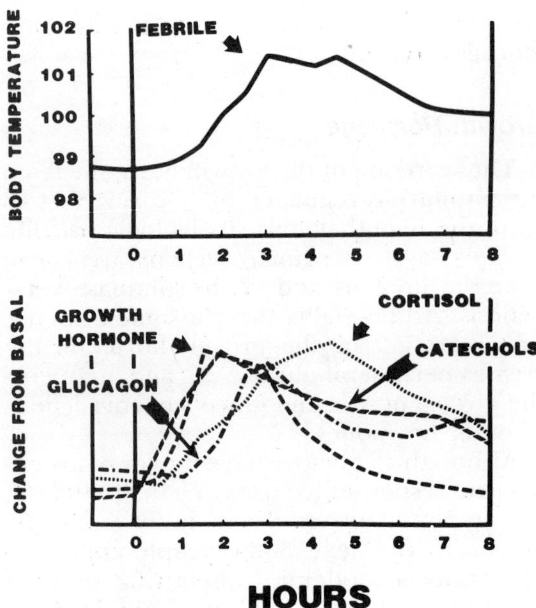

Figure 11–2. Stress hormone response to pyrogen-induced fever in six insulin-dependent diabetics. (Reprinted with permission from Schade D, Eaton P: "Hormonal relationships," in Ellenberg M, Rifkin H, eds.: *Diabetes Mellitus*. New Hyde Park, NY: Medical Examination Publishing Co., 1983.)

on continued absorption of insulin from the subcutaneous depot, there is no counter-regulatory rise in insulin levels. In fact, in many situations of stress, subcutaneous absorption of the insulin may be reduced owing to decreased blood flow to such sites. This is particularly true whenever dehydration or tissue hypoxia is present.

ACUTE STRESSFUL STIMULI

The list of stressful conditions associated with hyperglycemia is lengthy, some of the more common being noted in Table 11–1. As is obvious from this list, almost any malady affecting the body may be associated with stress hormone secretion, with resultant hyperglycemia and ketonemia. In our experience in children with diabetes, the two most common causes are those that are due to infections and those that follow emotional stress. These will be discussed in some detail here, with later chapters covering postsurgical problems (Chapter 17), diabetic ketoacidosis (Chapter 12), and hypoglycemia (Chapter 13) as etiologic factors.

Illnesses Associated with Infections

Various studies have demonstrated stress hormone release and hyperglycemia following severe infections, particularly those associated with septicemia. When an endotoxin-like substance (leukocyte-endogenous mediator, or LEM) has been given, there has been an increase in glucagon and ACTH secretion and a similar rise in growth hormone. Likewise, most severe infections are associated with significant febrile reactions, which, by themselves, may be responsible for such a stress hormone response.

Children are particularly susceptible to infection, but the majority of such infections are not severe or life threatening. At the same time, most children produce a significant febrile response, and in the child with diabetes, these infections, mostly viral, can significantly alter metabolic control. The following example is typical of such a case:

R.P., an 8-year-old boy with Type I diabetes of 13 months' duration, was in his usual state of health. Normally, he received two doses of insulin per day (12 NPH/4 Regular in AM: 3 NPH/3 Regular in PM) and was monitored by HBGM. He had been seen two months previously when his level of glycosylated hemoglobin was 9.2 percent (normal in our laboratory at this time was 5 to 8 percent). For the past month, his prebreakfast blood glucose values ranged between 60 and 150 mg/dl, whereas those before the evening meal ranged between 60 and 240 mg/dl (75 percent less than 180 mg/dl).

On Tuesday of the week in focus, R.P. felt well, and blood glucose values before breakfast and supper were 94 and 146 mg/dl, respectively. On Wednesday morning, he was noted to have a cold and had nasal congestion and red eyes. He did not have a fever. His blood glucose was 130 mg/dl, and urine did not demonstrate ketones. He received his usual insulin and went to school. Upon return from school in the afternoon, R.P. felt worse and had a temperature of 38.6°C or 101.6°F. Blood glucose was 240 mg/dl and urine ketones were "small."

By 8:00 PM, R.P.'s temperature had reached 39.4°C, or 103°F, and blood glucose values had increased to 310 mg/dl, despite the fact that the afternoon snack and supper had been poorly eaten and the usual dose of insulin had been taken. Urine ketones were now "moderate to heavy." The parents instituted appropriate supportive therapy, which included antipyretic treatment, increased fluid intake, and supplemental doses of Regular insulin at two- to three-hour intervals.

By the next morning, the boy's blood glucose was at 180 mg/dl, and the urine ketones had

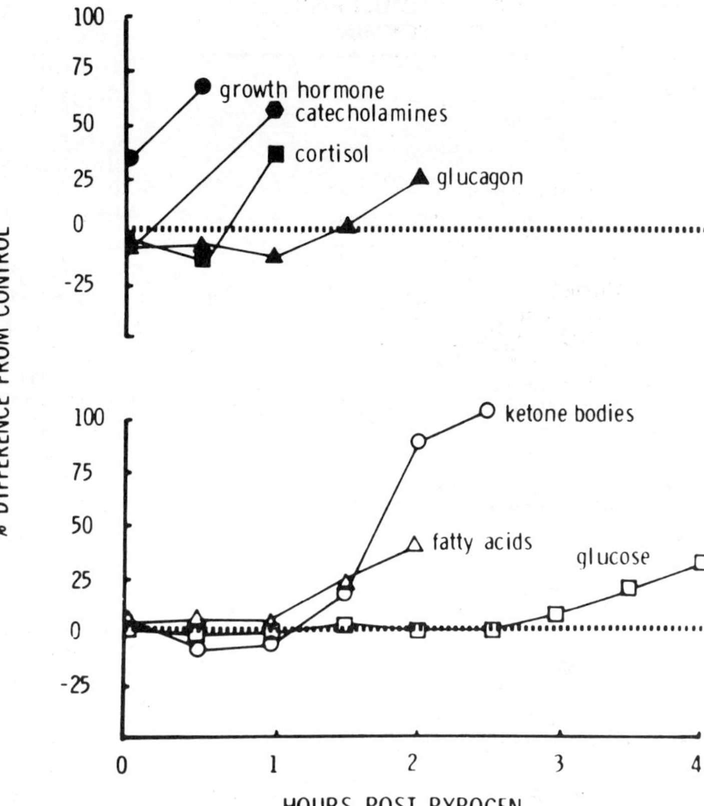

Figure 11–3. Response of blood glucose and fat to stress hormone secretion. (Reprinted with permission from Schade D, Eaton P: "Hormonal relationships," in Ellenberg M, Rifkin H, eds.: *Diabetes Mellitus*. New Hyde Park, NY: Medical Examination Publishing Co., 1983.)

resolved. Examination by his physician revealed a nonstreptococcal pharyngitis, and symptomatic treatment was continued. The child had some fever and continued the same symptoms for two days, during which a few additional doses of Regular insulin were administered. He returned to school on the following Monday, and his subsequent course was uneventful.

This child's experience with infection-related hyperglycemia and ketonemia is commonly seen. In this instance, the situation was appropriately managed by the parents, and the boy's convalescence was not compromised; he missed no more school than he would have, had diabetes not been present. But consider for a moment another child in a similar situation, in which the parents' and physician's responses were not as appropriate:

S.L., a 7-year-old girl, had been diabetic for 17 months. She was receiving a dosage of 9 NPH/3 Regular insulin in the morning and 5 NPH/3 Regular with the evening meal. Her blood glucose values in the morning were generally between 60 and 120 mg/dl. Seventy-five percent of her urine sugars were negative for glucose. Her last glyco-

sylated hemoglobin was performed three months earlier and was 10.1 percent (normal in our laboratory at this time was 5 to 8 percent).

The patient developed nasal congestion, fever, and a cough at school one day. Upon arriving at home after school, her temperature was 38.8° C, or 102°F, and she felt and looked "bad." She was not hungry for dinner, and thus her dose of Regular insulin was not given (she did, however, receive the NPH dosage). A prebedtime urine sample revealed 5 percent glycosuria, but the urine sample was not checked for ketones. She was treated with acetaminophen and rest.

On the following morning her cold was unchanged, but the cough was worse. Temperature was 37.7°C, or 100.8°F. Her morning blood glucose level was 320 mg/dl. She took her usual morning dose of insulin. An appointment was made to see the physician that afternoon, and when seen the child appeared somewhat lethargic and had signs of an upper respiratory infection. Her blood glucose level was 460 mg/dl, and her ketone levels were strongly positive.

The child was immediately admitted to the hospital for fluid and insulin therapy. Her course was uneventful, and after three days she was discharged from the hospital with a diagnosis of "brittle" diabetes and upper respiratory infection.

Table 11–1. STRESS STIMULI PRODUCING HYPERGLYCEMIA

Illness
- A. Infectious
  1. Sepsis
  2. Meningitis
  3. Others
- B. Noninfectious
  1. Myocardial infarction
  2. Cerebrovascular accidents

Metabolic
- A. Fasting
- B. Hypoglycemia
- C. Diabetic ketoacidosis
- D. Hypoxia
- E. Dehydration

Trauma
- A. Usual trauma
- B. Burns

Surgery

Non-specific
- A. Fever
- B. Hypothermia
- C. Pain

Psychologic or Emotional

S.L. appears also to have had infection-precipitated hyperglycemia and ketosis. The ultimate outcome of her illness was similar to that of R.P. (both had full recovery), but the course of each was quite dissimilar. The stress-associated syndrome was recognized by R.P.'s parents, and early intervention shortened the period of his morbidity, allowing the child to be managed at home at minimal extra expense. The parents of S.L. failed to recognize the potential of her stress-induced problems and the likelihood that she would require extra insulin. By the time S.L. was seen by the physician, ketosis was more significant. Even then, however, since the child was still able to retain fluids orally, it is very likely that the child could have been managed as an outpatient, thus significantly reducing the cost for care and preventing much of the emotional upheaval attendant to hospitalization.

Trauma and Injury

Hyperglycemia has been causally related to trauma or injury, or both, in the diabetic and the nondiabetic individual. As in the case of infection-related stress, the nondiabetic generally experiences hyperglycemia alone, whereas the person with IDDM is likely to experience both hyperglycemia and ketosis, reflecting the significance of a more marked decrease in insulin action in the latter.

K.F., an 8-year-old with IDDM of three years' duration was in excellent health, receiving two injections of a mixed insulin regimen per day. His blood glucose values were between 60 and 180 mg/dl.

On the way home from a ballgame, an automobile accident occurred. The boy's mother was killed, and K.F. received multiple injuries, including several fractures and other contusions and abrasions. On arrival at the hospital his blood glucose was over 400 mg/dl, and during the next four days he required almost three times his usual maintenance insulin therapy.

Numerous examples of a similar nature are detailed in the literature; and in some cases, such traumatic episodes appear to precipitate the onset of diabetes. In children who have sustained significant burns, this is rather commonly seen, and studies in these children have demonstrated marked elevations in the serum concentrations of catecholamines and cortisol. In the nondiabetic who lacks the genetic predisposition, the hyperglycemia is usually transient, lasting from 1 to 14 days. Whenever genetic factors are favorable, trauma-induced stress may precipitate "permanent" diabetes.

Emotional or Psychologic Stress

The literature is replete with instances of hyperglycemia occurring as a consequence of psychologic stress. A number of reports from several decades ago incriminate emotions or personality states or both as etiologic factors in the generation of diabetes. Even more recent literature discusses the prospect of the existence of a "diabetic personality."

Hinkle and his co-workers (1949, 1950) documented the role that psychologic stress plays in the day-to-day life of the diabetic and described the frequency with which emotional outbursts were associated with loss of carbohydrate control. The profound effect that emotions have on disordering diabetes is exemplified by the following case summary:

N.H., an 18-year-old young woman with a 12-year history of Type I diabetes, had been in good diabetic control for approximately three years. She was adherent to diet, and her insulin regimen consisted of two to three injections of NPH or

Regular insulin or both per day. She monitored blood glucose at home three times daily and over 80 percent of her test results were between 60 and 150 mg/dl. Her last two measurements of glycosylated hemoglobin 1.5 and 4.5 months earlier had been 7.8 percent and 8.2 percent, respectively (normal 5 to 8 percent).

She was engaged to be married on a Saturday, but approximately 36 hours before the wedding, she and her fiancé had a severe disagreement that resulted in cancellation of the wedding. Within four hours of the argument, she noticed increased thirst and polyuria; and within six hours, her breathing was noted to be labored. Measurement of blood sugar showed values of 280 mg/dl (values had been 130 mg/dl only two hours before the argument), and urine ketones were positive. She administered extra Regular insulin, but the symptoms persisted; and soon she developed abdominal discomfort and vomiting. Twelve hours after the emotional episode, she was admitted to the hospital with moderately severe ketoacidosis: blood glucose 640 mg/dl, plasma pH 7.10, plasma bicarbonate 8 mEq/L, and strongly positive urine ketones.

Her hospital course following intravenous fluid therapy and insulin administration was uneventful.

This history vividly demonstrates the role of emotional stress in the pathogenesis of diabetic ketoacidosis. Despite the fact that diabetes was previously in good balance and the amount of insulin given was higher than usual, significant ketosis occurred as a result of the stressful episode. Obviously, persons with poorly controlled diabetes, and consequently diminished resistance are at even greater risk for the development of stress-related ketosis.

The degree of stress necessary to produce hyperglycemia in persons with Type I diabetes is variable, but the effect is consistent. Figure 11–4 demonstrates the hyperglycemic effect of moderate emotional stress on seven children with IDDM (ages 9 to 14 years) who were housed in our Clinical Research Center at various times for a variety of investigations not pertaining to stress-induced hyperglycemia. All children were on two or more injections of insulin per day and were receiving a constant carbohydrate diet. All were felt to be in relatively good carbohydrate control. From each child, an unannounced venous blood sample was obtained prior to breakfast on the third, seventh, and ninth hospital days. The prebreakfast venous blood sample on the 12th day was preannounced on several occasions: on the preceding afternoon by the physician; in the evening by one

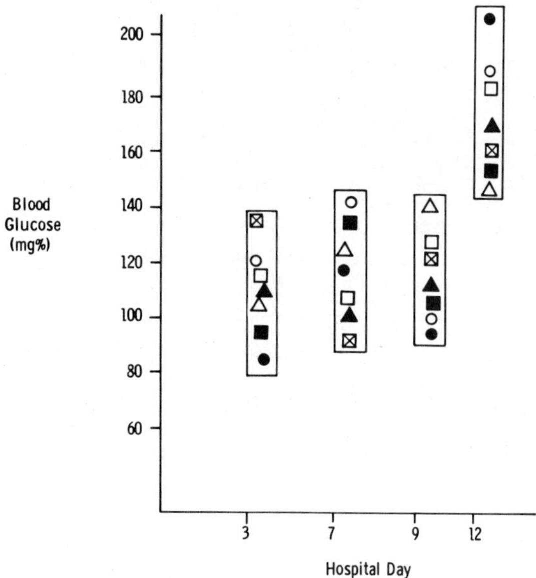

Figure 11–4. Response of patients with IDDM to minor stress (see text).

or more nurses; and at 6:00 AM, when the child was awakened. At 7:00 AM, the technician appeared with syringe and tubes but then placed these on the bedside table while excusing herself for a few moments. She returned 15 minutes later to obtain the sample. In every instance, the blood glucose on this sample was higher than had been demonstrated on any of the preceding days. Ketonuria was not detected in any of the children.

Data such as these suggest that milder degrees of anxiety also provoke stress. They raise the question as to the validity of blood glucose concentrations that are obtained in the physician's office, particularly if the child is aware that blood-letting is always part of the visit.

INTERVENTIONS IN ACUTE STRESS-RELATED HYPERGLYCEMIA AND KETOSIS

As noted earlier, children with diabetes are at risk to develop the hyperglycemia-ketosis syndrome (HKS). In the young child, the risk is usually associated with an infectious illness, purely because of the frequency of these in this age group. In the adolescent and young adult, the inciting event is more likely to be emotional or to result from common life stresses. Whatever the precipitating event,

Table 11–2. INTERVENTIONS IN ACUTE HKS

I. *Identify and initiate management of cause*
  A. Specific
  B. Symptomatic
      Relieve anxiety
      Manage fever and other symptoms
II. *Maintain hydration*
  A. Prevent or treat vomiting
      Antiemetics
  B. Oral fluid therapy
        3 to 5 ml/kg pound body weight/hour
        Glucose or nonglucose-containing (dependent
          on need)
  C. Intravenous fluid therapy
        If above fails to maintain hydration
III. *Supplemental Insulin Administration*
  A. Type: Regular, crystalline
  B. Amount: 20% or 1/5 of total daily dose of insulin
  C. Frequency: Every 2 hours until blood glucose
        falls to below 150 mg/dl

appropriate intervention consists of eradicating or neutralizing the cause of the stress, maintaining fluid balance, and counteracting the effect of the stress-hormone secretion by administering supplemental insulin. As demonstrated in one of the case examples earlier, early and appropriate intervention decreases morbidity and allows the young person to recover in a timely fashion. Delayed or inappropriate intervention, on the other hand, prolongs the recovery process. Table 11–2 summarizes our management program.

Neutralizing the Cause

As noted, infection is the more common initiator of HKS. At times, HKS may precede obvious clinical signs of the infection by a few hours, but rarely is this more than a day. Some more subtle infections (sinusitis, urinary tract infection, tuberculosis, and so forth) may escape initial detection and should be considered if the cause of HKS is either not discernible or if there is slow clearing or resolution of the syndrome.

Although it is obvious that bacterial infections will require appropriate antimicrobial therapy, it is equally apparent that most infections of childhood are viral in nature. With either cause (bacterial or viral), it appears that nonspecific, or symptomatic, therapy (rest, antipyretics, fluid replacement, and so forth) is more important for the diabetic than is more specific therapy. The demonstration of parental concern and the child's realization of parental closeness and support relieves anxiety and apprehension. Moreover, the relief of fever by the judicious use of antipyretics relieves another known cause of stress-hormone release. Maintenance of fluid balance for the prevention of dehydration is another supportive measure of immense importance. The use of other medications to relieve symptoms (for example, nasal decongestants and antitussive medications) may have mixed results. Although they may remove the symptomatic stress, they may also contribute to the hyperglycemia. This latter effect relates more to the fact that many of these products contain ephedrine or adrenergic-like agents than to the fact that their base is generally lactose. In general, we do not feel that these agents are harmful if used judiciously.

Noninfectious illnesses may also create similar stress-related episodes. Two of the more notable illnesses in childhood that may produce or create problems are asthma and the migraine syndrome. Not only these illnesses but also medications used in their management are capable of producing HKS. This is readily apparent in the following synopsis:

F.D., a 7-year-old HLA-identical sibling of a child with known IDDM, had multiple environmental allergies with frequent episodes of mild to moderate asthma. When the usual management did not abort an episode of asthma, a short course of prednisone was instituted. On the fourth day of management, polyuria, polydipsia, and malaise were noted. Blood glucose values were found to be elevated to above 300 mg/dl and did not immediately abate when prednisone was tapered and stopped. Insulin was required for approximately four weeks, before normal glucose tolerance was again achieved.

Several weeks later, another asthma attack was treated in the traditional manner (that is, no prednisone), but hyperglycemia was soon noted. Insulin therapy was restarted. The diabetes did not abate following either insulin therapy or resolution of the asthma.

Acute emotional stress commonly precipitates HKS. Removing the child from the environmental stress, even temporarily, is helpful in reducing the tension. Fortunately, the memory of the young child is so poor that the cause of the stress is quickly forgotten. Not so in the older child and young adult, for whom time alone may be the only healing factor. Chronic emotional stresses, such as those seen in dysfunctional families, are common causes of HKS and require more prolonged intervention. These are discussed later.

Maintaining Hydration

Anorexia, decreased fluid intake, or vomiting, or any combination of these, is frequently associated with stressful situations, particularly those secondary to infectious illnesses. When such occurs, the stress is worsened and the potential for developing dehydration is present. Dehydration occurs more rapidly in the person with diabetes than in a nondiabetic peer because of the continuing high rate of urine water loss as a consequence of hyperglycemia. As dehydration progresses, renal function declines and the ability of the body to eliminate hydrogen ion is compromised. Progression to ketonemia and early metabolic decompensation occurs.

Ketonemia itself is often responsible for further anorexia, vomiting, and an exaggerated stress reaction. The cycle is thus established for the development of DKA. Experience has shown that intervention early in the cycle (that is, when hyperglycemia and mild ketonuria are present) can prevent its worsening in a significant number of persons. Specific attention must be directed to maintenance of hydration. Our practice has been to develop with the child and family an anticipatory program for body fluid maintenance. The family will have received a liquid exchange diet prepared from the liquid exchange list (see Chapter 7) and is encouraged to initiate this for the anorectic child. The amount of fluid consumed is more important than its composition, however. A minimum is essential, but too much at once may precipitate vomiting. The amount we recommend is 3 to 5 ml/kg body weight per hour. Most parents are well aware of the types of liquids their child will consume during such periods, and they are encouraged to use their judgment. Many children seem to handle carbonated beverages well during this time. The decision as to whether to provide sugar-containing or dietetic beverages is best made according to the child's needs at the time. If the child's blood glucose is over 250 mg/dl, sugar-free fluids seem indicated; whereas with blood glucose values in the low or normal range, sugar-containing beverages are more appropriate.

Vomiting is of particular concern; for if oral intake is curtailed for long periods, there is no protection from the ensuing dehydration. All families discharged from our institution are given a small supply of antiemetic suppositories, with specific anticipatory instructions on the manner of their use. We have generally used either trimethobenzamide hydrochloride (Tigan) or promethazine hydrochloride (Phenergan). We have also enjoyed some success with the simultaneous oral administration of Emetrol. This is a phosphate-buffered, glucose-fructose–containing liquid with some antiemetic properties. At times, parents will have discovered other effective home remedies to curtail vomiting. Usually we will make repeated attempts to stop the vomiting for periods of 6 to 12 hours in the home situation. During this time, the family must have ready access to the diabetes team and remain in telephone contact. Needless to say, if the condition worsens or if the vomiting cannot be stopped, intravenous fluid replacement is mandated. In most instances, however, this is not required and a physician visit is prevented. If vomiting does persist, intravenous fluids must be initiated. If the child is only mildly dehydrated, this can be accomplished in the office or clinic without resorting to hospitalization. In these instances, the intravenous fluid replacment is given according to principles outlined in Chapter 12.

Supplemental Insulin Administration

As is apparent, HKS is caused by the unbalanced effect of the stress hormones. While attempts are being made to correct the cause of the stress hormone response, insulin need is immediate and, it is hoped, of short duration. The use of Regular, crystalline insulin is appropriate. The patient and family are instructed to initiate such therapy whenever both hyperglycemia and ketonuria are present and to continue its administration at two-hour intervals until a blood glucose value of 150 mg/dl or lower is achieved.

The dosage of insulin that is effective varies with the situation, but the schedule we recommend has been effective with several thousand episodes of HKS over the past 25 years. The child is instructed to take one fifth, or 20 percent, of the total morning dosage of insulin and to administer this dose subcutaneously or intramuscularly every two hours. Some authors have recommended a standard dose of insulin (for example, 5 or 10 units every one or two hours), but it is our belief that such a set dosage schedule undertreats some children and overtreats others. Other authors have recommended dosages of 0.1 unit per kilogram body weight per hour (0.05 unit per pound per hour) in a fashion similar to the initial management of diabetic ketoacidosis. Althouth certainly effective, this requires calculations that are beyond the grasp of some families.

An example of our recommended management obtained from the records of one of our children at camp seems warranted:

L.C., an 11-year-old with diabetes of three years' duration, usually received 20 NPH/6 Regular in the morning along with 6 NPH/6 Regular with the evening meal. Her control was considered acceptable.

At noon on the day of observation, she complained of headache, abdominal discomfort, nausea, and "feeling bad." Her blood glucose at 7:00 AM that day had been 184 mg/dl, and she had taken her usual insulin and had eaten breakfast. She did not want lunch and was brought to the camp infirmary; a temperature of 100.8°F (38.2°C) was recorded and diffuse abdominal tenderness noted. Her pharynx was moderately inflamed, and no other abnormalities were found. Her blood glucose concentration was 322 mg/dl, and urine demonstrated moderate ketonuria. Her blood glucose and urine ketone records and the insulin therapy received during the next 24 hours are detailed below:

TIME (hr)	BLOOD GLUCOSE (mg/dl)	URINE KETONES	INSULIN ADMINISTRATION (units)
1200	322	Mod	6 Reg
1400	268	Mod–Lg	6 Reg
1600	158	Mod	—
1800	183	Mod	6 NPH/6 Reg
2000	288	Sm–Mod	6 Reg
2200	140	Sm–Mod	—
2400	190	Sm	—
0400	300	Sm–Mod	6 Reg
0600	160	Sm	—
0800	90	Sm	20 NPH/6 Reg
1000	154	Neg	—
1200	168	Neg	—

Throughout this time, L.C. was able to keep up her fluid intake orally and continued to participate in most camp activities.

In general, we recommend that suitably trained families follow this regimen for up to 12 hours independently. After that time, most families welcome the opportunity to interact with a member of the team, even if that conversation merely affirms what they have been doing. As long as the patient is improving, the general pattern of therapy may continue.

It seems important to state that a "sliding scale" method of management is not recommended. In this method, the dosage of insulin given each time is varied depending on the level of the blood glucose obtained. Our experience with such a sliding scale is that most patients receive an inappropriate dosage of insulin and many have significant problems, notably hypoglycemia.

SUMMARY

The syndrome of hyperglycemia and ketonemia secondary to stress is common in the young person with Type I diabetes. If not appropriately managed, HKS will lead to a more serious metabolic state culminating in hospitalization. Most acute episodes can be managed at home by the well-trained patient and family, using the diabetes team as consultants. Based on comparative data from other families whom we see at camp and who have not been so trained, it is estimated by our team that through patient and family training several hundred potential hospitalizations are prevented each year. The dosages of insulin given appear effective yet safe, and problems with significant hypoglycemia have not occurred.

12

Diabetic Ketoacidosis

Diabetic ketoacidosis (DKA) is the most common serious complication of diabetes in the young person and is the major cause of hospitalizations: over 60 per cent of diabetic admissions are due to this single consequence. Data from both the United States and Europe suggest that approximately 14 per cent of all persons with IDDM are hospitalized yearly for DKA.

Prior to the availability of exogenous insulin, DKA was almost always fatal and accounted for over three fourths of all diabetes-associated deaths. During the first 30 years of insulin therapy (1920s to 1950s), the mortality rate in this country dropped significantly to about 10 percent; but there has been minimal, if any, further reduction over the last 30 years (1950s to 1980s). Depending on which medical center or general hospital is surveyed, the current mortality rate for DKA is said to range from 0 to 18 percent, with an overall average of about 10 percent. The rate in most tertiary hospitals for children is about 2 percent, with a range from 0 to 5 percent. Some community hospitals have similar rates, but others report figures much higher when both children and adults are included. The comparison of mortality statistics between children's hospitals and general hospitals is not appropriate, though, since the person at greatest risk of a fatal outcome is the adult with pre-existing coronary artery disease. However, even if one considers the average child mortality from the "best" centers only, the 2 percent figure is still unacceptably high, particularly considering the frequency of DKA. Since many children with DKA do not have immediate access to a specialized hospital, therapy for DKA must usually be given or at least initiated in community hospitals or emergency clinics. It is thus imperative that the generalist (for example, pediatrician, internist, family practitioner, or emergency room physician) have an understanding of the pathophysiology of DKA, a working knowledge of its appropriate management, and an appreciation of the potential consequences.

As discussed in Chapter 11, the majority of instances of DKA can be prevented by a combination of (1) public and patient education, (2) early recognition of ketosis, and (3) appropriate ambulatory management. This is the only certain way of reducing the unacceptable mortality rate.

PATHOGENESIS AND PATHOPHYSIOLOGY

The reader may wish to review the chapter on stress, hyperglycemia, and ketosis (Chapter 11), as the mechanisms of the development of DKA are covered there and will be merely amplified in this section.

DKA is the metabolic consequence of a

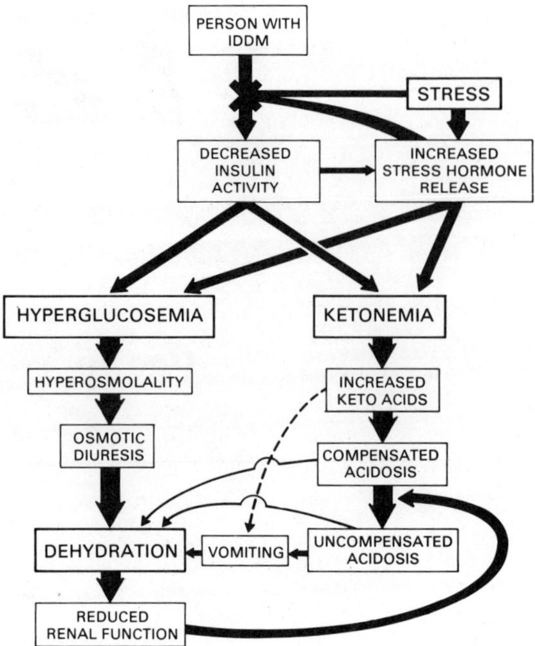

Figure 12–1. Pathogenesis of DKA. As indicated, the major factor initiating the metabolic derangement is stress, with its attendant effects on glucose, fat, and protein metabolism.

severe but usually relative deficiency of insulin. In actuality, it is a decrease in the action or activity of insulin that is paramount, rather than an absolute absence of the hormone. Metabolic or carbohydrate homeostasis is the result of a balance among the actions of the anabolic hormone insulin and the catabolic hormones glucagon, epinephrine, norepinephrine, cortisol, and the growth hormone. The amounts of these catabolic hormones are greatly increased during stress (see Fig. 12–1). Gluconeogenesis and glycogenolysis are stimulated by these stress hormones, and the hepatic concentration of insulin is not sufficient to overcome this effect. Hepatic glucose production increases from about 150 mg/min to levels as high as 600 mg/min. Ketonemia occurs because this unbalanced hormonal interaction produces increased lipolysis and ketogenesis. It is the body's response to these perturbations that creates the clinical picture of DKA. In order to manage the condition appropriately, an understanding of the various facets involved in its production is necessary. The overall disturbance is summarized in Figure 12–1 and will be discussed here as separate but inter-relating processes.

Hyperglycemia and Hyperosmolality

Hyperglycemia is the result primarily of increased hepatic glucose production and, to a lesser degree, of its decreased peripheral use. Since glucose is an osmotically active substance that is predominantly confined to the extracellular fluid, there is a resultant alteration in the solute-to-water ratio. Figure 12–2 illustrates body water shifts between fluid compartments, as these occur in dehydration associated with DKA (*B*) contrasted with those that occur when the dehydration is caused by other disorders (*A*). In usual conditions, the movement of water between the intracellular fluid (ICF) and the extracellular fluid (ECF) compartments is balanced. When the nondiabetic (*A*) experiences abnormal losses of water, as result from vomiting, diarrhea, or curtailment of intake, the ECF volume decreases and the solutes (osmoles or milliosmoles) within the compartment become concentrated. This creates a solute or osmotic drag, forcing free water to move from the ICF to the ECF, once again equalizing osmolality. In contrast, the person who becomes dehydrated and has coexistent hyperglycemia maintains a high ECF osmolality, keeping the ECF volume relatively expanded at the expense of the ICF volume (*B*).

The free water extracted from the ICF dilutes the solutes of the ECF. Thus, there is a progressive decrease in concentrations of ECF ions, such as sodium. Although total body sodium is in fact decreased (owing to mechanisms discussed later), the serum concentration usually suggests a deficit more marked than that which actually exists. Consequently, if the serum sodium concentration in the person with DKA is found to be either normal or increased, a more severe degree of dehydration is strongly suggested. In such instances, the magnitude of the dehydration could be ascertained by either measuring or estimating plasma osmolality. Plasma (or ECF) osmolality (P_{Osm}) can be closely approximated by applying the following equation:

$$P_{Osm} = 2[Na^+] + \frac{\text{blood glucose (mg/dl)}}{18} + \frac{\text{BUN (mg/dl)}}{2.8}$$

Normal plasma osmolality is approximately 285 mOsm/kg (275 to 290 mOsm/kg). If the measured or estimated osmolality in a patient is found to be 314 mOsm/kg, this indicates a 10 percent increase in the solute concentra-

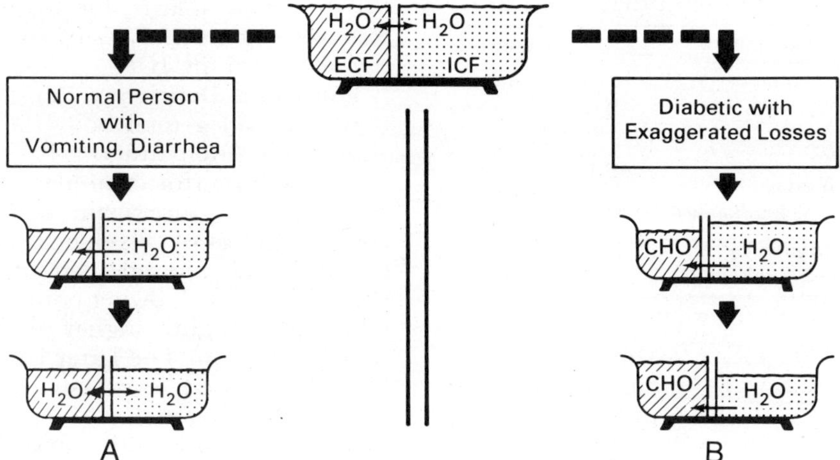

Figure 12–2. Development of dehydration. Both the nondiabetic (*A*) and the diabetic (*B*) individual lose fluids from the extracellular fluid (ECF) with reduction in volume and concentration of solutes. In the nondiabetic, equilibration between compartments is again reached by the movement of free water from the intracellular fluid (ICF). In the diabetic with high concentrations of the carbohydrate (CHO, as glucose) in the ECF, there is relatively greater extraction of water from the ICF. This tends to maintain ECF volume despite the fact that total body water is severely diminished.

tion (for example, 285 + 28.5 = 313.5). Furthermore, this translates to a reduction of approximately 10 percent in total body water. Similarly, an ECF osmolality of 328 mOsm/kg corresponds to a 15 percent increase in solute concentration and to a similar decrease in total body water. Such calculations and data can be of real benefit in establishing the degree of dehydration and, consequently, in aiding the physician to estimate the severity of the process. Additionally, they are useful in estimating the volume of fluid necessary for replacement and in determining its rate of administration. The following is an example:

C.J. is admitted with DKA and is found to have the following chemical values: glucose—720 mg/dl, sodium—128 mEq/l, BUN—18 mg/dl.
Estimated plasma osmolality therefore, is:

$$P_{Osm} = 2\,(128) + \frac{720}{18} + \frac{18}{2.8}$$

$$P_{Osm} = 256 + 40 + 6 = 302 \text{ mOsm/kg}$$

This value indicates about a 6 percent increase over the "normal" and suggests a dehydration of approximately that magnitude. If the weight of C.J. was 20 kg, this 6 percent would indicate an approximate fluid deficit of 1200 ml (20 kg × 6 percent).

In our experience, this calculated amount of deficit is usually smaller than the amount generally required to restore hydration, but it does serve as a useful guide to the minimum amount of fluid deficit. Often, replacement amounts are 25 to 50 percent higher.

Dehydration

The dehydration of DKA is primarily the result of the osmotic diuresis created by the hyperglycemia. Part of this increased urine volume relates to an actual increase in the glomerular filtration rate (GFR), but mostly it relates to the increased concentration of glucose in the glomerular filtrate (that is, filtered load). This increased filtered load of glucose exceeds the reabsorptive capacity of the proximal tubule, and, because of its osmotic properties, a greater volume of water escapes reabsorption in this proximal nephron. At all of the more distal sites within the nephron, this increased volume and concentration reduces normal reabsorptive processes. As a consequence, other solute is swept out into the urine, leading to deficits in many areas.

Two other factors augment development of dehydration: increased insensible water loss and vomiting. The increase in water loss from the body through insensible processes relates mostly to the hyperpnea and tachypnea associated with development of metabolic acidosis. Evidence suggests that the water volume lost through this route is two to three times the normal rate and may be as much

Table 12–1. **BODY FLUID DEFICITS IN DKA**

Substance	Magnitude	Cause
Water	50–100 ml/kg (1500–3000 ml/m²)	Osmotic diuresis Hyperventilation Vomiting Absence of intake
Sodium	4–9 mEq/kg (120–240 mEq/m²)	Urinary losses Vomiting
Potassium	3–10 mEq/kg (90–300 mEq/m²)	Urinary losses Vomiting

as 1500 to 2000 ml/m²/24 hrs. Vomiting is often associated with ketonemia and with metabolic acidosis, but its precise pathogenesis is unknown. The volume or amount of vomitus lost from the body is not as great a factor in the pathogenesis of the dehydration as is the fact that vomiting almost guarantees a decrease in fluid intake. Deprived of intake, the body's defenses against dehydration are limited.

Degree of Dehydration. The magnitude of water loss is variable, depending on a number of factors. Table 12–1 provides data on the range of pre-existing losses observed in patients hospitalized with DKA. For water, this amounts to from 50 to 100 ml/kg of body weight (approximately 1500 to 3000 ml/m² body surface area [BSA]). Once the volume of water loss reaches an amount equal to 6 to 10 percent of body weight, there is reduction in renal blood flow and glomerular function. As indicated in Figure 12–1, this complicates the metabolic situation, making it increasingly difficult for the kidney to moderate or restore acid-base balance successfully.

Sodium Deficiency. In dehydration there is virtually always a total body sodium deficit, amounting in hospitalized patients to between 4 and 8 mEq/kg body weight. Much of this deficit is the result of exaggerated urinary losses, with smaller amounts being lost in vomitus. In early stages of DKA, the urinary concentrations of sodium are often in the range of 50 to 100 mEq/l. As sodium deficiency develops and extracellular volume decreases, there is an accelerated synthesis and secretion of aldosterone, the primary renal effect of which is reduced sodium excretion and enhanced urinary loss of potassium.

Serum sodium values are often in the range of 120 to 130 mEq/l, but, as noted earlier, the serum concentration does not accurately reflect sodium balance. Most of this hyponatremia is due to dilution of the extracellular electrolytes by solute-free water derived from the ICF.

Potassium Deficiency. Most studies have demonstrated a total body deficit of potassium during dehydration that approximates that of sodium (for example, 3 to 10 mEq/kg body weight). Once again, urinary losses account for most of this deficit. In early stages of DKA, the filtered load of potassium is slightly increased, owing both to the elevated GFR and to slightly higher serum concentrations of this ion. The latter is brought about by (1) increased lean-tissue catabolism, (2) increased glycogenolysis, and (3) developing metabolic acidosis with intracellular buffering of hydrogen ion. Figure 12–3 depicts the effects of increased extracellular hydrogen ions (acidosis) on potassium dynamics. Approximately 50 percent of the hydrogen ion load is buffered within the cell. In order to maintain electrical neutrality, potassium leaves the cell, thereby raising the ECF concentration. As dehydration and sodium depletion progress and hypersecretion of aldosterone occurs, hyperkaluria is the result.

As with sodium, the serum level of potassium does not accurately reflect total body balance. Whereas there is virtually always a significant total body deficit, the serum concentration is variable. Values may be low, normal, or high, depending on the relative magnitude of factors tending to raise the level (tissue catabolism, glycogenolysis, metabolic acidosis and cellular buffering, decrease in renal function) and those tending to lower it (degree of deficit prior to reduction in renal function, cumulative urinary losses, vomiting). The electrocardiogram provides a much better index of potassium balance than does the level of serum potassium.

Ketonemia and Acidosis

Increased plasma levels of free fatty acids (FFA) are derived from adipose tissue by their conversion from triglycerides. This conversion is facilitated by activation of lipase, an enzyme that is enhanced by the stress hormones epinephrine and cortisol as well as by a reduction in insulin activity. Circulating FFA is rapidly metabolized by the liver; a small portion is converted to triglycerides and phospholipids, while the larger portion is transported to the mitochrondria where it is oxidized to acetylcoenzyme A (acetyl-CoA).

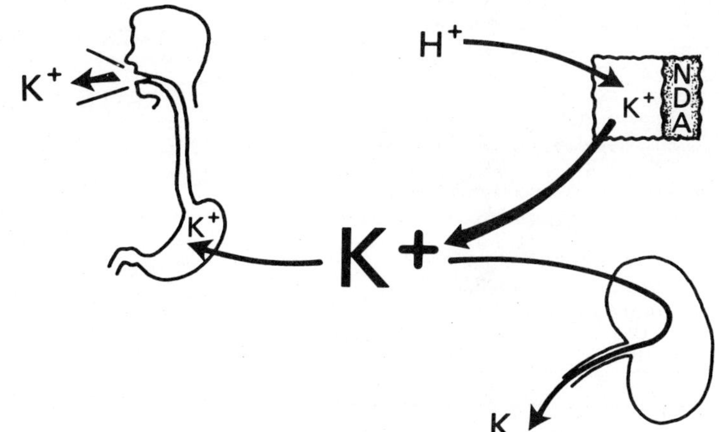

Figure 12–3. The extracellular potassium (K$^+$) concentration rises as the acidosis develops and hydrogen (H$^+$) is buffered in the cell by nondiffusible anions (NDA). This leads to kaluresis. Potassium is also lost in vomitus.

POTASSIUM DYNAMICS IN ACIDOSIS

Further metabolism of acetyl-CoA occurs either by conversion to carbon dioxide and water via the tricarboxylic acid or Krebs cycle or by other pathways to keto acids. Several potential factors in DKA favor the production of keto acids: (1) alterations in other enzymes of the Krebs cycle caused by the insulin deficiency; (2) the high availability of the substrate acetyl-CoA; and (3) perhaps, the action of glucagon on stimluation of ketogenesis.

Acetoacetic acid is the first ketone formed from acetyl-CoA, and this is slowly decarboxylated to acetone. Whereas acetoacetic acid is a stong acid, acetone is not and consequently has little or no effect on plasma pH. Acetoacetic acid can be reduced to beta-hydroxybutyric acid, another strong acid. These two ketones are interconvertible, their relative concentrations depending on several variables. The keto acids are taken up by peripheral tissues (mostly muscle and kidney) and oxidized to carbon dioxide and water. There is some evidence that peripheral uptake of these keto acids may be reduced in DKA.

Metabolic Acidosis

As the ketoacids are released into the ECF and initiate a change in the hydrogen ion concentraton, the body's intricate buffer systems are activated. These systems include both extracellular and intracellular mechanisms, all designed to minimize significant shifts in body pH. Approximately 50 percent of the acid load is initially buffered within the cell by nondiffusible anions. Extracellular buffering is carried out by both bicarbonate and nonbicarbonate systems (for example, albumin, hemoglobin, and phosphate), but it is the bicarbonate system that is most important and most easily measured. This system is measured by the equation:

$$H^+ \cdot A^- + B^+ \cdot HCO_3^- \leftrightarrows B^+ \cdot A^- + H^+ \cdot HCO_3 \leftrightarrows H_2CO_3 \leftrightarrows H_2O + CO_2$$

As acetoacetic acid and beta-hydroxybutyric acid (H$^+$ · A$^-$) enter the ECF, they are buffered, mostly by the sodium salt of bicarbonate (B$^+$ · HCO$_3^-$), and converted to the salt of the keto acid (B$_1$ · A$^-$) and to the weak acid carbonic acid (H$^+$ · HCO$_3^-$); the latter is quickly disassociated to CO$_2$ and H$_2$O and excreted by the lungs. In the process, the concentration of B$^+$ · HCO$_3^-$ falls, and there is a reciprocal rise in the concentration of the anions of acetoacetate and beta-hydrobutyrate. The latter are usually not measured and are referred to as the R-fraction, unmeasured anions, or *anion gap*. This R-fraction is expressed as:

$$R\text{-fraction} = [Na^+] - ([HCO_3^-] + [Cl^-])$$

Normally, the difference between the sum of the concentrations of chloride and bicarbonate and the concentration of sodium is between 8 and 12 mEq/l; but in classic DKA, there is a significant fall in the HCO$_3^-$ and a reciprocal rise in R$^-$ fraction.

The buffering of the keto acids moderates the fall in plasma pH, but values in the range of 7.00 to 7.25 are common. This acidemia

Table 12–2. **CLINICAL FEATURES OF DKA AND CAUSES OF THE VARIABLE PRESENTATIONS**

I. Newly Diagnosed Diabetic
  A. Etiologic factors (see Chapter 2)
  B. Awareness of disease and its features
  C. Precipitating stress—severity
  D. Residual beta-cell function
II. Known Diabetic Under Management
  A. Degree of carbohydrate control
  B. Residual beta-cell function
  C. Current insulin regimen
  D. Precipitating stress—type and severity
  E. Appropriate knowledge, skills, and attitudes—survival skills
  F. Status of hydration

stimulates the respiratory center, resulting in increased rate and depth of respirations. Through this increase in respirations, the volatile acid $H^+ \cdot HCO_3$ is removed from the body, thus further compensating for the alteration in the usual 20:1 ratio of $B^+ \cdot HCO_3^-$ to $H^+ \cdot HCO_3^- \rightarrow H_2CO_3$.

The other component of the bicarbonate buffer system is the kidney. The appropriate renal response is to (1) reabsorb all of the filtered bicarbonate, (2) excrete the keto acid, and (3) reconstitute or regenerate (more) bicarbonate. Both proximal and distal nephrons are involved in this process, which consists of (1) reduction in urine pH to the lowest possible value of around 4.5; (2) buffering of the excess hydrogen ion by filtrate buffers, mostly phosphates; and (3) the synthesis and secretion of the buffer ammonia. The latter system is the most efficient in removing H^+ but requires two to three days before it is fully operative.

As long as the renal system is reconstituting new bicarbonate and excreting the keto acids, the acidosis can usually be stabilized. On the other hand, if dehydration compromises renal function and thus restricts these tubular functions, the acidosis can quickly decompensate. Fortunately, the osmotic load in the ECF tends to protect renal function longer than would be seen with comparable degrees of dehydration from other causes.

CLINICAL ILLNESS

The clinical features of DKA are quite variable and depend on a number of factors. Some of these factors are noted in Table 12–2 and are discussed below.

Variable Presentations: Signs and Symptoms

Newly Diagnosed Diabetic

In past decades, almost all children with IDDM presented with DKA. In a review of a 10-year experience published in 1962, one of the authors (LBT) noted that almost 70 percent of children seen in his institution presented initially with DKA. This is in marked contrast to the current situation, in which less than 25 percent have DKA at onset. This change in presentation characteristics has been noted by other authors, with the general consensus being that this is related to an increased public awareness concerning diabetes. It also appears that physicians are more apt to consider a diagnosis of diabetes now than they were two decades ago. Even among those presenting with DKA, there is variability still in how early the symptoms and signs are recognized and acted on.

The type and severity of the precipitating stress is another key factor in determining early characteristics, as are etiologic factors (Chapter 2) and the functional status of the beta cells.

Usual Symptoms and Signs. These have been covered in Chapter 3 and will only briefly be restated here. Polyuria, polydipsia, and weight loss occur in virtually all patients who have the diagnosis of DKA. Either anorexia or polyphagia may have been present earlier, but by the time the patient comes to medical attention in DKA anorexia is almost always present. This symptom may be accompanied by nausea, abdominal discomfort or pain, and vomiting. The child may have also had leg cramps, headaches, weakness, personality changes, or intermittent breathlessness. Examination usually reveals loss of fatty tissue and, if symptomatic for long periods, loss of lean body mass. The abdomen is often protuberant and distended. There may be a mild generalized tenderness, much worse in the right hypochrondrium, where the liver may be enlarged. Varying degrees of hyperpnea and tachypnea may be present, and invariably there is tachycardia. The skin is usually warm and may be cherry-red. Only rarely is the skin cold or pale and then only as a late sign associated with peripheral vascular collapse secondary to marked dehydration. The clinical features of extracellular dehydration (skin tenting, dry mucous membranes, and so forth) are usually minimal to moderate in degree, and the examiner may underestimate the degree of fluid loss accordingly. The saliva is usually viscid, and urine output may be high. The sensorum is variously depressed, ranging from lethargy to coma; and a fruity odor to the breath may be apparent.

Known Diabetic Under Management

Here again, the clinical features are variable, but the potential causes for this variability are more numerous (Table 12–2).

Degree of Pre-existing Diabetic Control. The person who is in optimal metabolic control has more resilience than the person in poor metabolic control. Thus, the person under optimum control may be able to withstand considerably more stress before succumbing to DKA. Unless the stress is sudden and severe, such persons may gradually slip out of control, developing DKA slowly over a longer period of time. In contrast, the person who is in poor metabolic control may develop DKA suddenly, precipitated by only a moderate degree of stress.

Residual Beta-cell Functions. Various studies have demonstrated that patients with IDDM who retain some beta-cell function, as evidenced by persisting levels of C-peptide, are not as susceptible to the development of DKA. Thus, such children may have a reduced tendency of sudden decompensation accompanying episodes of moderate stress.

Current Insulin Regimens. Ordinarily, with persons receiving intermediate-acting insulins (with or without associated Regular), a single forgotten or missed insulin injection is rarely the cause of DKA. There is sufficient depot-effect to prevent this occurrence; this is particularly true in those persons receiving two injections per day. Whether the person who misses his or her sole daily dose develops DKA is contigent on the prior level of glucose control and the degree of the associated stress. Conversely, those persons whose diabetes is controlled solely or predominantly by Regular insulin may develop DKA within an 8- to 15-hour period of time. This has been apparent with increased experience with the external insulin pump and is evident from the following:

R.B., a 13-year-old, had been placed on an external insulin pump one year earlier because of hyperlability and recurrent DKA. During this time, her hopsitalizations had dropped from an average of 16 per year over the preceding two years to one (for routine reassessment). Her glycosylated hemoglobin had dropped from 13.2 percent to 6.1 percent, and HBGM indicated good control.

After feeling well the previous day, R.B. awakened at 7:00 AM feeling unwell. She was tired, thirsty, and nauseated, with mild abdominal discomfort. Her blood glucose was in excess of 400 mg/dl, and her urine contained large ketone levels. Because of her appearance (she was sick, listless, and breathing heavily) she was taken to the local emergency room and there admitted to the hospital. In addition to having clinical DKA, she was found to have a pharyngitis and left otitis media. Significant laboratory studies showed: blood glucose 660 mg/dl; pH 7.18; and bicarbonate 8 mEq/l. The pump tubing was discovered to be plugged, and inspection of the pump's accumulated dose indicated that she probably had received no insulin since about 4:00 PM the previous day (about 15 hours earlier). Blood glucose had been 168 mg/dl at 6:30 PM and one had not been obtained prior to sleep.

Persons receiving only Regular insulin are at considerable risk if such therapy is abruptly discontinued, particularly when there is an associated stress-provoking condition. In R.B.'s case, the pharyngitis and otitis were apparently sufficient to elicit this stress response and, when coupled with insulin withdrawal, to produce DKA.

Precipitating Stress. This subject has been explored in Chapter 11 and will not be repeated here. Both the type and severity of the stress are significant factors.

Appropriate Knowledge, Skills, and Attitudes. Persons who have appropriate knowledge, adequate skills, and a mature, responsible attitude toward diabetes will rarely develop DKA. Alterations in their normal health are recognized and treated early, and only unusual degrees of stress provoke DKA. The "uneducated" diabetic may have as profound an episode of DKA as that noted in the section on the newly diagnosed diabetic. Additionally, the clinical picture may be confused by manipulative behaviors. We have observed a number of teenage girls who have purposely undercontrolled their diabetes in order to lose weight without dietary restriction. Such persons developing the hyperglycemia-ketosis syndrome have minimal resilience and, with minimal stress, develop DKA.

Status of Hydration. This is one of the most important, if not the most important, determinants of symptomatology in DKA. As noted earlier, the dehydration is predominantly an intracellular one, with the volume

Table 12–3. DIABETIC KETOACIDOSIS: INITIAL LABORATORY RESULTS IN 100 CHILDREN

Examination	Normal Range	Mean (and Range)
Blood glucose (random) (mg/dl)	60–130	458 (298–1670)
Arterial pH	7.35–7.45	7.11 (6.88–7.24)
$B^+ \cdot HCO_3^-$ (mM/l)	22–25	9.8 (2.0–15.0)
Serum sodium (mEq/l)	138–142	128 (119–146)
Serum potassium (mEq/l)	3.8–4.5	5.4 (2.2–7.5)
WBC (cells/mm³)	5–15,000	19,200 (11,200–54,000)

of the ECF being relatively well maintained. Only when dehydration becomes extreme does the blood pressure drop and typical signs of ECF dehydration occur. As also noted, adequate renal function is necessary for correction of the acidosis to occur spontaneously.

It is appropriate to re-emphasize that the degree of dehydration is often underestimated in the diabetic with DKA. The reason for this underestimation by the physician observer seems obvious: most of the clinical signs that the practitioner uses to calculate the degree of dehydration are extracellular signs (poor skin turgor, dry mucous membranes, pallor, tachycardia, drop in blood pressure, and so forth), while the dehydration of DKA is predominantly intracellular.

Laboratory Features

As with the clinical features, the initial laboratory study results vary with the duration and severity of the disease state. In the subsequent discussion of individual examinations, we focus on the usual results and give estimates of the range of variables. Results in our hospital obtained from 100 consecutive patients admitted for DKA are noted in Table 12–3 and are expanded on in this section.

Blood and Urine Glucose

Hyperglycemia is a uniform feature of DKA, and initial values from the last 100 children with DKA in our institution have ranged from 298 to 1670 mg/dl, with a mean of 458 mg/dl. These values are generally comparable to those reported elsewhere, although the other ranges may be even broader. In this series, the height of the blood glucose correlated directly neither with the physician's impression of clinical severity nor with the rapidity of response to therapy. For instance, the child with the blood glucose of 1670 mg/dl had a markedly depressed sensorium but was not felt to be "semicomatose" by any of three examiners. His plasma pH was only 7.21, and his bicarbonate level 14 mM/l. Within 24 hours, he was alert and consuming a normal diet; intravenous fluids were discontinued at 34 hours of therapy. The lack of a direct correlation between the level of hyperglycemia and clinical status has been repeatedly noted by others.

Urine glucose, on the other hand, will usually reflect the degree of hyperglycemia and is almost always at the 5 percent level by standard testing in patients with DKA. The marked glycosuria is associated with a urine osmolality of between 300 and 500 mOsm/kg but with a urinary specific gravity in excess of 1.035.

Arterial pH and $B^+ \cdot HCO_3^-$

In our group of 100 children, the admitting arterial pH ranged from 6.88 to 7.24, whereas the plasma bicarbonate concentration ranged from 2.0 to 15.0 mM/l, with a mean of 9.8 mM/l. As might be expected, the physician's assessment of clinical severity was closely correlated with the degree of metabolic acidosis. The clinical findings most nearly associated with the most extreme acidosis were central nervous system (CNS) depression, pallor, hypotension, and hyperpnea. One child from this group expired secondary to cerebral edema; her pH and bicarbonate concentration on admission were 7.02 and 5.6 mM/l, respectively. In the remaining 99 children, the rapidity of response to therapy did not significantly correlate with the degree of acidosis.

Serum Sodium and Potassium

The mean serum sodium concentration was 10 mEq/l below the normal range, the lowest value being 119 mEq/l. This latter value occurred in a 6-year-old child whose blood glucose concentration at onset was 1540 mg/dl. The estimated serum osmolality of 323 mOsm/kg seen in this child was not the highest detected, however, as eight children had initial values over 330 mOsm/kg. The response to therapy was not significantly different in these very hyperosmolar children, but in each there was a more cautious approach to reduction of blood glucose.

The serum concentration of potassium was quite variable at the time of initial hospitalization, with values ranging from 2.2 mEq/l to 7.5 mEq/l, the mean being 5.4 mEq/l. In general, the potassium concentration varied inversely with the arterial pH (r = 0.78), but there was no uniform association. For instance, the serum potassium concentration was 2.8 mEq/l in the child with the most severe depression of arterial pH. This new diabetic teenager with a blood glucose of 1100 mg/dl had a brief period of significant symptomatology but had sustained a 35-pound weight loss over the preceding 8 to 10 weeks. The electrocardiogram revealed striking hypokalemic changes that only slowly returned to normal despite the intravenous administration of potassium salts in concentrations exceeding 120 mEq/l of fluids.

Other Laboratory Studies

The initial *white blood cell count* (WBC) averaged 19,200 cells/mm^3 with a range of 11,200 to 54,000. The majority of these patients did not demonstrate evidence of associated infection, a bacterial infection being documented in only 11 of the 81 cases in which such was investigated. The leukocytosis was predominantly polymorphonuclear in type, and this is in agreement with reports from others. The explanation for the profound leukocytosis is incomplete, but the acute metabolic stress is thought to play a major role.

Serum *creatinine* concentrations, generally measured by the AutoAnalyzer, averaged 2.4 mg/dl (normal 0.4 to 0.8 mg/dl) and seemed to correlate directly with the degree of acidosis (that is, ketonemia). Various studies have demonstrated that keto acids interfere with the analysis of creatinine; thus, these elevations do not reflect renal function. Blood concentrations of urea nitrogen *(BUN)* ranged from 13 mg/dl to 38 mg/dl, with a mean value of 18.5 mg/dl.

Serum lipids were obtained in 24 instances and were elevated in 19 of these. *Cholesterol,* on the other hand, was found to be normal in 36 of the 51 determinations. Total serum

Table 12–4. **LABORATORY STUDIES OBTAINED ON ADMISSION**

Essential	Useful	Optional
Blood glucose	Arterial pH	Serum calcium
Serum sodium	Arterial gases	Serum phosphorus
Serum chloride	Urine glucose	Serum magnesium
Serum potassium	Electrocardiogram	Serum creatinine
Serum bicarbonate	Complete blood count	Serum lipids
Urine ketones	Serum osmolality	Serum ketones
Blood urea		Urine culture
nitrogen		Chest
		roentgenogram
		Liver profile
		Glycosylated
		hemoglobin

calcium averaged 8.8 mg/dl (range 7.4 to 11.1 mg/dl); whereas initial serum *phosphorus* ranged from 2.0 to 4.9 mg/dl (mean 3.2), with normal values ranging from 3.5 to 5.5 mg/dl. Serum *magnesium* was below 2.0 mg/dl in 10 of the 14 samples evaluated.

The initial laboratory studies noted earlier for our most recent 100 children are representative of studies reported elsewhere. Consequently, it is perhaps appropriate to identify those laboratory studies that are essential to obtain and those that are useful additions but are not mandatory. These are noted in Table 12–4. Also listed are other studies that are frequently obtained but are rarely used in the management of persons with DKA.

MANAGEMENT OF DKA

The first goal of therapy is to reiterate the principle of prevention established in Chapter 11 . As noted, better public awareness and a heightened index of suspicion among professionals have resulted in fewer persons presenting initially with DKA. Efforts toward this end should be intensified by continued measures toward public education and by earlier identification of those who are most susceptible.

Among those who have Type I diabetes, the frequency with which decompensated ketosis occurs is totally unacceptable. Two factors are known to lessen the frequency of this complication: appropriate patient education and better blood glucose control. To these, one additional factor should be added: the early recognition and management of symptomatic hyperglycemia and ketosis. This has been reviewed in the previous chapter and will not be further elaborated on here.

This chapter will deal with the management of those patients with DKA who require intravenous fluid therapy or hospitalization or both. Attention to these more severe cases will certainly lessen the unacceptably high mortality attendant to this problem. The four major areas of (1) ambiance, (2) general supportive care, (3) intravenous fluid therapy, and (4) insulin management will be addressed here.

Ambiance

Setting

The setting in which DKA is managed is an important consideration. Although initial therapy may be given in any setting, some thought should be given to the location for overall management. Since DKA is a serious problem with dire potential consequences, it might seem most appropriate to admit all such persons to an intensive care unit. Unfortunately, such units are not always available, and even when they are, the staffs of many general ICUs are inexperienced in dealing with children, as well as with diabetes. The physician must select the patient care unit where the most experienced, observant, and clinically competent nursing is practiced. In many centers, this may mean placing a child with DKA in a general pediatric nursing unit in preference to an ICU. If at all possible, the parents should be in attendance with the child.

Facilities

The patient must be in an area that can be closely observed by the nursing and medical staff. The ability to monitor the rates of intravenous fluids and medications carefully is of paramount importance. Blood glucose monitoring by one of the optical methods (Glucometer, Accu-Chek, Glucoscan, and so on) as well as by visual estimation (Chemstrip bG) is an essential on-site necessity. The hospital laboratory must be continuously operational and must have the capability of performing the appropriate blood studies with a turnaround time of less than one hour. The availability of a sophisticated laboratory and the ability to monitor vital functions mechanically are desirable but not always essential.

Medical and Nursing Personnel

A competent medical and nursing staff accustomed to working together is highly desirable. The nursing staff should consist of skilled professionals who are careful and accurate observers. In addition to their technical skills, they should demonstrate a supportive and caring attitude, as both patient and family are usually in a state of extreme psychologic stress.

Documentation: Flow Sheets

Therapy of DKA results in varied and sometimes rapid changes in clinical and biochemical parameters. The trend of such events is often more informative than is the patient's condition at any single point in time. A flow sheet is, perhaps, the most important facilitator and gauge of proper management and should always be at the bedside. This flow sheet should incorporate clinical data about the patient (status of sensorium, vital signs, and so forth), about intake and output, and about biochemical parameters.

General Supportive Care

Causative Factors

Search for and elimination of causative factors is an important aspect of optimum care. Chapter 11, in addressing the issue of stress as a causative factor, is very relevant. In most instances, the physical basis for the decompensation will be obvious (for example, vomiting, febrile illness, and stressful circumstances), but the true etiology may not be discerned. Only rarely will a treatable bacterial infection be found, but the thoughtful practitioner will always exclude such causes. At times, "hidden" causal infections of the urinary tract or of the paranasal sinuses will be discovered. More frequently, the precipitating infection is viral, and no specific therapy will be indicated. Although some writers have advocated the routine use of antimicrobials, we do not find this practice to be warranted.

Urethral Catheterization (Indwelling)

We believe that urethral catheterization is to be resisted, even though it is advocated by some diabetologists and is an accepted practice in some institutions. Some investigators, in their zeal to acquire accurate data concerning urinary output, seem to forget about the potential consequences of such a routine practice. An indwelling urethral catheter, regardless of how well cared for, is associated with an unacceptably high nosocomial infection rate. Once such an infection has occurred, there is a high recurrence rate, and chronic urinary tract infections may become a lasting problem. In the end, the short-term gain (that is, better data collection) may be a long-term loss.

Oral Fluids and Gastric Aspiration

In most children admitted to the hospital, the CNS depression and frequent occurrence of vomiting preclude administration of oral fluids. Despite intense thirst, it seems best to withhold oral intake during the first several hours of therapy or, at the most, to limit this to ice chips. In most persons, even those with moderately severe DKA, it is possible to institute oral fluids into the management protocol after six to eight hours.

Gastric dilatation is often present and is occasionally marked. If this situation prevails, and particularly if the sensorium is depressed, it may be appropriate to consider gastric aspiration. In our experience, it is not often necessary to continue such aspiration, but if vomiting persists after initiation of therapy, this action might be considered.

Hyperventilation and Anxiety

Anxiety on the part of the patient with DKA may be extreme and may parallel the severity of the acidosis and of the rate and depth of respirations. The hyperpnea and tachypnea are not secondary to the anxiety but are compensatory responses of the body designed to moderate the metabolic acidosis. Although this statement may appear unnecessary to most readers and even trite to some, the authors are aware of two recent instances of severe DKA in which professionals promoted rebreathing of carbon dioxide by application of a paper bag over the face in the mistaken belief that this would help the condition. Whereas this practice is accepted for purely anxiety-provoked hyperventilation, it is contraindicated in persons with metabolic acidosis, since it further increases the plasma hydrogen ion concentration (that is, reduces arterial pH) by adding a respiratory component to the already existing acidosis.

Intravenous Fluid Therapy

Appropriate fluid therapy is almost as important to successful management as is insulin therapy. In fact, many investigators have demonstrated dramatic early improvement in the clinical state of patients merely by the institution of rehydration therapy. For this reason, it seems prudent to mention that, should a child with DKA need emergency transport from a primary center to a tertiary center, initiation of intravenous fluid therapy is always indicated.

It is important to restate the characteristics of the dehydration of DKA, for this will assist in deciding on correct replacement therapy: DKA dehydration is predominantly an intracellular deficit during which the volume of the ECF is relatively well maintained.

Fluid Volume

The volume of fluid necessary for replacement will obviously vary from patient to patient, and, in contrast to other forms of dehydration, the clinical findings may not as closely predict the appropriate volume. In our experience, the volume that is predicted at onset is usually less than that which is found to be necessary for rehydration.

The principles of selecting an amount for rehydration therapy in patients with DKA are similar to those in patients with other forms of dehydration: (1) estimate the antecedent deficit, (2) estimate an amount for maintenance fluids during the time of rehydration, and (3) estimate concurrent losses during the period of rehydration.

Antecedent deficit can be estimated from averages of similar patients, as indicated in Table 12–1. The range of volume necessary for replacement of these losses varies between 50 and 100 mg/kg body weight (that is, between 1500 and 3000 ml/m²). Alternatively, this deficit may be estimated by measuring the ECF osmolality (either determined or calculated) and calculating the fluid deficit necessary to produce that osmolality.

Maintenance fluid replacement, the water necessary to replace normal losses (that is, insensible and renal water losses) can be estimated to range between 1500 and 2500 ml/m²/24 hours (or between 50 and 80 ml/kg body weight/24 hours). These losses are slightly higher than would be considered usual, owing to the presence of hyperventilation and the persisting osmotic diuresis. In actuality, these estimates anticipate and include some of the concurrent losses.

The "starting " fluid volume is thus the sum of these two estimates. In practice, the physician must exercise judgment in deciding the correct volume for a given patient within these ranges. The following child is an example:

K.L., a 7-year-old girl, is admitted with DKA. A newly diagnosed diabetic, she has been acutely symptomatic for only 24 hours; but anorexia, polyuria, and weight loss have been present for about four weeks. On admission, her weight is 20 kg (S.A. = 0.8 m^2); she has a moderately depressed sensorium, a respiratory rate of 42 breaths per minute, and thickened saliva and slightly dry mucous membranes. Her initial laboratory studies reveal glucose 518 mg/dl; sodium, 134 mEq/l; potassium, 5.8 mEq/l; chloride, 98 mEq/l; bicarbonate, 6 mM/l; arterial pH, 7.01; BUN, 22 mg/dl; and plasma osmolality, 304 mOsm/kg (calculated).

Her antecedent deficit (from Table 12–1) is estimated to be 2500 ml/m^2, or 2000 ml. If this estimate had been made on the basis of K.L.'s plasma osmolality, the anticipated volume would have only been 1300 ml. Because of the comments made earlier, we usually choose the first method (see Table 12–1) or increase the calculated amount by 25 to 50 percent (that is, bringing the total to between 1600 and 1950 ml). If the maintenance fluid is chosen as 2500 ml/m^2/24 hr (or 2000 ml), then the total "first 24 hour" fluid volume is estimated at about 4000 ml (about 5000 ml/m^2/24 hr).

Once again, it is necessary to remind the reader that these figures represent mere estimates but that such steps are essential if one is to arrive at a starting place from which modifications can then take place. In this context, one can appreciate the fact that a starting estimate of either 4000 ml (from Table 12–1) or 3300 ml (from the calculation of 1300 + 2000) will probably not make a great deal of difference in the eventual course of the DKA, if the patient is adequately monitored and fluids are altered appropriately.

Rates of Fluid Administration

An acceptable rule of thumb is to administer approximately one half of the total estimated amount of fluid during the first eight hours, the other half being distributed over the remaining portion of the 24-hour period (16 hours). Likewise, it seems prudent to administer a similar portion of the first eight-hour volume estimate during the early part of this time (for instance, perhaps one half

the eight-hour volume in the first 2½ hours, or 150 minutes). This replaces the majority of the antecedent deficit early when the need is greatest. In the preceding example of K.L., the following program was followed:

Total estimated fluids/24 hr: 4000
Amount given:
    Hours 0 to 2.5: 1000 or 400 ml/hr
    Hours 2.5 to 9.0: 1000 or 150 ml/hr
    Hours 9.0 to 24: 2000 or 125 ml/hr

As is obvious, the initial 2½ hours of fluid is given, in this example, at a rate of between 6 and 8 ml/m^2/min (between 12 and 16 ml/kg/hr), a safe rate of fluid administration for periods like this if renal and cardiac problems are not severe. It is unlikely that more rapid administration of fluids will shorten the recovery time. The rate of infusion will, of course, be reduced in the third hour of management, under most circumstances.

Types of Fluid Administered

Several principles of fluid and electrolyte management that represent considerations relative to the type of fluid or concentration of solutes to be administered include (1) The overall need for water exceeds that of solute, and thus the 24-hour combined volume should be hypotonic with respect to that of the ECF; (2) there is a total body deficit of sodium, but much of the hyponatremia is dilutional; (3) sudden shifts in volume of the body fluid compartments are not desirable and may be harmful; (4) there is an absolute deficit of potassium even if not reflected in plasma determinations; and (5) an absolute maxim of fluid therapy is "to do no harm." Specifically, the latter means that the kidney, when function is restored, can modulate body fluid and solute changes more successfully than can the practitioner.

Initial Two to Three Hours. During the first two to three hours, maintenance of ECF volume is of prime importance. Additionally, beginning rehydration of the ICF is an important consideration. The optimum fluid composition appears to be one with an effective osmolality close to normal isotonicity (approximately 280 to 290 mOsm/kg). When one considers the average child presenting with DKA (see Table 12–3), the ECF osmolality is 284 mOsm/kg and thus does not differ significantly from the normal osmolality. Isotonic sodium chloride has an osmolality of approximately 310 mOsm/kg and would seem suitable only for those patients with more marked hyperosmolality. On the other hand, in our experience and in those of most diabetologists, isotonic sodium chloride solution is the fluid most commonly used as the initial infusate. In our center, all patients receive this fluid for the first one to three hours, and our experience in mortality rates demonstrates only two deaths in 384 treatment regimens over 24 years, both deaths secondary to cerebral edema. Additionally, we have seen only one other child develop significant neurologic sequelae.

Perhaps the ideal initial solution would have the following characteristics: osmolality of 280 to 290 mOsm/kg; sodium of 130 to 145 mEq/l; chloride of 105 to 115 mEq/l; and bicarbonate of 25 to 30 mM/l. A seemingly good fluid would consist of three-quarters isotonic sodium chloride, to which is added 25 mEq/l of sodium bicarbonate. This amount of bicarbonate (approximately 25 mEq of $NaHCO_3$ added to each liter of fluid) is not sufficient to produce an alkalosis but does provide some additional ECF buffering capacity. This would give a fluid composition of osmolality, 282 mOsm/kg; sodium, 141 mEq/l; chloride, 116 mEq/l; and bicarbonate, 25 mEq/l. Such a fluid would be sufficiently near isotonicity to protect the ECF and prevent sudden shifts of water into the ICF, particularly that of the central nervous system. At the same time, this would provide some free water to begin hydration of the ICF. Such a fluid is not routinely available and would need to be prepared. This is a major limitation.

Third through Eighth Hours. During this period, primary rehydration of the ICF should occur, and fluids with more free water are indicated. Our practice is to use 0.45 percent sodium chloride to which is added 25 mEq/l of $NaHCO_3$ during hours three to four, and then to go to a more dilute fluid for hours five through eight. This latter fluid is usually 0.33 percent sodium chloride, to which is added 25 mEq/l of sodium bicarbonate. In children under age 4, because of their greater need for free water, we occasionally progress to somewhat more dilute fluids at an earlier time.

Ninth through 24th Hours. At the beginning of the ninth hour, we usually recommend a complete reassessment to determine if rehydration is proceeding according to plan (see section on monitoring later in this chapter). If rehydration appears to be progressing well, most children are either continued at 0.33 percent or converted to 0.25 percent sodium chloride solution, to which is added 25 mEq/l of sodium bicarbonate. Unless chemical or clinical findings indicate otherwise, this fluid composition is continued until hydration is complete.

Glucose Administration. Some authors advocate the addition of 5 percent glucose even to the initial fluids, reasoning that the insulin administration can easily compensate for this relatively small amount of excess glucose. While this may be true in some instances, the routine addition of glucose to initial fluid replacement adds needlessly to the hyperosmolar state and further reduces the ICF fluid volume. Thus, it is our belief that early addition of glucose could potentially create more problems. Consequently, it is our practice to add 5 percent glucose to the infusate when the blood glucose concentration approaches 250 mg/dl. If the decline in glucose concentration reaches a value of 150 mg/dl, it is more prudent to add additional glucose (that is, up to 10 percent), rather than to stop or decrease the insulin administration.

Potassium Administration. Based on previous discussions, the need for potassium administration should be obvious. Three factors warrant consideration: (1) the type of potassium salt, (2) its concentration, and (3) the time of initial administration. In our unit, the phosphate salt of potassium has been used almost exclusively since the early 1960s, and none of the patients have experienced clinically detectable problems. The rationale for using potassium phosphate rather than the chloride salt is threefold: (1) phosphates are lost during the osmotic diuresis in almost equimolar concentrations to those of potassium, and total body phosphate content is diminished; (2) the phosphate buffer system of the ECF is very effective in binding free hydrogen ions and is compromised in deficit states; and (3) a primary method of eliminating hydrogen ion during acidosis is by the formation of titratable acid by renal tubular cells. Titratable acid is predominantly a phosphate buffer system allowing excretion of hydrogen ion without significant reduction in urinary pH. The first rationale may not be a practical reason; the second may be of little consequence because of the small amount of this particular buffer system in the ECF (less than 1 mM/l); but the third reason is both real and important, since potassium phosphate infusions significantly increase urinary phosphate and titratable acidity. This does allow for a quantitatively greater hydrogen ion excretion.

While none of our patients have had clinical problems with such infusions, other clinicians have reported development of significant hypocalcemia and clinical tetany during such therapy. This has predominantly been a problem of the adult patient with DKA, but it does bear consideration. Consequently, a number of authors currently recommend that one half of the potassium be given as phosphate and the other half as chloride.

The *concentration of potassium* administered will vary with the degree of hypokalemia, the clinical features, and the stage of management. The standard method is the use of potassium in a concentration of 40 mEq/l of fluids unless there are indications to do otherwise. Not infrequently, it will be necessary to increase the concentration to 60, 80, or even 100 mEq/l, but such must be done only with careful monitoring by the electrocardiogram and chemical values.

Initiation of potassium therapy should, in most instances, be withheld for the first one to two hours of therapy until renal function is ensured. This is particularly true if the initial value for serum potassium is elevated above 6.0 mEq/l. It is usually not appropriate to withhold potassium, until the potassium level begins to fall or until the acidosis is improved. Some persons may be benefited by potassium added to the initial fluids, and those are persons whose initial acidosis is associated with hypokalemia (that is, values below 4.0 mEq/l). This is particularly important if there are electrocardiographic changes.

Administration of Bicarbonate. Prior to the mid-1970s, there was controversy regarding the bolus administration of sodium bicarbonate in the severely acidotic diabetic. Proponents of *bolus therapy* (relatively rapid, "push" infusions of $NaHCO_3$ in amounts usually varying from 1.0 to 3.0 mEq/kg/dose) noted that, in response to such therapy, patients experienced immediate slowing of respirations, had "better" peripheral coloring, enjoyed a more restful state, and had improvement in the blood gas profile. Opponents of such therapy noted occasional incidences of cerebral edema, serious hypokalemia, and cardiorespiratory arrest. A number of experimental and clinical studies, in which the physiologic mechanisms were clearly defined, demonstrated that such bolus bicarbonate therapy was attended by unwarranted risks. Studies have clearly shown that bolus bicarbonate (1) worsens the intracellular acidosis, (2) lowers the pH of cerebrospinal fluid (CSF), (3) increases the lactate content of CSF, and (4) decreases oxygen availability to the CNS. Such therapy has been demonstrated to decrease the level of consciousness and to be a factor in the development of cerebral edema. Thus, such therapy is no longer warranted and is generally discouraged.

But, as discussed earlier, our recommendations are that intravenous fluids be adjusted by the addition of sodium bicarbonate in concentrations of about 25 mEq/l of infusate. Does this method aid in clinical recovery? Does this contribute to problems similar to those alluded to with bolus therapy? The evidence supporting its usefulness (as contrasted to fluids containing sodium chloride alone) is not strong, but there is a great deal of circumstantial evidence attesting to its safety. It seems logical that the addition of this extra buffering capacity would help moderate the acidosis. Thus, its use seems reasonable, particularly in those whose pH is below 7.20 and whose bicarbonate concentration is below 10 mM/l.

Some clinicians prefer to use a sodium lactate solution (Ringer's lactate solution). In the majority of patients, this solution, roughly equivalent to three-fourths isotonicity, is satisfactory in the first two to four hours, and its more diluted form (half-strength Ringer's lactate solution) may be fine for maintenance. Some patients, particularly those with profound acidosis, may have a significant component of lactic acidosis, and these persons would be compromised by use of sodium lactate–containing fluids.

Insulin Management

Insulin is obviously the most important single aspect of therapy for DKA, and its clinical usage has changed markedly over the past decade. Insulin therapy today is based on more physiologic evidence than in the past, and few meaningful controversies currently exist. We will briefly discuss recommendations on the dosage of insulin and the appropriate method or route of administration. Obviously Regular or crystalline insulin must be used in order to gain an immediate effect.

Dosage of Regular Insulin

Prior to the mid-1970s, the standard insulin dose varied markedly from center to center. Given a patient with moderately severe DKA, recommendations for the initial insulin dose ranged from 2.0 to 5.0 units per kilogram of body weight. Complicated schemes utilizing blood glucose or ketone concentrations or both were occasionally used to arrive at initial dosage, but, despite the scientific façade, all were based on totally empirical conclusions. In defense of this empiricism, such strategies were partially, if not totally, responsible for a significant reduction in mortality. However, such high doses produced unphysiologic concentrations of circulating insulin (often in excess of 2000 to 3000 μU/ml); and, on occasion, certain clinical problems were felt to be directly related to these excessive insulin concentrations: hypoglycemia, cerebral edema, and the potassium-depletion syndrome. Some investigators theorized that many if not all of these problems would abate if insulin were administered in more physiologic amounts. Thus was born the era of low-dose insulin therapy; and over the last 12 years, this has generally become the standard management regimen. Multiple side-by-side and random-allocation studies have been conducted and, almost without exception, all attest to a more predictable clinical and blood glucose response to these more physiologic concentrations.

Although we adopted low-dose insulin therapy over a decade ago and are now confirmed advocates, questions still exist in our minds as to whether blaming high-dose therapy for the problems that occurred was in fact justified. Stated differently, one must still question whether the problems of hypoglycemia, cerebral edema, and hypokalemia have been significantly reduced in either number or degree.

Low-dose insulin therapy essentially uses doses of insulin that are 10 to 50 times less than those used routinely a decade ago. The most widely used current individual dose schedule recommends amounts of 0.1 unit per kilogram of body weight. Plasma insulin levels achieved with this dose are usually in the range of 100 to 200 μU/ml, and the glucose lowering effects of this dosage are

Table 12–5. INSULIN ADMINISTRATION IN DKA

Initial Dose
→0.1 U/kg body weight IV
and
→0.1 U/kg body weight IM

Subsequent Doses*
→0.1 U/kg body weight IM (or SC) *Hourly*

*If smooth fall in blood glucose of approximately 100 mg/hr does not occur, either dose should be increased to 0.2 U/kg/hr *or* route should be changed to IV.

If rate of fall of blood glucose exceeds 150 mg/hr for two consecutive hours, either dose of insulin should be reduced to 0.05 U/kg/hr or additional glucose should be added to IV fluids.

generally comparable to those achieved with high-dose therapy.

Our standard regimen for insulin administration is depicted in Table 12–5. We routinely give 0.2 U/kg body weight of Regular insulin initially (one-half by the intravenous route) and follow this with 0.1 U/kg/hr. The route of administration will be discussed subsequently.

In our last 100 cases of DKA treated by these doses, only one child did not have the desired glucose response. This child was one whose DKA was associated with a severe lobar pneumonia with an initial plasma pH of 6.90. This child required doses of about 0.3 U/kg/hr over the first three to four hours. There are a few anecdotes in the literature describing certain patients who did not respond to such low doses of insulin, but these appear to be unusual.

Route of Administration

Insulin may be given by one (or more) of three routes—intravenously (IV), intramuscularly (IM), or subcutaneously (SC)—and all three routes have been demonstrated to be effective. Fisher, Shahshahani, and Kitabchi published in 1977 a most enlightening article on this subject. Forty-five subjects with DKA were randomly allocated to one of three low-dose insulin treatment groups. After receiving a loading dose to achieve a 10 percent fall in plasma glucose, all patients received a standard dosage of 7 units Regular insulin hourly by their respective routes (approximately 0.1 U/kg body weight). All patients received similar supportive care. Figure 12–4, taken from this report, demonstrates the findings of this group with relation to plasma glucose and ketone bodies. The continuous IV insulin produced the greatest initial fall in both glucose and ketones, significantly

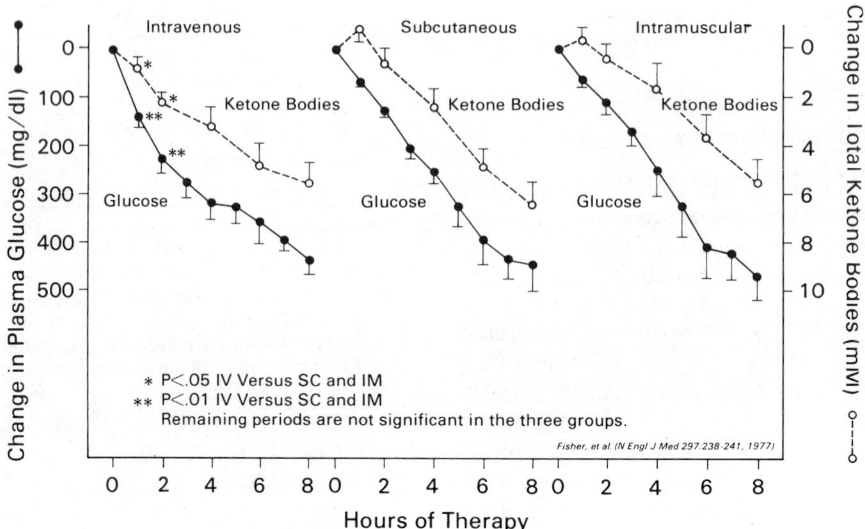

Figure 12–4. Low-dose insulin therapy in DKA. Intravenous administration of insulin produced a more dramatic fall in both glucose and ketone bodies in the first two hours of therapy. Thereafter, the rate of decline was similar in all groups with similar levels of glucose at the end of the study period. (Reprinted with permission form Fisher J, Shahshahani M, Kitabchi A: Diabetic ketoacidosis: Low dose insulin therapy by various routes. N. Engl. J. Med. 297:238, 1977.)

different in the first two hours. Thereafter, the rate of fall of blood glucose and ketones was comparable regardless of the route of administration. By the end of the third hour, the actual values were identical in all three groups, and the rate of clinical and chemical improvement was the same. Doses of approximately 0.1 U/kg at 0 and 1 hours produced drops in blood glucose at the second hour of about 225 mg/dl, 100 mg/dl, and 100 mg/dl in the persons given insulin by intravenous, subcutaneous, and intramuscular routes, respectively. The initial drop in plasma ketone bodies was even more dramatic in those treated by the intravenous route. Thus, it might appear that the best therapy would either be continuous IV therapy throughout, or an initial dose of IV therapy followed by either SC or IM doses at hourly intervals.

The *choice of route*, therefore, would seem to relate more to other factors than to response. The only absolute criterion for intravenous administration is the person who has marked contraction of peripheral vasculature in which absorption of either IM or SC insulin may be hindered. Other factors that influence this decision are past experience of the practitioner and his or her comfort with the regimen; the experience and comfort of the nursing team with the regimen; the availability of an intensive care unit; and the adequacy of peripheral veins. The first two

factors are obvious, but the latter two require brief explanation. Whereas continuous IV insulin may be the superior route for experienced personnel practicing one-on-one care in an ICU, there are potential problems of great significance if the infusion is left unattended. First, insulin delivered IV must be given using a reliable insulin pump. Even then, a worrisome problem is that insulin delivery will be interrupted: the needle may come out, the intravenous line may clog, the pump may malfunction. Because of the short half-life of insulin and the fact that insulin is being delivered in small amounts continuously (that is, 0.0017 U/kg/min), rather than in depot amounts, a person whose delivery is interrupted will be without *any* insulin after about 12 to 15 minutes. If this were not detected for some time (30 to 90 minutes), the outcome could be serious. Thus, it is our belief that *continuous IV insulin should not be used unless the person is under intensive or continuous observation.* Obviously, intensive observation can occur in areas that are not defined as ICUs, but this is more difficult to achieve.

The fourth point is the adequacy of venous access. Although this may appear superficially obvious, the point to be made is that *an intravenous access that is separate from that used for fluid therapy and blood drawing is absolutely essential.* In young children particularly, this is an important consideration.

Recommendations on Insulin Therapy

The general insulin therapy recommendations of the Children's Diabetes Management Team are noted in Table 12–5. We recommend that the initial dose be 0.2 units of Regular insulin per kilogram of body weight and that one half of this dose be given IV, the remainder being given IM (or SC). This initial dose schedule seems to have the best aspects of both routes: the IV dose establishes the initial response, and the IM (or SC) dose provides the depot effect.

Subsequent dosages of Regular insulin are advised at 0.1 unit per kilogram body weight per hour. Blood glucose values are obtained at hourly intervals at the bedside on blood taken from either fingerstick or a venous access. The optimum rate of fall of blood glucose is approximately 100 to 150 mg/hr, until the blood glucose reaches values around 250 mg/dl. If the rate of fall is significantly less than this (that is, 0 to 70 mg/hr), then either the IM dosage can be increased to 0.2 U/kg/hr or the insulin can be changed to an IV route. A blood glucose level that falls too rapidly puts the patient at greater risk for development of cerebral edema (see later) and should be seen as a cause for concern. If the rate of glucose fall exceeds 150 mg/hr, then one should either consider altering the insulin dosage or adding glucose to the infusate. If such a fall occurs for two consecutive hours, such an alteration is mandatory.

As noted earlier, glucose as a 5 percent solution should be added to the intravenous fluids when the blood glucose reaches levels around 250 mg/dl. This will aid in preventing reductions in blood gluose below 150 mg/dl, but a cut-back in the hourly insulin dosage to an equivalent of 0.05 U/kg/hr may be necessary. Alternatively, the amount of glucose may be increased to a 10 percent solution. The physician should be extremely cautious about further decreases in insulin as long as ketonuria persists, for the patient at this stage is quite susceptible to a secondary "starvation ketosis."

Monitoring

Careful monitoring and recording of sequential data on the clinical and chemical recovery process are among the most important aspects of management. A specially pre-

Table 12–6. MONITORING TREATMENT OF DKA

Parameter Monitored	Recommended Times
1. Clinical features	
a. Sensorium	a. Every 15 to 30 min
b. Vital signs	b. Every 15 to 30 min
c. Weight	c. Admission, 8 hrs, 16 hrs, 24 hrs, and then daily
2. Fluid balance	Precise recordings for
a. Intake (IV/Oral)	only those hours when IV
b. Output (urinary/GI)	fluids are being given
3. Chemical analyses	
a. Arterial blood gases*	a. Admission
b. Venous blood gases*	b. 2, 6, 10, 24 hrs
c. Na^+, K^+, Cl^-, Osm	c. Admission, 2, 6, 10, 24 hrs
d. Glucose (lab)	d. Hourly until glucose falls below 400 mg/dl; then at 4 to 6-hr intervals
e. BUN	e. Admission, 6, 24 hrs
f. Urinary Ketones	f. Admission, 6, 10, 24 hrs
4. Capillary blood glucose (bedside)	At least hourly for first 24 hrs
5. Electrocardiogram	Admission, 2, 6 hrs (continuous if admission K^+ under 3.5 mEq/l or over 7.0 mEq/l)

*See text for discussion.

pared flow sheet, inherent in most hospital programs, is essential. The main items to be monitored are noted in Table 12–6 and are discussed below.

Clinical Features

The most important item to evaluate is the condition of the child, particularly the status of the sensorium. Children who may be wide awake and conversant at initiation of therapy frequently become sleepy or more lethargic after intravenous fluid therapy is started. This may be attributed to normal relaxation as anxiety and apprehension are relieved. These children should be easily arousable. On the other hand, a child who is not arousable except with painful stimulation (that is, semicomatose) should be suspected of having worsening cerebral edema. Return to a normal level of cerebral functioning may be delayed for 12 to 24 hours.

The initial blood pressure is often slightly elevated, secondary to the massive sympathetic response with peripheral vascular constriction and tachycardia. Only with extreme dehydration will the initial blood pressure be low, and this is often an ominous finding. With optimum therapy, the pulse usually begins to gradually slow after two to three hours and blood pressure returns to normal. Sudden decreases in heart rate, particularly if coupled with a rise in blood pressure are suggestive of impending problems with cerebral edema. The slowing of the respiratory rate parallels improvement in the degree of metabolic acidosis. Minimal slowing may occur in the first hour as anxiety lessens, but Kussmaul's respirations may not abate for four to six hours. A completely normal respiratory rhythm may not return for 12 to 18 hours. Sudden changes in the respiratory rhythm—particularly brief periods of choking or apneic episodes—are bothersome and may also suggest cerebral edema.

Weight measurements can provide the best overall estimate of improvement in hydration or of underhydration or overhydration, but to be useful, the weighing technique must be meticulous and precise. The initial weight should be obtained *after* all tubes, monitors, and catheters (venous) are attached to the patient. Eight hours after starting therapy, the child should have increased weight by 6 to 8 percent. If a weight-gain of 6 percent has not been achieved, it suggests that fluid administration should be increased. On the other hand, a weight gain of 9 percent or more in this first period suggests that the rate of infusion is excessive and the child is accumulating too much fluid. Thus, the usual 20-kilogram child with DKA should gain between 1.2 and 1.6 kilograms in the first eight hours. A gain of only 0.5 kilogram would suggest that concurrent losses are greater than anticipated. A gain of 2.0 kilograms would suggest that the initial assessment of the degree of hydration was excessive. Both would dictate a recalculation of fluids for the next time period.

Most children with DKA will have increased their weight by 10 to 12 percent at the end of 16 hours and by 12 to 15 percent at the end of 24 hours. A number of children may have mild clinical edema, detected at either 24 or 48 hours. This is usually transient and is thought to be due to salt and water retention secondary to increased secretions of aldosterone and antidiuretic hormone.

Fluid Balance

We believe that the best estimate of cumulative fluid balance is weight data. Most physicians also feel a need for some formative data between these eight-hour blocks of time. Thus, measurements of intake and output are traditional, and, when viewed in the context of other parameters, may be useful. To be meaningful, however, the basic characteristics of intake and output data must be appreciated. Several points are worth noting: (1) The aim is for the ratio of intake:output to be positive, indicating that the patient is retaining fluids; (2) intravenous fluid intake is easily measured, but all oral intake (that is, fluids, ice chips, water content of foodstuffs) must also be closely measured; (3) only urinary output is easily measured, and even this may be immeasurably lost owing to uncontrolled voiding; (4) the amount of emesis or gastric aspirant should be either measured or carefully estimated; and (5) one of the major losses of water from the body is insensible, that loss during breathing as the ambient air is warmed and humidified. (This latter loss may be quite high in the person with deep, pauseless respirations.) These points indicate the intrinsic difficulties with using this system as the sole means of monitoring hydration status.

Chemical Analyses

Monitoring of *arterial blood gases* (pH, P_{CO_2} bicarbonate), if available, is desirable at the time of admission, for it gives a definitive estimate of the severity of the situation. But even if the technology to perform blood gases is present, the ability to obtain an arterial puncture may be a limiting factor, particularly for repeated assessments. On the other hand, therapy is rarely if ever modified on the basis of the arterial pH but on the basis of the bicarbonate concentration. Since the concentration of bicarbonate in venous blood is rarely more than 1.0 to 1.5 mM/l different from arterial blood bicarbonate, it seems superfluous to perform serial arterial punctures.

We recommend *venous blood gas* determinations to be performed at 2, 6, 10, and 24 hours after admission. Additional samples are not generally helpful. There is rarely a significant improvement between zero and two hours, but a worsening of the acidosis would not be desirable. Usually, by the time of the six-hour sample, the initial bicarbonate value should have roughly doubled or be approaching 10 mM/l. Even in the most severe case, the plasma bicarbonate should be around 15 mM/l by 10 hours of treatment. A rate of improvement significantly less than this suggests one or more of the following: (1) inadequate insulin effect in blocking ketogenosis; (2) inadequate return of renal function; (3) insufficient buffering capacity of the ECF. Alterations in therapy designed to correct the deficiency are appropriate.

Electrolyte (Na^+, K^+, Cl^-) determinations should be performed at admission and at 2, 6, 10, and 24 hours, if the clinical progress of management is proceeding smoothly. *Osmolality* also should either be measured or calculated on admission and at 2 and 6 hours. Reduction in plasma osmolality should be between 3 mOsm/hr and 8 to 10 mOsm/hr during the first six hours and should not fall more rapidly than 8 to 10 mOsm/hr. This will moderate a shift of free water into the ICF and lessen the likelihood of cerebral edema.

Glucose (hospital lab), BUN, and urinary ketones are three additional studies that we consider routine. Venous or capillary blood glucose is measured hourly in the hospital laboratory until the value falls below 400 mg/dl. This practice is due to the fact that bedside methods are very inexact at levels over 400 mg/dl. The BUN gives a rough measure of renal function, but one must remember that renal function can decline by 50 percent or more before the BUN will rise above normal levels. Urinary ketones are monitored in order to have another check on the adequacy of therapy. Ketonuria should generally clear between 12 and 24 hours. We see no benefit in the routine measurement of plasma or serum ketones.

Capillary Blood Glucose Determinations

These should be performed hourly at the bedside by use of glucose-oxidase strips, either read visually or by an optical instrument. Control samples should be checked at the beginning and end of each nursing shift, and the machine should be recalibrated according to the manufacturers' recommendations.

Electrocardiograms

These should be performed at onset, and, if normal, a rhythm strip (lead II, at least) should be obtained at two hours. If there are abnormalities in the QRS or T-wave complexes or if the initial serum potassium is below 3.5 mEq/l or above 7.0 mEq/l, constant monitoring should be performed.

Other Studies

Additional studies that might occasionally be performed during the course of DKA are monitoring of serum concentrations of calcium, phosphorus, and magnesium. We do not generally consider these as essential unless the initial value is low. Even then, determinations at 0 and 24 hours are all that is necessary unless symptoms arise.

Expected Outcome

The expected outcome is a prompt return to health. Except in unusual circumstances (see later), the hyperglycemic syndrome and the serious acidosis should be corrected within 8 to 12 hours after initiation of therapy. Intravenous fluids are usually discontinued sometime between 18 and 36 hours, depending mostly on the child's alertness and willingness to consume oral fluids, which are usually started after 8 to 12 hours.

Conversion to Intermediate-Acting Insulins

This is a matter of some concern to many, and there are a number of ways of effecting this conversion. Our plan for the newly diagnosed diabetic differs from that for the diabetic with an established disease.

For the newly diagnosed diabetic, the precise amount of insulin needed for the maintenance of metabolic balance is unknown, and we usually keep the child on Regular insulin for two to four days while establishing the required total daily dose. Our general plan is initiated as soon as the IV is discontinued and the child is placed on a three-meal, two- or three-snack regimen. The total amount of insulin required during the previous four hours is then given subcutaneously before each of the three regular meals. At bedtime (about 10:00 PM), this same dosage is given as either NPH or Lente insulin. The children at this stage have their capillary blood glucose levels monitored seven or eight times daily (that is, before each meal, two hours after each meal, at bedtime, and at 3:00 AM) and modifications in insulin are made as necessary. After three to four days, most children are converted to a two-shot or three-shot per day regimen.

For the established diabetic recovering from DKA, our plan may be the same as the aforementioned, if we believe that recent control was poor. Otherwise, the child is returned to his or her standard dosage and schedule as soon as possible.

POSSIBLE COMPLICATIONS

The possible complications of DKA are multiple, and some will not even receive mention here. Instead, we will concentrate briefly on those complications that are most common and most likely to be encountered. These are listed neither in order of frequency nor in order of severity.

Hypoglycemia

Hypoglycemia, particularly of the severe variety, is no longer reported as frequently with low-dose insulin therapy as it was formerly with higher-dose therapy. This may be attributed to dosage but is more probably a factor of less-frequent (and bigger) doses given in the past and of better patient monitoring achieved today with bedside techniques.

Mild hypoglycemia is occasionally observed in patients on low-dose therapy, and the physician must aggressively act to prevent its worsening. Whenever we have observed this, the patients' conditions have always been similar. The physician should be attuned to such possible events as those in the following typical case:

G.J., a 14-year-old girl with IDDM of six years' duration, was in only fair carbohydrate control (HbA$_{1C}$ 13 per cent) when she developed a respiratory illness with fever, sore throat, and anorexia. She developed ketonuria on the second day of the illness and began Regular insulin supplementation at 8 units every two hours. When her blood glucose remained over 400 mg/dl, she increased the dose to 15 units every two hours. She remained anorexic and did not take fluids. Thirty-six hours into the illness, she developed vomiting. Her blood glucose and urinary ketones remained high, and during the 24 hours prior to admission she had received her usual NPH insulin dose (48 units) plus a total of 92 units of Regular insulin.

On admission, G.J. had severe DKA with blood glucose of 640 mg/dl and plasma pH of 6.86. She had marked tachycardia and marked peripheral vascular constriction.

Therapy was instituted in the usual fashion, and she responded appropriately. Six hours into this treatment, her blood glucose was between 150 and 200 mg/dl, her bicarbonate was 12 mM/l, and her appearance was good. She had 5 percent glucose in the infusate, and she had received her last dose of IM insulin (5 units) at 3:00 PM. At 4:00 PM, the blood glucose was 180; at 5:00 PM, it was 140 mg/dl; at 6:00 PM, it was 90 mg/dl, and 10 per cent glucose was then started. At 6:30 PM, blood glucose had dropped to 65 mg/dl, and the glucose concentration was increased to 15 percent. Between 7:00 PM and midnight, the level varied between 80 and 130 mg/dl despite continued 15 percent glucose infusions. By 3:00 AM, the blood glucose had risen to 160 mg/dl and ultimately stabilized around 200 mg/dl, and the infusate was then changed to 5 percent glucose.

It is our supposition that this girl had not absorbed much of the Regular insulin that had been given at home. Then, as her hydration and circulation improved, this insulin was mobilized.

Persistent Acidosis–Lactic Acidosis

Acidosis with bicarbonate values of less than 10 mM/l that persists for longer than six to eight hours should be evaluated as to cause. The most common cause of this condition is inadequately treated DKA. Specifically, this means too little insulin effect, and this is characterized by persisting hyperglycemia and ketonemia. The causes for this condition might be too little insulin to counteract the stress hormone production, decreased peripheral absorption of injected insulin (either SQ or IM), or some other cause of relative insulin resistance. Appropriate action is to (1) change insulin administration to continuous intravenous administration and (2) increase the dose to 0.2 unit per kilogram body weight per hour for the next one to two hours. Occasionally there have been patients in whom usual doses of insulin, even when given intravenously, are not effective. A step-wise increase in hourly dosage is the correct procedure.

In severely dehydrated persons with DKA, and particularly in those who have had an episode of either hypotension or apnea, a superimposed lactic acidosis may be present. Many of these patients have already shown a glycemic response to insulin. Their lactate-to-pyruvate ratio is increased. Management

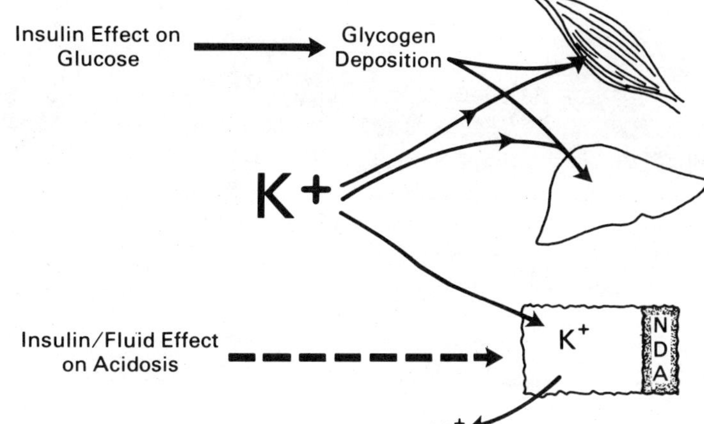

Figure 12–5. Effect of treatment on potassium.

consists of ensuring adequate tissue hydration and oxygenation. Judicious increases in the rate of bicarbonate infusion are appropriate, but even in these cases, bolus infusions are not indicated.

Another cause of persistent acidosis is inadequate renal compensation. This generally occurs only in those children who have experienced a shocklike episode and have acquired a degree of acute tubular necrosis. Management is conservative with adequate hydration and judicious administration of bicarbonate in a slightly increased concentration.

Hypokalemic Syndrome

The person with DKA who has an initial serum potassium at or below 4 mEq/l is at risk, and that risk increases as the level of potassium falls. Extracellular potassium concentrations regularly fall as therapy is initiated (Fig. 12–5). This drop in potassium is due to (1) deposition of potassium with the increased synthesis and formation of glycogen, and (2) re-entry of potassium into cells as the acidosis is corrected. Thus, the most basic aspect of therapy, insulin, is the primary cause of this fall. Most investigators recommend waiting until renal functional status is determined to be adequate before starting potassium therapy. Others recommend starting potassium replacement with the initial bottle of fluid if the initial potassium value is less than 3.0 mEq/l. Based on experience, we agree with the latter approach, and in fact might go one step further. In patients whose initial potassium value is at or below 3.0 mEq/l, we would recommend vigorous administration of hydration fluids containing potassium *before* administration of insulin. In such cases, a delay of insulin administration for one to two hours will not be detrimental and may be much safer.

The consequences of significant hypokalemia include, most importantly, myocardial conduction defects with arrythmias. Cardiac arrest may occur. An additional consequence is marked muscular weakness, in its worse state manifested as muscular paralysis. Therapy, obviously, involves the administration of potassium intravenously in amounts needed to restore the patient's muscle contractility to normal. Concentrations in excess of 100 mEq/l have occasionally been necessary. Continuous EKG monitoring is also essential.

Cerebral Edema

This is the most serious consequence of DKA and of its therapy. The etiology of cerebral edema is multifactorial. Accumulation of idiogenetic osmols in the CNS, mostly polyols, are felt to be largely responsible. These sugar alcohols accumulate under the influence of the massive transport of glucose into the CNS during hyperglycemia. Figure 12–6 graphically demonstrates one mechanism by which these osmotically active substances create a water drag from the ECF, as blood glucose and ECF osmolality decline under treatment. Additional factors contributing to cerebral edema are severe acidosis, anoxia, and other less-well defined etiologies.

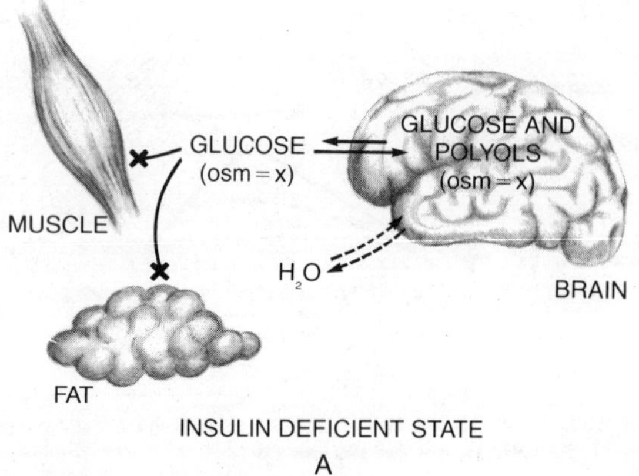

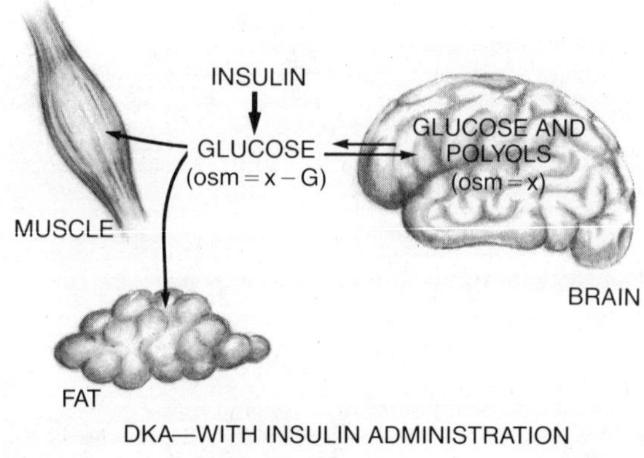

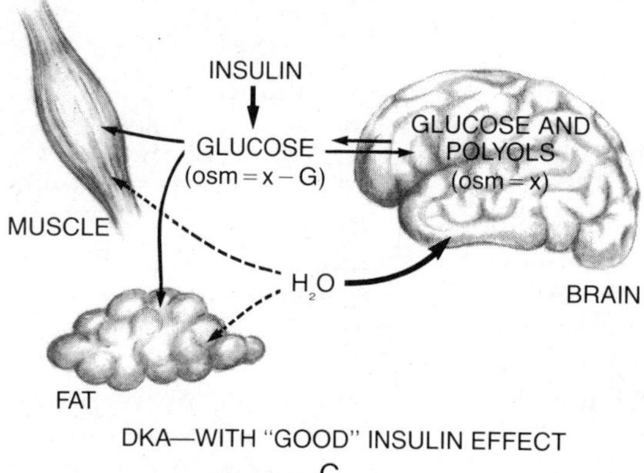

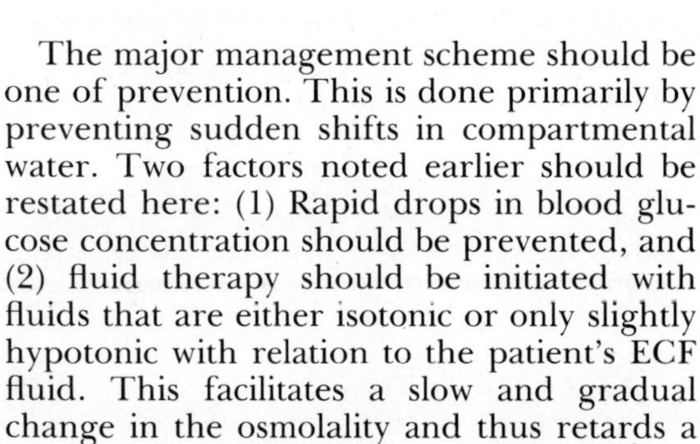

Figure 12–6. *A*, In the insulin-deficient state, glucose transport into insulin-sensitive tissues is limited, but entry into the brain is by mass action. Glucose undergoes slow metabolic processing within the CNS and the osmolality in the ECF and ICF (that is, brain) are equal (here noted as X). *B*, When insulin is given, glucose transport into insulin-sensitive tissues is facilitated and plasma glucose falls. This drop in glucose is reflected in a drop in ECF osmolality where Osm = X − G (G represents fall in glucose). Brain osmolality remains unchanged. *C*, Because there is now a disproportionate osmolality between the ICF and ECF, water moves readily into the ICF, producing edema.

The major management scheme should be one of prevention. This is done primarily by preventing sudden shifts in compartmental water. Two factors noted earlier should be restated here: (1) Rapid drops in blood glucose concentration should be prevented, and (2) fluid therapy should be initiated with fluids that are either isotonic or only slightly hypotonic with relation to the patient's ECF fluid. This facilitates a slow and gradual change in the osmolality and thus retards a rapid shift in intracellular water content.

If cerebral edema becomes marked, cerebral functioning declines, the first clinical evidence of which may be worsened somnolence, bradycardia, and/or apnea. Cardiorespiratory arrest may occur and ophthalmoscopic examination may reveal classic evidence of papilledema. In such cases, the prognosis is often grave and specific therapy may not be helpful. On the other hand, some children with very serious cerebral edema do survive and have restored mental and motor functioning. Aggressive therapy is not likely to be harmful if the diagnosis is certain. Such therapy should include intravenous dexametha-

sone and a mannitol infusion (1.0 to 1.5 g/kg body weight), as well as the judicious use of anticonvulsants. A neurologic consultant is often of immense assistance.

SUMMARY

DKA is a serious complication of Type I diabetes. The mortality rate in this country is still unacceptably high. To reduce this rate, two items are essential: earlier recognition and better treatment.

Early recognition allows the physician to treat the condition in its milder form before severe dehydration develops. Once the latter occurs, it is imperative to initiate hydrating fluid therapy and to blunt the glucose and ketone body production with insulin supplementation.

The hospitalized child with DKA is at risk and should be carefully observed and monitored until oral fluids can be restarted and intravenous fluids discontinued. Cerebral edema is the worst of several complications of DKA.

13

Hypoglycemia

Hypoglycemia is the most common acute complication occurring in the person with IDDM. Whereas in the nondiabetic, hypoglycemia is defined as a blood glucose concentration of less than 40 mg/dl, the definition of hypoglycemia in the diabetic is often determined by the clinical picture as well as by the level of blood glucose.

Hypoglycemia is a common accompaniment of the patient with well-controlled diabetes, and it may be impossible with current management tools adequately to control hyperglycemia without periodically incurring hypoglycemia. This is one reason why many physicians and some young patients are hesitant about the attainment of "tight" control. Hypoglycemia is disliked by diabetic patients, for it tends to make them feel unwell and to produce symptoms that set them apart from peers. Many young persons seem willing to risk the potential complications related to hyperglycemia, in order to avoid the immediate inconvenience of symptomatic hypoglycemia. This represents one of the most important challenges for the diabetes team.

Hypoglycemia can produce disorientation, convulsions, or unconsciousness, or any combination of these. It may be mistaken by the layman for results of either drug or alcohol abuse. Such a mistake can have dire consequences. For this reason, the Medic Alert bracelet or necklace is recommended and may be life saving. One of these can be obtained from Medic Alert (PO Box 1009, Turlock, California 95381). The emblem or insignia is widely known and recognized. On the reverse side of the insignia, the wearer's medical problem is identified, along with the member's identification number and the Medic Alert toll-free answering service number.

PATHOGENESIS AND PREDISPOSING CAUSES

Simply stated, hypoglycemia is usually the consequence of a relative excess of insulin action. Table 13–1 outlines the usual mechanisms. Hypoglycemia may be produced by various factors that lead to absolute increases in circulating free insulin, increased utilization of glucose by insulin-dependent tissues, or an inadequate glucose-regulatory response.

The ability to measure free insulin levels is a relatively recent tool available to the investigator studying insulin-glucose dynamics. Various conditions have now been identified in which there is an absolute increase in the circulating level of free insulin. The result of this absolute increase is that more glucose is utilized by insulin-dependent tissues, with consequent lowering of the blood glucose and reduction of the amount available to the central nervous system. Some of these conditions are discussed in detail here.

Excessive Insulin Administration

Although this appears to be an obvious case of hypoglycemia, it may be erroneously

Table 13–1. **PATHOGENESIS OF HYPOGLYCEMIA**

A. Absolute Increase in Free-Insulin Levels
 1. Excess insulin administration
 2. Increased absorption of insulin from depot
  a. Exercise
  b. Warmth of site
  c. Massage of site
  d. Characteristics of either insulin or injection
 3. Alterations in antibody binding of circulating insulin
 4. Decreased destruction of insulin
B. Dietary
 1. Prolonged fasting
 2. Missed meals
 3. Decreased gastrointestinal absorption
C. Increased Utilization of Glucose
 1. Exercise
 2. Hypercatabolic states
D. Inadequate Glucoregulatory Response
 1. Neuroendocrine dysfunction
 2. Hepatic factors
 3. Metabolic
  a. Alcohol consumption
  b. Adrenergic blocking drugs

assumed that it is a rare or unusual occurrence. On an average of three or four times per year, a member of our team receives a call from a patient who has suddenly realized (after giving his or her insulin injection) that the doses of the Regular and intermediate-acting insulins were reversed. These calls come from the diabetic patient who recognizes that a mistake was made and is concerned about the consequences. One must wonder how often this mistake goes unrecognized.

On occasion, the reason for recurrent hypoglycemia may be unrecognized excessive insulin administration. The following case summary is an example:

P.T., a 14-month-old child, developed diabetes at 10 months of age. From the beginning, the control of blood glucose was erratic, despite much attention from the local physician and parents. At the time of her referral to the Children's Diabetes Management Center, P.T. was receiving two injections of U-100 insulin per day (3 NPH/1 Regular in the morning; 1 NPH at supper). She was experiencing three to five severe hypoglycemia episodes per week, but her average blood glucose values were "too high" and her HbA_{1C} was 10.6 percent. Her weight was 13 kg.

Upon admission, our first maneuver was to change P.T.'s insulin type to a U-25 insulin specifically diluted for her. The parents then administered this diluted insulin drawn into a U-100 syringe in the following amounts: 12 NPH/4 Regular in the morning; 2 NPH/2 Regular at supper. Despite the fact that this is the same insulin dosage, the extreme fluctuation in blood glucose

abated and severe hypoglycemia episodes disappeared. Some final manipulations were made before sending the child home, where relative stability of the diabetes has persisted.

Even when using the low-dose insulin syringe and while practicing extreme care in insulin withdrawal, it is difficult to be accurate when dealing with such small doses. A 0.5-unit mistake in either this child's morning Regular or evening NPH dose represented a 50 percent change in available insulin. Would anybody have been surprised if hypoglycemia occurred in a patient with tightly controlled diabetes whose evening NPH dose was suddenly increased from 10 to 15 units? Probably not; and yet an increase from 1 unit to 1½ units represents a change of the same magnitude.

Excessive insulin administration is also seen in persons who make a practice of treating already existing hyperglycemia, rather than attempting to prevent its occurrence. The following case example demonstrates this problem:

S.N., an 11-year-old boy, was first seen in our camp after two years of diabetes. He, his parents, and their diabetologist were making heroic attempts to precisely control his diabetes.

He was monitoring his blood glucose level four to seven times per day and was on a split-mixed insulin regimen (15 Lente/5 Regular in the morning; 5 Lente/5 Regular at supper). Additionally, he was instructed to administer:

1 unit Regular for any blood glucose level of 100 to 120 mg/dl
2 units Regular for any blood glucose level of 120 to 150 mg/dl
3 units Regular for any blood glucose level of 150 to 180 mg/dl
4 units Regular for any blood glucose level of 180 to 210 mg/dl
5 units Regular for any blood glucose level of 210 to 240 mg/dl

Precamp history revealed that this compulsive family spent almost two hours per day managing diabetes and that the boy averaged three extra shots of insulin per day. In the one-month period prior to camp, they had recorded 16 hypoglycemic episodes, all described as being mild. His HbA_{1C} was in the midnormal range.

One additional group of patients with excessive administration of insulin is worthy of mention. This group consists of children who intentionally administer extra Regular insulin as a means of gaining attention or as a "cry for help." These youngsters, mostly adolescents, are generally bright and seemingly motivated but usually have significant personality disorders. Profound hyperlability without apparent cause is the usual indication.

As the desire to achieve normal glycemia has become more common, so too has the occurrence of significant hypoglycemia. In a prospective study of symptomatic hypoglycemia in children with IDDM, Goldstein and Massry (1978) studied 147 children during an 18-month period. Of these, 53 percent did not experience hypoglycemia; 33 percent had mild, infrequent hypoglycemia episodes; 10 percent had mild, frequent episodes; and 4 percent had severe episodes associated with altered levels of consciousness. The level of diabetic control in the group was assessed by measurement of glycosylated hemoglobin and found to be 9.5 percent, 7.9 percent, 7.5 percent, and 7 percent, respectively, with normal values of 5.4 percent. Thus, patients whose diabetes was in better biochemical control had more frequent and more severe hypoglycemia. Indeed, several investigators have emphasized the risk of hypoglycemia for patients attempting to achieve consistent euglycemia.

Increased Absorption of Depot Insulin

As noted in Chapter 8, exercise of the extremity in which an injection of depot insulin has been administered accelerates the absorption and subsequent action of that insulin. This results in a transient period of hyperinsulinemia and a later period when there is inadequate insulin action. Injection of insulin in sites that are removed from the areas of vigorous activity decreases this effect. Other investigators have noted that the temperature at the injection site influences insulin absorption (heat accelerates absorption, whereas cold retards it). Additionally, massage of the site of injection accelerates absorption.

Insulin absorption, even when not influenced by these factors, is not uniform from day to day. There are minor variations in the rate of absorption so that the insulin action curve varies slightly. In most persons, this does not significantly affect blood glucose control, but, in the person who is rigidly controlled, such variations may be significant and may lead to occasional episodes of hypoglycemia.

Alterations in Antibody Binding of Circulating Insulin

Beef and pork insulin elicit an antibody response, and a certain percentage of injected insulin binds to the antibody and thus has no hypoglycemic effect. This antibody-bound insulin is later taken up and destroyed by the reticuloendothelial system. In general, the percentage of insulin bound to antibody is relatively constant from day to day, but minor variations (amounting to several percent) are regularly observed. Whether this represents true differences in the day-to-day binding or whether the variations relate to technical problems with the assay is not certain. In the diabetic who is only partially controlled, these differences of four to six percent are probably inconsequential, but in the rigidly controlled diabetic, such differences in the level of free insulin may be critical and lead to symptomatic hypoglycemia.

Dietary Variations

Hypoglycemia is frequently associated with missed or delayed meals, particularly when the patient is receiving intermediate-acting insulins and the control of diabetes is tight. This is of great significance in the very young child whose central nervous system has a high demand for glucose but in whom less glucose is available from storage sites. An overnight fast may deplete glycogen stores and make the child particularly susceptible to early morning hypoglycemia.

Increased Utilization of Glucose

This subject has been discussed extensively in Chapter 8 and will not be discussed further here. The effect of exercise on lowering of blood glucose is probably multifactorial, including increased insulin absorption, increased number of insulin receptors, increased affinity of the receptors for insulin, and other factors.

Inadequate Glucoregulatory Response

This general term takes into account many of the poorly explained hypoglycemic episodes that are known to occur.

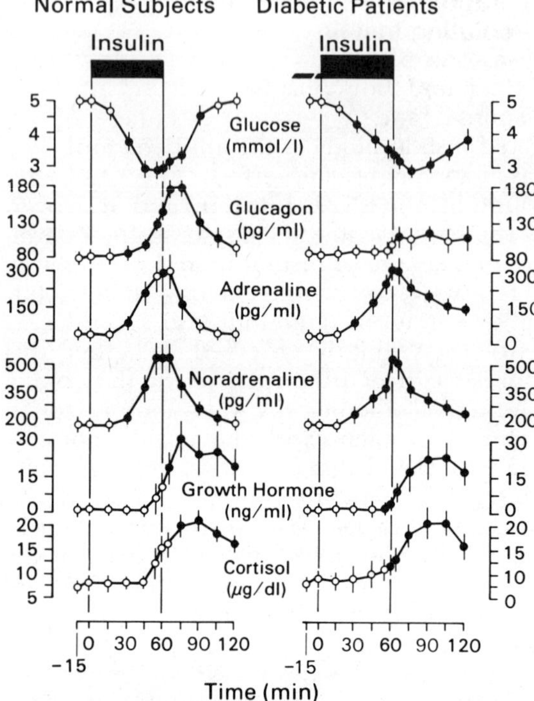

Figure 13–1. The counter-regulatory response to insulin-induced hypoglycemia in normal subjects and in diabetic patients. The diabetic patients fail to exhibit a normal glucagon response to hypoglycemia, whereas their adrenalin, noradrenalin, growth hormone, and cortisol responses are normal. (Reprinted with permission from Bolli G, Calabrese G, DeFeo P, et al.: Lack of glucagon response in glucose counter-regulation in type I diabetics: Absence of recovery after prolonged optimal insulin therapy. Diabetologia 22:100, 1982.)

Neuroendocrine Dysfunction

Various investigators have demonstrated a poor catecholamine response to insulin-induced hypoglycemia in those persons with autonomic neuropathy. More recently, investigators in St. Louis (Santiago and co-workers, 1984) have also demonstrated a diminished catecholamine response in some children who had no other evidence of autonomic neuropathy. They propose that such persons be identified by specific testing in order that the insulin-food regimens can be sufficiently modified so as to prevent severe hypoglycemia.

Bolli and associates (1982) have also noted poor glucagon response in some persons with insulin-induced hypoglycemia (Fig. 13–1). A more common occurrence, however, is a reduced glycogenolysis in response to an adequate hormonal stimulus. This occurs most frequently in the poorly controlled diabetic who has diminished glycogen stores. As noted earlier, the infant whose diabetes is in good control may demonstrate diminished glycogen stores even after an overnight fast. Unger and Orci (1981) also have suggested that those patients with hyperinsulinemia (and tight control) have such marked inhibition of hepatic glucose production that even maximum counter-regulatory responses are inadequate.

Alcohol Consumption

Alcohol consumption in patients with diabetes may also be associated with hypoglycemia. This is most commonly seen in persons who have previously depleted their glycogen stores through poor intake and through fasting. The effect of alcohol is most likely an inhibitory one of gluconeogenesis, but other mechanisms have also been postulated. Other aspects are covered in Chapter 21.

CLINICAL MANIFESTATIONS

The symptoms and signs of hypoglycemia are not exclusively dependent on the absolute level of blood glucose. Although it is true that diabetics and nondiabetics alike will have symptoms of hypoglycemia if their blood glucose levels are under 40 mg/dl, rapid and significant drops in blood glucose levels may also elicit a symptomatic response, even when the lower glucose level is still in the hyperglycemic range. DeFronzo and associates (1980) have conclusively shown that, in patients with long-standing hyperglycemia (that is, those whose diabetes is in poor control), an acute lowering of blood glucose from levels around 300 to 400 mg/dl to levels around 150 mg/dl will be associated with a counter-regulatory response and symptomatic "hypoglycemia."

The manifestations of hypoglycemia are both neurologic (CNS, or "brain" symptoms) and neuroendocrine (counter-regulatory). The nervous system, both central and peripheral, consists of non-insulin-dependent tissue; and yet glucose may be looked upon as its sole metabolic nutrient. Normal metabolic function and oxygen utilization is intimately tied to glucose transport and utilization. Glucose entry into nervous system tissue appears to be most clearly related to its extracellular concentration, and both active and passive transport mechanisms are postulated. Because of this unique dependence on glucose, it is not surprising that brain function

Table 13–2. CLINICAL CATEGORIES OF HYPOGLYCEMIA

A. Nervous System Manifestations (Primary)
1. Disorientation
2. Confusion
3. Dizziness
4. Personality or Behavior Change
5. Hunger
6. Visual Changes
7. Nerve Palsy
8. Alterations in Consciousness
  Lethargy
  Somnolence
  Convulsions
  Coma
B. Neuroendocrine Manifestations (Secondary)
1. Shakiness
2. Tremors
3. Hot or cold sensations
4. Tachycardia, palpitations
5. Palor
6. Sweating
7. Abdominal discomfort
8. Nausea, vomiting

Table 13–3. SYMPTOMATIC HYPOGLYCEMIA—CLINICAL FEATURES

A. Mild
1. Weakness, tiredness
2. Shakiness, tremors, anxiety
3. Increased hunger
B. Moderate
1. Altered consciousness (sleepy, lethargic)
2. Change in personality (inappropriate behaviors)
3. Tachycardia
4. Pale, cold skin
5. Hot or cold feelings
6. Hypothermia
7. Inappropriate sweating
C. Severe
1. Unconsciousness (coma)
2. Convulsions

is significantly altered when blood values fall below certain critical levels. Actual and irreversible brain damage has been reported with severe and prolonged hypoglycemia, and this has also been suspected following recurrent episodes of hypoglycemia in the infant.

Usual Clinical Features

Table 13–2 divides the clinical features of hypoglycemia into those that represent pure nervous system dysfunction (primary) and those that are generated by the outpouring of counter-regulatory hormones (secondary). For reasons considered below, this distinction has profound clinical significance.

As noted earlier, brain functioning deteriorates in the face of hypoglycemia, and there are specific symptoms and signs of this dysfunctional state. Generally, the primary features are more closely tied to the presence of absolute hypoglycemia than are the secondary clinical features (i.e., those occurring as a result of the neuroendocrine hyper-responsiveness). The primary, or brain, symptoms and signs may be more difficult for the individual with diabetes to identify. Mental confusion occurs early, and this confusion may not only prevent personal recognition of hypoglycemia but may also promote actual rejection and denial of the idea. For the observer, the changes in behavior represent the most reliable indicator of hypoglycemia, but the casual acquaintance or uninitiated observer may not consider that such altered behavior is an indication of hypoglycemia.

As blood sugar approaches the level of absolute hypoglycemia or when there is a sudden drop in blood glucose concentration, neuroendocrine activity increases. This elicits signs and symptoms that are more easily recognized both by the person with diabetes and the observer. When these features are observed, the recovery process is already in operation. Usually, the person with diabetes is taught to respond to these symptoms with food ingestion; but these symptoms are nonspecific as to causative factors. Similar neuroendocrine symptoms and signs occur with anxiety and with fear of exercise. Consequently, the person with diabetes may mistakenly and inappropriately treat such symptoms when blood glucose values are actually normal to high.

As overall diabetic control approaches optimal levels, it is more likely that the primary symptoms will predominate early. Only later, after mental confusion may have occurred, will the secondary features become evident; and by this time, they may not be recognized. Thus, it is more likely that the patient with well-controlled diabetes will experience unrecognized hypoglycemia than it is for the patient with poorly controlled diabetes.

In Table 13–3, the clinical features of hypoglycemia are tabulated on the basis of their clinical severity. Such a classification is helpful when the physician considers whether or not to intervene in an attempt to alter either the frequency or the severity of episodes. Mild episodes are common in the patient with well-controlled diabetes and may not require intervention. To be appropriately labeled "mild," episodes should also be easily recognized by the individual and quickly relieved by appropriate food ingestion. Those listed as "moderate" should not generally occur with a frequency of more than once per month without consideration being given to alterations in therapy. "Severe" episodes are to be avoided, and the frequency of their occurrences dictates preventative measures.

Nighttime Hypoglycemia

Hypoglycemia occurring at night carries a greater potential risk for the person, since spontaneous awakening may not occur during the early decline of blood glucose to hypoglycemia levels. Thus, the presence of nighttime hypoglycemia may be first suspected when the child has a seizure or when attempts are made to awaken him or her the next morning. There is often great concern and anxiety among parents relative to this potential problem, and many take extreme measures to prevent such occurrences, sometimes to the detriment of both child and family. Fortunately, it would appear that the anxiety or agitation phase of hypoglycemia most often awakens the person, and he or she either seeks or is given sufficient carbohydrate to recover without consequence. Additionally, if adequate glycogen stores are available and if the person is normally responsive, there will be an endogenous correction of the hypoglycemia.

When one considers the diurnal pattern of blood glucose in either the nondiabetic or the diabetic who is treated by virtually any insulin regimen, the occurrence of nighttime hypoglycemia is not surprising. Blood glucose values are normally lowest between 2:00 and 4:00 AM, and this corresponds with the time of greatest frequency of severe nighttime hypoglycemia in the diabetic. After 4:00 AM, normal increases in cortisol and other stress hormones tend to cause a rise in blood glucose by the time of usual awakening. Many diabetologists, particularly those advocating tight control, recommend that periodic blood sugars be obtained between 2:00 and 4:00 AM. This seems mandatory when the pre-breakfast blood glucose is consistently low.

Because nighttime hypoglycemia is of considerable importance and because it may go undetected based on the usual criteria, some common predisposing factors and outlines of those occurrences that should provoke sus-

Table 13–4. HYPOGLYCEMIA OCCURRING AT NIGHT

A. Conditions That May Predispose
  1. Attempts to consistently achieve normoglycemia
  2. Missed or inadequate evening meal
  3. Missed or inadequate before-bed snack (if usual)
  4. Unusual or vigorous activity between supper and bedtime
  5. Hypoglycemia episode occurring earlier in day
B. Occurrences That Produce Suspicions
  1. Recurrent nightmares
  2. Recurrent nightsweats
  3. "Feeling bad" on arising (i.e., morning headaches, drugged look, "hung-over" appearance)
  4. Hypoglycemia before breakfast
  5. Blood glucose values in the morning that are
    a. Consistently below 80 mg/dl
    b. Often below 60 mg/dl
  6. Normoglycemia before breakfast with ketonuria
  7. Morning blood glucose consistently higher than bedtime glucose (particularly if the latter is in normal range)
C. Confirmation
  Blood glucose values below 60 mg/dl between 2:00 and 4:00 A.M.

picions are shown in Table 13–4. Nighttime hypoglycemia should be confirmed by the determination of low blood glucose values, obtained on several occasions. The finding of documented levels below 60 mg/dl confirms the diagnosis. The inability to detect such low values does not refute the diagnosis, nor should it necessarily remove the suspicion. Several investigators have recommended the use of urinary cortisol values obtained on overnight samples as indicators of asymptomatic nocturnal hypoglycemia. Whereas early studies demonstrated a rise in the urinary cortisol/creatinine ratio, some more recent studies have questioned the usefulness of such a procedure. These later studies suggest that the urine collection must be obtained within three hours of a hypoglycemic episode in order to be valid. Clinical testing of a wristwatch-like instrument, the Sleep Sentry (Teledyne Avionics), is encouraging. This instrument detects changes in skin temperature and conductivity (sweating) and signals an alarm. It may be useful in certain children. The false-negative rate is low, but the false-positive rate may be a problem.

Behavioral Responses

Parental fear of hypoglycemia and its consequences is often so intense that there is a reluctance to control hyperglycemia adequately. Children object to the feelings of being "out of control" during hypoglycemic episodes and have concerns about the embarrassment that is occasionally associated with it. This latter fear is of particular concern to the adolescent who does not wish to be singled out by peers if strange or unusual behaviors are manifest. The responses of the parent and child represent barriers to good carbohydrate control. The young person may try to prevent hypoglycemia by purposeful overeating. Still others are so attuned to the nonspecific secondary symptoms that they misinterpret feelings of fatigue and anxiety and treat these as hypoglycemia. As previously noted, some of the symptoms of hypoglycemia are, in themselves, behavioral and striking changes may occur in the child's personality. These may appear as acting-out behaviors such as fluctuating mood changes, emotional outbursts, temper tantrums, and so forth. Parents sometimes have difficulty in deciding whether such symptoms are pure behavioral reactions or are secondary to hypoglycemia. Because of their inherent concerns, most parents think first of hypoglycemia and react (or overreact) to this fear. Children quickly sense this parental concern, and manipulative behaviors often follow. At its worse, the child may gain control over parents by "feeling shaky," "feeling faint," or attempting to obtain an excuse for unacceptable behaviors. Many parents seem willing participants in this charade.

Another common manipulative behavior observed in children is the result of inappropriate patient education. Usually, the family is instructed to manage hypoglycemic episodes by administration of simple sugars. Often, they choose forms of sugar that are generally recognized as "treats" (candy, soft drinks, mints, juice, and so forth). These are items that are highly desirable to many children but that are usually restricted from the diabetic diet. It is no wonder that some children fake hypoglycemia in order to obtain these forbidden items.

The occurrence of a severe hypoglycemic episode produces great stress for the family as well as for the child. Seizures are particularly disturbing. Afterward, many parents seem to lose the self-confidence built up over time and may revert to a more dependent state. The possibility of the parents' reverting to a more overprotective stance with relation to the child is real and must be addressed by the diabetes team.

MANAGEMENT

Prevention of Significant Hypoglycemia

Mild hypoglycemia is virtually unavoidable, if control of hyperglycemia is to be accomplished. In the patient with tightly controlled diabetes, it is not unusual for there to be several mild hypoglycemic episodes per week. Thus, by prevention, we mean (1) ensuring that the frequency of mild hypoglycemia does not significantly interfere with lifestyle, (2) interrupting the progression of mild episodes to more severe ones, (3) anticipating those situations likely to precipitate significant hypoglycemia, and (4) taking steps to ensure prompt recovery from an episode of any severity.

Limiting the Frequency of Mild Hypoglycemia

Obviously, the optimum therapeutic plan is one that will produce euglycemia without hypoglycemia. Until such time as our therapeutic modalities include a glucose sensor, most patients will not reach this optimum level. Thus, as attempts are made to normalize blood glucose, the prospects for significant hypoglycemia increase. The solution to this dilemma with present therapies is to seek a compromise, or balance of control, wherein the frequency and severity of hypoglycemia does not adversely affect lifestyle. Many factors must be involved in arriving at such a balance for each individual.

Interrupting Progression. This is primarily an educational objective involving two basic components. The first essential component is enabling the individual to be aware of the earliest symptoms of hypoglycemia. It is not sufficient merely to be aware of "rebound symptoms." Most persons with diabetes have subtle changes in mental processing prior to onset of rebound symptomatology. These subtle changes have been described by some perceptive persons with diabetes as unexpected drowsiness, loss of attentiveness to surrounding events, loss of concentrating abilities, visual images or sounds that are slightly out of focus or distorted, and fatigue or weakness. Since many of these are normal occurrences in the young child, it is obvious that they may be missed in such patients. It is essential, however, that the older child and the adult learn to recognize these subtle signals. Immediately after experiencing a recognized and documented episode of hypoglycemia, the person should be asked to recall preceding events. Often, the brain has emitted subtle messages that were missed or went unrecognized. Repeated recall sessions may assist the person in eventual early recognition.

The second essential component to this process is a prompt response to the early warnings. The first requirement of this component is that the diabetic person be willing to keep a source of rapid-acting carbohydrate with him or her at all times. We prefer the use of sugar cubes (wrapped in foil), packets of sugar, or glucose wafers. The second requirement is the person's willingness to take the nutrient. One barrier to this is a form of denial ("It's probably not hypoglycemia, and if I just ignore it, it will go away," or "It's almost dinnertime, and I can wait until then"). Another barrier to management is fear of embarrassment from peers or recriminations from teachers if the carbohydrate is consumed.

Anticipation of Precipitating Events. As noted in Chapter 8, exercise is more likely to precipitate hypoglycemia (1) when the activity occurs at the peak of insulin action, (2) when glucose control is very tight, or (3) when meals or snacks are missed. With this knowledge, it is possible for the person to preplan certain events. The probability of exercise-induced hypoglycemia can be lessened either by reduction in the insulin that is scheduled to be most operative at the time of exercise, by administration of extra food prior to the event, or both.

Reduction in the amount of insulin (in order to be most effective at the time of activity) and administration of the insulin in a site removed from the most marked activity (abdomen or arm) are the desired methods with preplanned exercise. The following represents such a problem and plan:

Problem: R. J., a 10-year-old boy with diabetes receives doses of 14 NPH/6 Regular insulin with breakfast and 4 NPH/4 Regular insulin with supper. His diabetes is under excellent control. A soccer practice is scheduled for 11:00 AM, with a game to follow.

Analysis: The morning dose of NPH will be the insulin most likely to produce hypoglycemia if the morning injection is given prior to 8:00 AM. Its administration in the thigh would enhance its uptake during running.

Proposed Solution: (1) Reduce the NPH dose on this day to 10 units (about a 25 percent reduction);

(2) give the injection of 10 NPH/6 Regular in the abdomen; (3) perform a blood glucose prior to the start of practice, and decide whether to give an extra starch exchange or protein exchange, or both; and (4) provide another starch and/or protein exchange after every 30 to 45 minutes of play.

Other solutions for this example are possible, but this approach will work for most. Similar manipulations could be made in the Regular insulin if the practice were to begin at 8:00 AM. If the event or exercise occurred after the evening meal, alterations in nighttime Regular insulin would be appropriate.

Administration of extra food is another alternative to be considered. Our experience has shown that if a starch and protein exchange can be given for about every 30 to 45 minutes of activity, this will prevent most episodes of exercise-induced hypoglycemia. One problem exists in attempting to enforce this practice. Extreme activity coupled with pregame anxiety, particularly in hot and humid areas of the country, produces nausea or vomiting or both. Additionally, some athletes feel sluggish when such food intake is consumed. Coaches and trainers do not favor this practice for others, and it may tend to set the diabetic child apart. Consequently, despite the fact that such a practice will prevent hypoglycemia, a reduction in insulin dosage may be the preferred method in all prescheduled events. Extra food intake can be reserved for those events that are not preplanned.

Insurance of Prompt Recovery and Prevention of Relapse. Spontaneous resolution of most hypoglycemic episodes will occur if there is pre-existing good carbohydrate control. Administration of carbohydrate at the time merely augments the normal process of recovery, but consumption of food has another important benefit. It replenishes liver glycogen that was released during the recovery process and aids in the prevention of later hypoglycemia—a second episode that occurs several hours after the first, most notably during the ensuing night.

Treatment of Hypoglycemia

Table 8–4 outlines appropriate care of hypoglycemia in the home, school, or work setting. Such therapy will fully correct the vast majority of all hypoglycemic episodes. Table 13–5 lists a number of helpful prod-

Table 13–5. PRODUCTS FOR HOME MANAGEMENT OF HYPOGLYCEMIA

Product	Amount	Manufacturer
Monojel	25 g/packet	Monoject Dept. T.I. 1831 Olive St. St. Louis, MO 63103
Insta-glucose	12.4 g/dose	Brado Health Care P.O. Box 76 Orangeburg, NY 10962
Glutose	32 g/2 oz bottle	Paddock Laboratories 2744 Lyndale Ave. S Minneapolis, MN 55408
Glucose tablets	15 g/tab	Becton-Dickinson 365 W. Passaic St. Rochelle Park, NJ 07662
Reactose	32 g/2 oz bottle	Bennett Pharmaceutical Corp. 251 Portlane Ave. S Minneapolis, MN 55451
Cakemate gel	12 g/tube (61% carbo-hydrate)	
Cakemate icing	10 gm/0.5 oz (78% carbo-hydrate)	
Glucagon injection	1 mg/1 cc	Eli Lilly and Co. (by prescription from pharmacist)

ucts for such therapy and identifies their sources. It is our belief that all families should have one of the oral preparations and glucagon (for injection) at their disposal and at all places where hypoglycemia is likely to occur (that is, home, weekend cabin, trailer, automobile, boat, school, athletic field, work, and so forth). Glucagon is supplied with two vials: 1 mg of the solid glucagon and 1 ml of sterile diluent. It must be mixed shortly before its use, since glucagon has a limited biologic shelf-life after being put into solution. Fifteen to 30 minutes are generally required before a significant rise in blood glucose occurs.

Severe Hypoglycemia Therapy

The treatment of choice for severe hypoglycemia (seizures, unresponsiveness) is the intravenous administration of glucose. A push infusion of 50 percent glucose (0.5 g/ml) in a dose of approximately 0.5 g/kg of body weight (1 ml of 50 percent glucose per kilogram body weight) is usually sufficient. This amount will usually raise the blood glucose to well above 200 mg/dl. Additional amounts are rarely required and should be given only when measured blood glucose concentrations demonstrate a subsequent fall to hypoglycemic levels. As soon as consciousness has

returned, and provided that nausea and vomiting are not present (see later), the person should be encouraged to ingest complex carbohydrates (starch exchanges) and protein.

Recovery Time

The recovery time from mild and moderate hypoglycemia is almost immediate, and after 15 to 20 minutes of rest, the person can usually resume normal activity. A mild headache may persist for some hours before spontaneous resolution. With more severe episodes of hypoglycemia, the response time varies directly with both the degree of hypoglycemia and its duration, the latter appearing to be a more important determinant. We have observed children who convulsed with blood glucose levels below 10 mg/dl who were returned to a relatively normal state of consciousness within minutes of receiving intravenous glucose. However, other young persons have been found to be unresponsive with blood glucose values at or above this range, in whom normal cerebral functioning did not return for several days. Our impression is that in a few of these latter cases, return of CNS function was delayed by overly aggressive initial management with 50 percent glucose. In a local emergency room, one child had received almost 5 g/kg of intravenous glucose, and her blood glucose upon referral to our institution was over 1500 mg/dl.

Consequences of Severe Hypoglycemia

Central and peripheral nervous system dysfunction is the usual consequence of severe hypoglycemia, and most of these conditions are transient. Peripheral nerve palsy, particularly of the sixth cranial nerve, is not uncommon. In this instance, transient blindness or diplopia is often observed. Permanent brain damage (cerebral palsy) is an occasional consequence and permanent motor neuropathies are also reported. Infants with diabetes mellitus appear more likely to develop permanent CNS injury. This is thought to be due to several factors: the brain is still undergoing extrauterine development and maturation, the occurrence of severe hypoglycemia is more likely, and hypoglycemia frequently goes unrecognized in infants. This group of children have been said ultimately to have a higher prevalence of nonhypoglycemic seizures (convulsive disorders) and specific learning disabilities. These observations have not been verified.

Vomiting, dehydration, and ketosis are occasional consequences. Nausea and vomiting are common aftermaths of severe hypoglycemia. Since both the injection of epinephrine and glucagon produce nausea and vomiting when given to nonhypoglycemic individuals, it is felt that this is a symptom of the counter-regulatory response. On most occasions, the vomiting is of short duration and easily managed; but at other times, the vomiting is more persistent and leads to dehydration. The stress hormone reactions naturally produce hyperglycemia and ketone-

mia. Our group has observed numerous young persons who develop typical diabetic ketoacidosis in the immediate aftermath of a severe episode of hypoglycemia.

SUMMARY

Hypoglycemia is a natural occurrence of Type I diabetes when this syndrome is appropriately treated with insulin. The more rigid the control, the more likely is the occurrence of hypoglycemia. More severe episodes of hypoglycemia are to be avoided. Early management of hypoglycemia is essential.

14

Hyperlabile Diabetes

The blood glucose excursion of the patient with IDDM varies directly with the degree of endogenous insulin secretion. Thus, the patient who has significant, albeit reduced, levels of C-peptide has a range of glucose fluctuation that is less extensive than that of the person without insulin secretion. However, it is well known that factors other than insulin secretion or even its exogenous administration are strong determinants of glucose excursion. In Chapter 11, attention was directed to the role of stress hormones in the regulation of carbohydrate, protein, and fat metabolism. That chapter was concerned primarily with acute alterations in secretion of these hormones rather than with situations of chronic or recurrent secretion. Yet in selected patients the metabolic responses to chronic stress are of major concern to the physician. Patients with such responses may have severe fluctuations in metabolic balance and are often spoken of as "hyperlabile" or "brittle."

Hyperlabile diabetes (HDM), as the name suggests, identifies a group of patients with insulin-dependent diabetes who have greater than normal lability of their diabetes. In such persons, plasma glucose values tend to fluctuate widely, and there are frequent episodes of either the hyperglycemia-ketosis syndrome, hypoglycemia, or both. An additional characteristic often noted in these persons is the ineffectiveness of traditional therapeutic interventions (for example, insulin or dietary changes). Such manipulations may, at times, even worsen the patient's hyperlability.

HDM is the result of a number of different causative factors, even though there may well be a commonality in the physiologic mechanisms responsible for the syndrome. Table 14–1 lists some of the causes that have been identified. Although all will not be considered in depth, a brief discussion of some of the more important ones appears appropriate. The reader will appreciate that there are obvious overlaps within this list and that other causative factors are possible.

ETIOLOGIC FACTORS

Management Related

Lability may be directly and specifically related to management of the disease, and Table 14–1 subcategorizes it as either being physiologic or behavioral in origin. At times, both factors appear to be involved.

Physiologic

In this section are considered those instances in which there is an altered balance between insulin activity and hyperglycemic factors (that is, either food intake or endogenous glucose production).

Table 14–1. FACTORS PROMOTING HYPERLABILITY IN IDDM

I. Management Related
  A. Physiologic
    1. Underinsulinization
    2. Altered insulin absorption or action
    3. Excessive insulin (rebound or Somogyi effect)
  B. Behavioral
    1. Educational
    2. Noncompliance/nonadherence
    3. Manipulative behaviors
II. Environmental
  A. Infections
    1. Acute, recurrent (coupled with poor control)
    2. Chronic
  B. Emotional
    1. Anxiety states—acute and chronic
    2. Family stresses
  C. Social
    1. School refusal syndrome
    2. Physical or sexual abuse
  D. Religious and Cultural
  E. Psychologic/psychiatric
  F. Hormonal
    1. Thyroid
    2. Menstrual
III. Other or Unknown

Underinsulinization. This occurs in a wide variety of situations and may be either absolute (too little insulin per kilogram of body weight) or relative (excessive food intake without compensatory increase in insulin administration). The result is often the same.

Failure to take or receive an adequate amount of insulin occurs with some regularity in persons with IDDM. In our experience, this is most often observed in the teenager who, although programmed to receive two shots of insulin per day, often "forgets" one of the injections, usually the evening one. As a result of this inconsistency, the day-to-day carbohydrate control is erratic. The following vignette is typical:

A.S., a 12-year-old sixth grader, had diabetes for two years and rarely had serious problems but never worked at controlling diabetes. She and her family moved to our area, and she was seen in consultation. Her height was in the 50th percentile and her weight was 50 kg. Her insulin dosage was 20 NPH/10 Regular in the morning and 10 NPH/10 Regular in the evening.

Blood glucose testing was initiated, revealing values always in excess of 240 mg/dl. Her HbA_{1c} was 14 per cent (normal 5 to 8 per cent).

Over the next three months, her dosage was increased progressively to 55 NPH/25 Regular in the morning and 25 NPH/25 Regular in the evening. Dietary management was emphasized, and her weight stayed around 50 kg. Despite these enormous increases in dosage (from 1.0 U/kg to 2.6 U/kg), her control did not improve. Instead, her glucose levels seemed to increase at unexpected times. She also had several episodes of moderately severe hypoglycemia and two episodes of ketosis.

Thinking that she might be demonstrating a Somogyi phenomenon, we admitted her to the Child Health Center in order to study her on the Biostator (Fig. 14–1). She was given her usual amount of subcutaneous insulin from the hospital unit. Almost immediately, her blood glucose began to fall. During the first 24 hours she had to be given (by the Biostator) large amounts of IV dextrose to maintain euglycemia.

Following the study, she admitted to withholding her insulin frequently over the preceding months—almost never giving the evening injection and occasionally omitting the morning dose as well. Her ultimate dose stabilized around 0.75 units/kg/day.

The person who is underinsulinized and hyperglycemic has been demonstrated to have elevated values for plasma cortisol, but it is not clear which is the primary incitor and which the responder. It is sufficient, but not surprising, to know that the erratic use of insulin is a factor leading to hyperlability.

Although the case of A.S. is dramatic, milder variations on this theme are quite common. Over half of an interviewed group of teenagers recently admitted that they probably miss one or more insulin shots per week, most often owing to simple forgetfulness. Some authors consider such behaviors as a form of continuing denial.

Reduction in Insulin Absorption. This has been discussed in Chapter 6 and will not be elaborated on here. Several patients have been reported in whom it is clear that local insulinase has destroyed the hormone prior to its absorption. In our experience, such cases are extremely unusual. Such persons respond dramatically to intravenous or intraperitoneal insulin.

Overinsulinization. This is usually spoken of as the Somogyi effect, or phenomenon, or as rebound hyperglycemia. That significant hypoglycemia can (and does) evoke a counter-regulatory response is clear from numerous studies. That such recurring events may lead to serious hyperlability is also clear. But there is a real difference of opinion among experts as to the frequency of this occurrence in actual practice. Rosenbloom and his colleagues (1981) found it to be the single most important cause of hyperlability in their patient group, but most investigators have found the phenomenon to be less prevalent than underinsulinization. The following

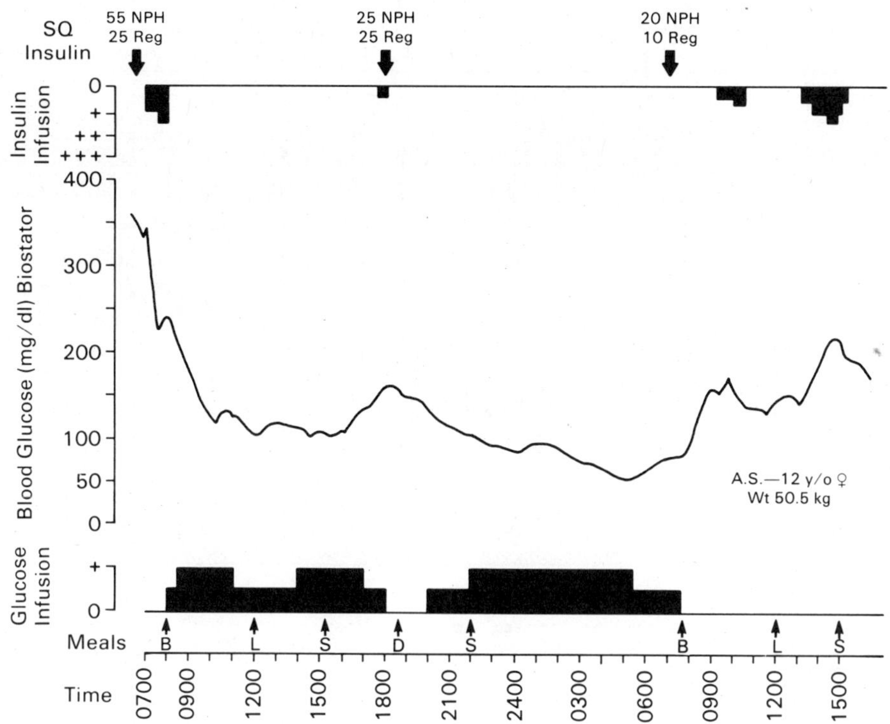

Figure 14–1. Patient A. S., described in detail in the text, was admitted and studied on the Biostator, a glucose-controlled insulin infusion pump. While receiving the insulin dosage that had been prescribed, she was found to be severely hypoglycemic and required glucose infusions. She later admitted to being noncompliant in the administration of insulin.

case represents a typical example of such a patient:

J.B., a 15-year-old young woman with a six-year history of IDDM, was in good diabetic control. All urine glucose levels were negative, and random blood glucose values in the physician's office varied between 100 mg/dl and 180 mg/dl. Insulin dose was approximately 0.8 U/kg/day, given in two doses (AM dose of 36 NPH/12 Regular; PM dose of 8 NPH/5 Regular).

She went to see her physician one afternoon following school for a regular health and diabetes visit. The examination was normal, and she was sent home to continue the "good work." By the time she reached home, a phone call was waiting, informing her that the blood glucose was in excess of 500 mg/dl and telling her to report to the hospital for admission. She did so.

She remained in the hospital for seven weeks before being transferred to our unit for "severe insulin resistance." Figure 14–2 demonstrates excerpts from those seven weeks as well as two in our hospital, three days of which are shown in detail.

Despite an increase in insulin dosage to over 200 U/day, she had persistent and severe hyperglycemia. She had lost weight (3.6 kg in 7 weeks), was ketotic, and felt very ill. She was receiving 65 NPH/25 Regular in AM and 50 NPH/25 Regular

in PM, with three or four Regular insulin supplements (10 to 20 units each).

For the first 24 hours in our hospital, we left J.B. on precisely the same regime as at home. Blood glucose values were performed every two to four hours. At the beginning of the second day, her insulin supplements were stopped, and her standard dose was reduced (45 NPH/15 Regular in AM; 30 NPH/10 Regular in PM). This was further reduced on the third day as severe hyperglycemia subsided and as ketonemia/ketonuria cleared. Small adjustments were subsequently made during the next 10 days as other studies were performed.

Although instances of profound overtreatment, similar to this, continue to occur, the frequency with which we see them has decreased considerably over the past 10 years. This decrease in incidence appears related to better professional and patient education.

The Somogyi phenomenon is a real event, appears related to excess counter-regulatory response, and is a cause for hyperlability. As an example, in the patient J.B., plasma cortisol levels on the first two days of her hospitalization at the University of Texas Medical Branch were 3.4 and 2.8 times higher than they were at the end of hospitalization.

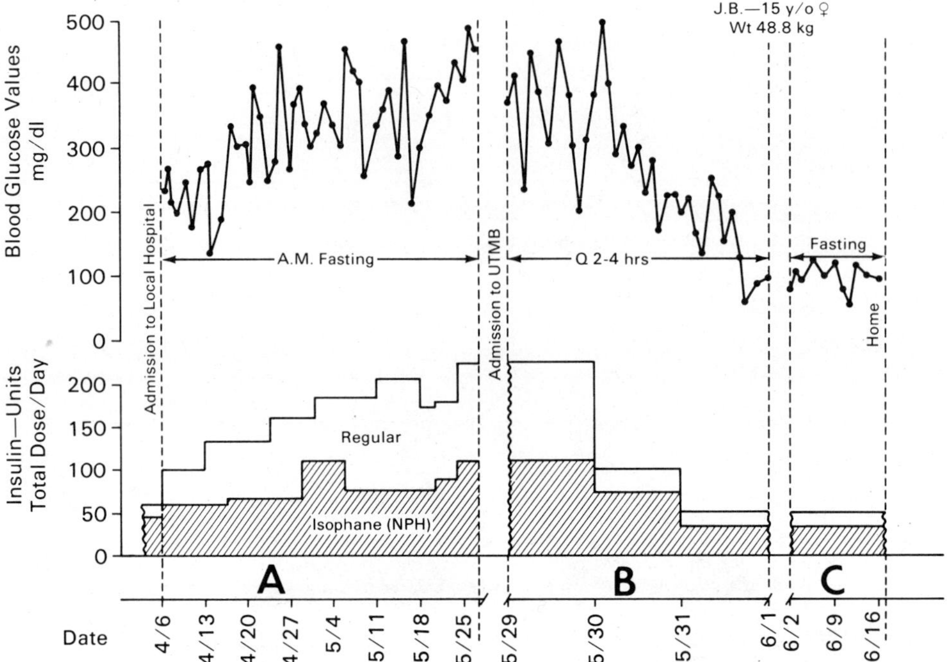

Figure 14–2. Patient J. B. (see text for complete case synopsis). *A*, Seven weeks' data from period of local hospitalization demonstrates marked morning hyperglycemia despite a marked increase in insulin dosage. *B*, Data from three days of hospitalization at UTMB are shown. Blood glucose values were obtained every two to four hours, and insulin was reduced on days 2 and 3. *C*, Data from last two weeks of UTMB hospitalization show glucose control re-established after reduction in insulin. No inciting cause was ever identified for the hyperglycemia.

It is surmised that comparable increases were present in plasma levels of growth hormone, glucagon, and catecholamines. But at least two factors confuse the issue: (1) Many patients experience excess insulin administration and hypoglycemia without notable or chronic rebounding; and (2) many of the patients who are diagnosed as having the phenomenon experience recurrent episodes over several years, and some of these have associated psychologic stress reactions. Thus, one might conclude that these persons are basically hyper-responders and that the excess insulin merely acts as one of many potential triggers to such a phenomenon.

Table 14–2 lists some of the clues that should alert the physician to the prospects of chronic overinsulinization as a cause for poor diabetes control. Blood glucose values often fluctuate widely from significant hyperglycemia to symptomatic hypoglycemia, although as seen earlier, evidence of hypoglycemia is sometimes missing. In most patients, the total insulin dose exceeds 1.0 U/kg/day, and often is in excess of 1.5 U/kg/day. A common finding is that significant increases in insulin dosage do not appreciably lower blood glucose.

Table 14–2. **CHARACTERISTICS SUGGESTING OVERINSULINIZATION**

A. Extreme Hyperlability
   1. Blood sugars fluctuating between hyperglycemia (>300 mg/dl) and hypoglycemia; particularly rapid variations
   2. Intermittent symptomatic hypoglycemia interspersed with hyperglycemia, ketonemia/ketonuria, or both
B. Insulin Dosage
   1. Dose significantly in excess of 1.0 U/kg (except during adolescent growth spurt)
   2. Usually in excess of 1.5 U/kg/day.
C. Insulin Effectiveness
   1. Increasing insulin dosage without appreciable effect on blood glucose
   2. Obesity occurring as a result of insulin-food-insulin cycle.

In patients whose cases are similar to this one, in whom the diagnosis is strongly suspected, the dosage of insulin can be reduced either abruptly or gradually to levels of approximately 1.0 U/kg/day. Abrupt reductions are best carried out during hospitalization, whereas a gradual reduction may be accomplished on an outpatient basis.

Behavioral

Hyperlability is frequently related to underinsulinization or overinsulinization, when the inciting cause is behavioral. Occasionally, such may be due to poor understanding on the part of the child or family, or both, but, in our experience, this is unusual. Noncompliant behaviors and manipulative behaviors are much more commonly encountered.

Environmental

All of the factors listed in Table 14–1 are potential causes of HDM. Most have in common the outpouring of anti-insulin hormones, which promote a catabolic effect on the host. Three of these deserve special mention and consideration.

School Refusal Syndrome (SRS)

In our experience, this is one of the more common associations: HDM and SRS. School anxiety reactions, school phobia, school refusal, separation anxiety states—these all occur in children, both diabetic and nondiabetic. But, in the person with diabetes, the school anxiety syndrome is much more difficult to manage, for the child can be extremely ill as a consequence of the stress-related events. Whereas it is relatively easy to get a parent to reintroduce his or her nondiabetic child with psychosomatic symptoms back into school, it is much more difficult if the child is actually ill. Since children with IDDM can become quite sick, parents may not wish to take them to school and leave them, and teachers and nurses often do not wish to take the responsibility into the classroom. It is often much easier for the child to be placed into a homebound program, in which personal tutoring in a nonthreatening environment can take place. Unfortunately, such children lose out on their socialization contacts, and they learn a maladaptive way of coping with day-to-day stresses. As seen in Figure 14–3 and in the following summary, the problems can be enormous and potential solutions quite costly in terms of both time and money.

T.N. was 13 years old and in seventh grade when he was diagnosed to have IDDM. The family underwent an educational program with T.N., and all quickly "adopted" diabetes with the boy being very involved in his own care. Two events during the initial hospitalization should have alerted observers to eventual problems: (1) the education nurse noted that T.N. was difficult to separate from his parents, both physically and emotionally; and (2) both T.N. and his parents chose for him not to attend summer diabetic camp three months later. Except for one episode of severe hypoglycemia with seizures about eight weeks after onset, he had no problems until September. During the eighth grade (last year of middle school), he had five hospitalizations for DKA; but they occurred at sufficient intervals that their association was missed.

In September 1979, he entered high school, a school approximately six to eight times the size of his middle school. On the third day, he was ill and could not attend school but returned for one-half day on the fourth and fifth days. On the Monday of the second week he was admitted with DKA. As noted in Figure 14–3, he then had 15 additional hospitalizations for DKA during the succeeding nine months. Although he was physically in school less than 100 days, he kept up and was promoted to 10th grade. During June 1980, he went to diabetic camp but became so ill on the third day that he spent most of the first week in the infirmary and was allowed to go home early.

In September 1981, the situation deteriorated once again and at the insistence of the school and with the consent and cooperation of the local physician and parents, he was placed in a homebound program, in which he excelled. In May 1981, he had a Mycoplasma pneumonia with DKA and was referred to our unit for evaluation. His school refusal syndrome was uncovered. He was also emotionally depressed. A stress management program was introduced and extensive psychologic counseling initiated. For a brief period just at the onset of school, he was treated with propranolol, but this was subsequently discontinued.

He is now a senior in full-time attendance and appears to have no remaining remnants of his earlier socialization problems.

This young man's course is not unusual, and this problem appears to be becoming more common. Children with diabetes are, of course, subject to more frequent school absenteeism than are children without chronic health problems. The child's re-entry into school after initial diagnosis may be particularly traumatic: the child's self-image has been altered because of the new disease; the child may not know how to explain his or her problem; the absence from school and playmates may have placed the child as an outsider with his or her previous group; other children may worry about the contagiousness of the problem and be hesitant in their acceptance of their former peer; teachers may handle the problems poorly. These stresses added to those usually experienced by the child produces an ideal situation for school refusal.

Perhaps the best treatment for school re-

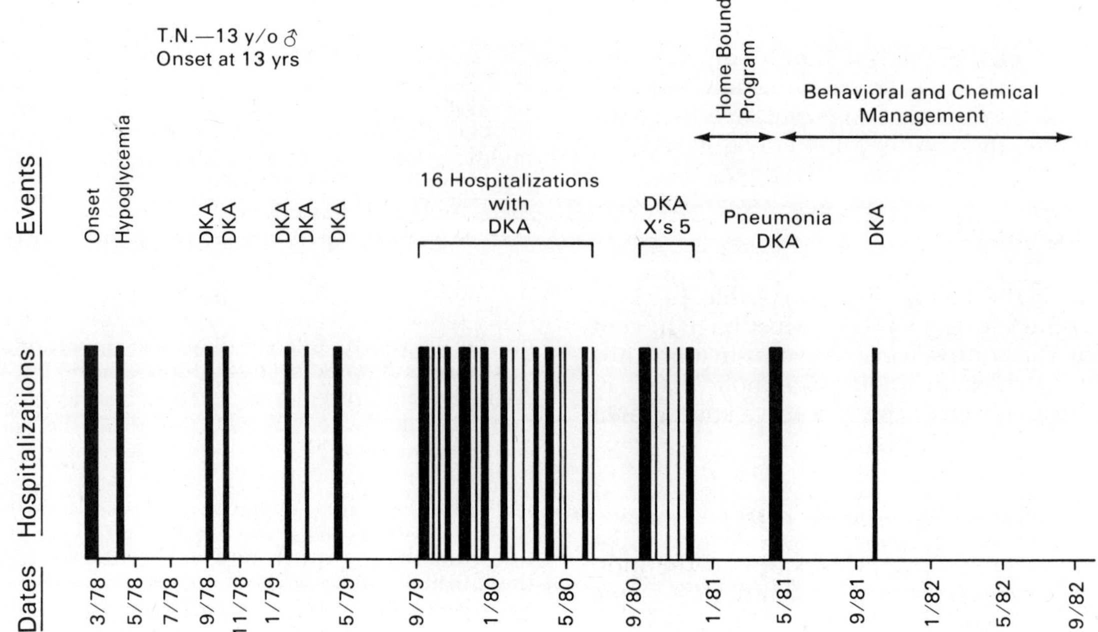

Figure 14–3. School refusal syndrome in patient T. N. (see text). Each line denotes a separate hospitalization, with the width of the line indicating the duration of each admission.

fusal is prevention. Part of the initial educational experience should focus on helping the child re-enter his or her school and social environment. This often involves role playing, allowing the child to experience some possible problems while in a nonthreatening situation. Contacts with the school nurse and teachers are also important in facilitating smooth re-entry into normal life.

When school refusal is present, the child, parents, and school personnel will require more care and attention than what is usually necessary for the nondiabetic in a similar situation. All adults involved must be committed to the same outcome; getting the child back in school. As many environmental stresses as possible should be identified and addressed individually. Empathetic support and understanding, along with continued counseling will usually resolve the problem.

If the child develops symptomatic ketosis, supplemental insulin and judicious use of fluids should be used. Antinausea agents may be helpful. Whenever possible the child should spend some time each day in school, the amount increasing weekly. On occasions when these measures are not fully successful, the use of a beta-blocking agent, like propranolol, may be tried. Studies by Baker and associates (1969) and others have demonstrated the occasional success of such therapy in moderating the rise in free fatty acids and ketone bodies initiated by stress. We have used such therapy in approximately two dozen children; in about 50 per cent there were some beneficial results. Propranolol therapy must be used with caution, because it also retards the sympathetic response to hypoglycemia.

Religious and Cultural

Strong religious and cultural customs can, on occasion, create management problems and may seriously compromise care. The following example is a tragic case in point.

N.S., diagnosed with IDDM at the age of 14 years, was the only son of well-educated, deeply religious parents. The entire family underwent initial education, and for nine months the boy did extremely well, with excellent carbohydrate control. He was then readmitted to the hospital with severe DKA and appeared almost cachectic, even after rehydration. The parents demonstrated appropriate concern. No cause for the DKA could be ascertained, and after four days he was again discharged.

Five months later, after re-establishing good control, he once again had an episode of DKA. In the recovery phase, N.S. admitted to having discontinued his insulin as a test of his religious faith. He believed that, through his religion and faith,

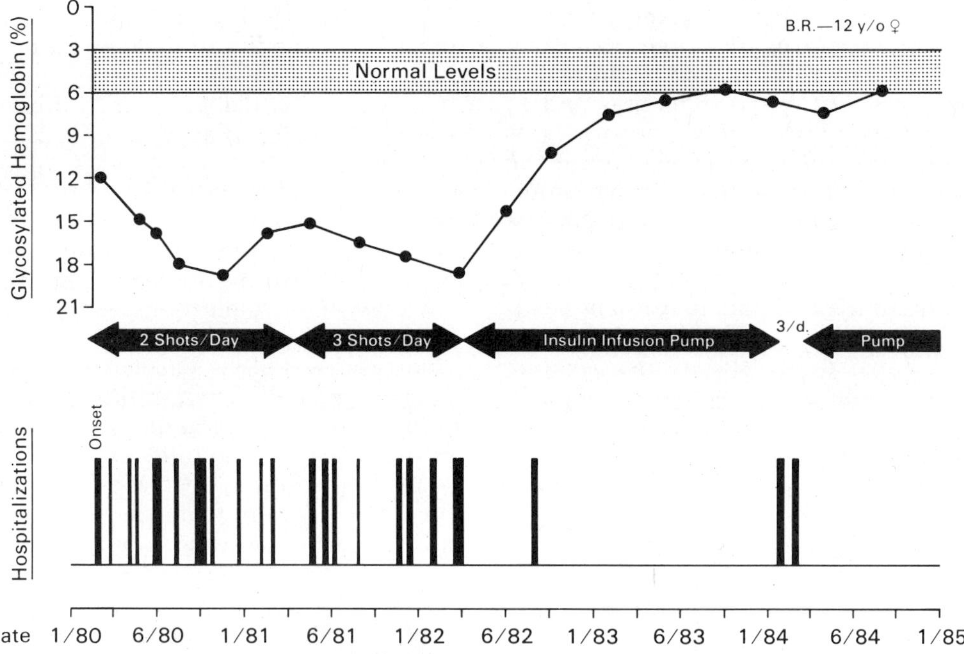

Figure 14–4. Hyperlabile patient B.R. had chronically poor control of diabetes with multiple hospitalizations for DKA. There were minimal psychosocial problems, none felt to be the causative factor for the hyperlability. Compliance with the medical regimen was determined to be good. A program of three shots per day produced no improvement, but dramatic improvement occurred in 1982 when the pump malfunctioned. In early 1984, B.R. was converted to a three shot per day program, but hyperlability recurred and two hospitalizations for DKA resulted, necessitating a return to CSII management.

he was healed. He and his parents were counseled and re-educated.

The situation repeated itself three months later, and the cause was the same. N.S.'s minister had told him that his inability to stop insulin was clearly a demonstration of his lack of sufficient faith; his faith would allow such to happen only when he believed, worked, and tested. The parents were concerned but did not feel that they should intervene in this process.

Extensive counseling occurred with all parties involved, including the minister, and an agreement was reached that no further pressure of this sort would be placed on N.S. Child Protective Services were involved, and the problems appeared to be resolving. Seven months later, he presented to another hospital with a pH of 6.90 and expired after three hours of aggressive treatment.

Following this episode several years ago, we have been more sensitive to the cultural and religious backgrounds of our patients and their families. Although we have not again witnessed as severe an episode as this one, we have been impressed with how such belief systems influence medical management. Faith healers, curanderos, charlatans, and cults abound; and persons with chronic illnesses are particularly susceptible to their appeals. The physician and health team need to incorporate these aspects of life into the management plan.

Other Causes of Hyperlability

Numerous causes of hyperlability have been described; the disease has been seen in patients with other hormonal problems. *Hyperthyroidism* may be associated with IDDM and, unless adequately treated, produces marked hyperlability. The person with *hypothyroidism* often has significant hyperglycemia but is not usually considered "brittle" or hyperlabile. Children who coincidentally have *hypoadrenocorticism* (Addison's disease) often have intense sensitivity to insulin; this condition should be considered in those children whose frequent hypoglycemic episodes persist even when insulin dosage is significantly reduced.

Young women are particularly subject to marked hyperlability during *menstrual periods*. Although not all young women experience marked fluctuations in blood glucose levels around the time of menses, some have significant problems during this time. The usual pattern is for hyperglycemia to begin one to three days prior to onset of menses and to persist for three to seven days. In some, this is associated with mild ketonemia and, if the young woman experiences other symptoms such as nausea, vomiting, or anorexia, the consequence may be symptomatic ketosis, or even DKA.

The cause of hyperlability may not be readily apparent and may not be clearly identified despite extensive investigations. As our knowledge of the many factors influencing carbohydrate metabolism increases, some of those unusual causes will be defined.

MANAGEMENT CONSIDERATION

The basic management philosophy must be to identify the cause of the hyperlability and then to modify or eliminate this etiologic factor. Too often, treatment is directed toward the hyperlability rather than toward its cause. Usually, such an approach is destined to fail.

As noted earlier, some children, like adults, hyper-respond to stress with excessive outpouring of one or more of the stress hormones. Thus, whatever its specific origin, the most common physiologic pathway is similar. Identification of stresses and modification of their effect on the subject is most important. Stress management may consist of such strategies as counseling, relaxation techniques, behavioral modification, biofeedback, self-hypnosis, and so forth. Most of these can be handled by the diabetes team, although psychologic and psychiatric back-up is essential.

Drug management is not generally recommended, although the temporary use of beta-blocking agents may be helpful. In a few adolescents, the judicious use of tranquilizers or mood elevators should be considered.

Occasionally, alterations in the method of insulin administration may produce remarkable results. This is particularly true of the patient who exhibits nighttime hypoglycemia with early morning hyperglycemia (that is, secondary to "rebound" as well as to the "dawn" phenomenon). Moving the nighttime NPH dosage from the time of the evening meal to bedtime (about 10:00 PM) is often successful. Hyperlability may sometimes be significantly modified by insulin pump management. Figure 14–4 demonstrates this dramatically in one hyperlabile diabetic.

SUMMARY

All children with IDDM are hyperlabile to some extent, and the degree of lability is partially related to the degree of insulin deficiency. The other major factor responsible for hyperlability is the subject's response to stress. The main objective in management is to identify the cause and either eliminate or modify its effect.

15

The Child Less Than 3 Years Old

Diabetes mellitus in any child poses many challenges to the health provider; but when the child is less than three years of age, even the most basic aspects of care become complex. Diabetes may take two forms in the early years of life: transient or permanent.

TRANSIENT DIABETES

Transient nonketotic diabetes in the neonate is uncommon but has been observed in the baby who is considered small for gestational age. The infant develops hyperglycemia, usually without ketonemia, within a few days of life. Persisting for weeks to months, the neonate may require insulin injections for a brief time. Authors suggest that the diabetic state is related to inadequate insulin production by the beta cell, but why this occurs remains obscure. However, one theory proposes that persistent maternal hypoglycemia during gestation and consequent low fetal blood glucose levels lead to inadequate beta-cell stimulation and thereby to decreased islet-cell growth. The underdeveloped or hypoplastic islet cells are then unable to keep pace with the infant's metabolic demands after birth. Whether an affected neonate will develop permanent diabetes can only be determined by the course of the disease, but the probability of this is low.

PERMANENT DIABETES

A relatively rare phenomenon, permanent diabetes in the child less than 3 years of age occurs in about 0.5 percent of all children with diabetes. Imerslund, in 1960, reported only 13 such children from 3847 juvenile diabetics followed in the Joslin Clinic between 1922 and 1956, a prevalence of 0.3 percent in this referral population. On the other hand, the prevalence of diabetes with onset in children less than 3 years of age in our young children's camp (6- to 12-year-olds) has been seemingly higher. During the past three years, 16 of 378 children had their onset at less than three years of age. In contrast, between 1975 and 1980, there were only 10 of 590 from this same population.

Onset of diabetes in the infant may differ from the classic picture. The child may present quite acutely with an abrupt illness manifest by fever, vomiting, and marked dehydration. Typically, the infant's symptoms are more likely to suggest a gastroenteritis or other alimentary disorder rather than a metabolic or endocrine problem. Polyuria is rarely noted, and excessive thirst is appreciated only as irritability and mostly in retrospect. To further hamper an early diagnosis, the infant may exhibit only mild glucosuria and no ketonuria at onset. These urinary findings are often interpreted as stress related or as a consequence of intravenous fluid therapy. Consequently, the usual clues to the diagnosis are often missing, and the diagnosis may be significantly delayed. This delay in recognition accounts for the severity of the infant's condition by the time insulin therapy is finally begun. Once insulin treatment is initiated, the infant's condition usually improves rapidly.

COURSE OF THE DISEASE

The infant or toddler with diabetes is often more sensitive to the blood glucose lowering and antiketogenic effects of insulin than is the older child. It is therefore not unusual to be able to manage these children quite effectively on amounts of insulin around 0.2 to 0.4 unit per kilogram of body weight, and these dosage levels may persist for years. The postonset remission, so common in older children, may be either nonexistent or extremely short in duration.

During infancy, there is a higher probability of episodic dehydration owing to the increased frequency of illness that compromises intake. These infants are more likely to have pure hyperosmolar dehydration than to have a typical ketotic form of diabetic acidosis. This is due in part to the infant's decreased ability to form ketones but also to the infants ability to utilize ketone bodies in energy metabolism more effectively than older persons. Only a few infants have been investigated as to persisting insulin production but in those studies the C-peptide response is either low or nonexistent, similar to that found in older children.

INTERVENTIONS

Planning an effective diabetes management program for the infant and family requires an understanding of general infant care measures and development needs, and, occasionally, a willingness to be unconventional in the approach to diabetes care. "Compromise" is the guideword. What one desires in diabetes control in the infant may have to give way to what is attainable. For example, the occasional hypoglycemia that is to be expected as a part of reasonable carbohydrate control in the older child is not an acceptable goal for the infant or toddler. Not only does the young child's nervous system require a constant and large supply of glu-

cose but also, since the brain and nervous system are still in a developmental stage (at least through the second year of life), cellular injury to the nervous system is more likely to occur with episodic hypoglycemia in the infant than in the older child. Preventing episodes of hypoglycemia is, thus, a major objective of therapy. To do this while still being able to maintain carbohydrate control in an acceptable range is extremely difficult, even in the most conscientious family.

PARENTS

Parents must always be included in setting overall goals and objectives for the child's care, but such sharing of goals may not be possible initially. At diagnosis, the parents may be shocked and confused, with manifestations ranging from anger to denial to quiet sadness. Such responses seem to be more pronounced in parents of infants. One explanation may be that such parents are generally younger and are still struggling with their own developmental issues as a couple and as new parents. They are saddened at the loss of their "perfect" child, they fear for the child's immediate health, and they feel guilty for not having sought help earlier. In the search for the cause or reason, they may blame themselves or each other for "passing on the diabetes." They fear for the health of their other children or for children yet unborn.

The parents should be encouraged to stay with their infant during the hospitalization. Obviously, the parent must be present to learn the necessary skills and information but equally important is the infant's need for the parent's nurturing presence. During the hospital stay, parents must be encouraged to assume increasing responsibility for their baby's diabetes care. Caring guidance and supervision permit the parents to try out their new skills and begin to exercise diabetes care decisions.

INSULIN

The infant or toddler with diabetes generally requires very small amounts of injected insulin. Even with the available low-dosage syringes, small amounts or portions of a unit are difficult to measure accurately even for the most experienced. Additionally, the infant is often quite sensitive to dose changes of as little as 0.5 unit. Diluting U-100 insulin to U-25 or U-50 insulin permits these small insulin doses to be more easily and safely measured. Parents are instructed to dilute their child's insulin as outlined in Figure 15–1 and Table 15–1. Careful attention is given to evaluating the parents' aseptic technique. Diluting fluids are available to physicians upon request from the manufacturers. Because of the manipulation with the insulin bottle, the diluted insulin should be refrigerated and then discarded in about two to three months, even if there is insulin still remaining.

Although the parents learn to think in terms of U-25 insulin, they must be cautioned to alert uninitiated medical professionals in emergency rooms, doctor's offices, and hospitals to this dilution. It is likely that the infant's drawn-up dose of 4 units of U-25 (actually 1 unit of U-100) may be unknowingly given as 4 units of U-100 by an unaware doctor or nurse.

Obviously, all types of insulin needed by the child must be diluted. Virtually all infants are best managed by a multiple dose regimen using NPH or Lente along with Regular insulin. The basic objections to a single dose of insulin are no different for the infant than for the older child, but they are more important in the former group, because (1) the infant changes too quickly to have much long-acting insulin in place; (2) the infant has

DILUTING INSULIN TO U-25

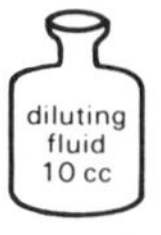

A new bottle of diluting fluid has 10 cc.

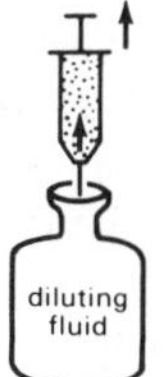

Take *out* 2.5 cc of diluting fluid and discard.

Figure 15–1. Instructions for diluting U-100 insulin for preparation of U-25 insulin. Procedure is necessary for those requiring very small amounts of insulin.

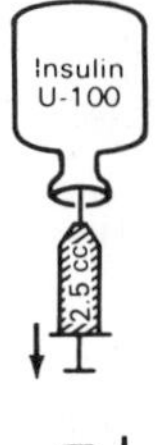

Next, take out 2.5 cc of *insulin* from a bottle of U-100 insulin.
(You may store the remainder in the refrigerator until you need to dilute again.)

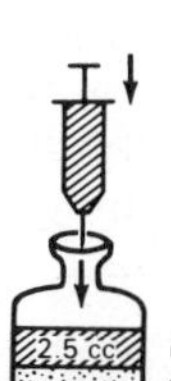

Add the 2.5 cc of insulin to the bottle of diluting fluid.

The resulting solution is 10 cc of U-25 insulin.

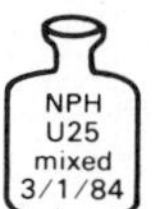

MARK the bottle: U25 insulin
                   Date Mixed________________
                   Date to Discard________________
Refrigerate this insulin and DISCARD in *2 months*.

Table 15–1. **CONVERSION CHART FOR PERSONS USING U-25 INSULIN**

U-25 Dose	Fill U-100 Syringe to This Mark
¼ unit	1-unit mark
½ unit	2-unit mark
¾ unit	3-unit mark
1 unit	4-unit mark
1½ units	6-unit mark
2 units	8-unit mark
2½ units	10-unit mark
3 units	12-unit mark
4 units	16-unit mark

an inordinate sensitivity to small dosage adjustments; and (3) the patterns of insulin action may not conform to meal or activity schedules as well in infants as with older persons. For these reasons, the infant should rarely be treated with a single-dose regimen. The child will usually be either overtreated or undertreated, and sometimes both can occur within the same day. Two doses per day provides a smoother pattern, but the potential for early-morning hypoglycemia persists. Consequently, many of these children are best treated with three injections per day. We have often converted these children to a three shot per day schedule by moving the suppertime NPH or Lente to 9:00 PM or 10:00 PM. Night-time hypoglycemia is far less frequent with this regimen.

Injections

Any injection site recommended for the older child is also acceptable for the infant and toddler. However, use of the buttocks is discouraged until the child is walking. Although the sciatic nerve is likely to be deeper than the needle's penetration, this nerve is not well stabilized in the infant. Alternative sites include upper outer arms, anterior thighs, and the little-used ventrogluteal sites.

Parents must be instructed in an injection technique that uses much care and reassurance. An underlying concern of the parent is that the baby will not understand and hence will learn to fear or hate the parent. Parents should not give the injections until their techniques are refined enough to permit early successes. Often parents will need to practice subcutaneous injections with each other or with a willing health professional.

Positioning and holding the squirming infant is an important aspect of the injection technique. Parents are taught to select sites that may be easily stabilized. To further the speed of the injection, aspiration after insertion is eliminated.

The parents are encouraged to hold and comfort the child after injection, but not to excess. Parents who are particularly anxious about injections are counseled and supported in relaxation exercises. Parents soon find that their calm, accepting attitude readily transmits to their child at injection time.

GOALS OF MANAGEMENT

Although the overall goals of good and lasting health are the same for diabetics of any age, the specific goals for the child under 3 years old are different in certain respects. The acceptable blood glucose levels must be liberalized a little in order to provide a relative buffer against hypoglycemia. At the same time, it is important that concern for glucose control not be abandoned, lest the child become growth retarded and have an increased likelihood of degenerative changes. We attempt to keep blood glucose values between 80 mg/dl and 180 mg/dl and aim to achieve more than 75 percent of blood glucose values greater than 80 mg/dl and less than 200 mg/dl. If urine samples are being monitored (and we believe this is a serious mistake, see Chapter 5), then a persistent trace to a 0.5 percent reaction seems more acceptable than aiming for consistently negative urine samples.

MONITORING

The advent of home monitoring of blood glucose has certainly made monitoring the infant's diabetes more practical. However, checking urine glucose levels may still be the method chosen by some parents. Checking each wet diaper probably gives the most information, yet this still may not have the reliability of twice daily blood glucose determinations. Parents may squeeze the diaper, place a few cotton balls in the diaper, or use test strips. Use of collection bags is strongly discouraged, as these bags easily lead to skin excoriation. Attempting to obtain urine samples for before-meal checks is nearly futile. Hence, parents must record both the time of day and the results.

Blood glucose testing may be done exclusively or as a periodic adjunct to urine testing. Even if urine testing is selected as the monitoring method, parents are encouraged to use blood glucose testing during times of illness or suspected hypoglycemia. Use of the Autolet (or a similar device) and lancets reduces the discomfort and time involved. Blood glucose testing sites for the infant include the earlobes, toes, and heel (parents must be cautioned to use only the outer aspects of the heel, as repeated punctures over the heel have been associated with osteomyelitis).

As with injections, having the supplies ready, working quickly, and holding the infant securely, increases the comfort of this task for both parent and child.

DIET

The capricious behavior of children toward food makes the diabetic meal plan difficult to implement. In planning the diet, one must consider normal growth requirements, normal developmental needs related to eating, prevention of hypoglycemia, normal wake and sleep patterns, and timing of insulin therapy.

The infant or toddler's meal plan should include at least six feedings per day planned around the child's sleep cycle. Even in the toddler and young child, this three-meal/three-snack pattern prevents prolonged periods without food, thus sparing the liver's glycogen stores and lessening the likelihood of serious hypoglycemia.

If a child is particularly finicky or unpredictable in food intake, the parent should consider giving the insulin during or after the meal. This change allows the parent to adjust the dose of Regular insulin to the child's food intake. Parents should be counseled regarding predictable changes in their child's eating behaviors. Parents become concerned when their toddler (1) refuses meals, (2) eats only one type of food, as in "food jags," or (3) eats less than expected. The professional should reassure parents by explaining that such responses to food are normal toddler behaviors and by verifying normal growth.

The conversion of baby foods and formulas for use in the exchange system has been provided by Benz and Kohler (1980).

EXERCISE

Although exercise is not easily planned for or regulated in the infant or toddler, it nonetheless affects diabetes control. Parents learn that the sedentary infant-turned-toddler usually requires a short-term decrease in insulin.

HYPOGLYCEMIA

Hypoglycemia is to be avoided in the infant or toddler, owing to the fact that early symptoms of this condition may not be recognized or interpreted, thus increasing the risks of more severe episodes. Yet, it is still a probable consequence, even in the most carefully monitored infant or toddler. Parents are taught to identify abrupt changes in the child's disposition or level of consciousness or to note signs of an adrenalin-glucagon outpouring: paleness, dilated pupils, tachycardia, or diaphoresis. They are further instructed, "When in doubt, check it out," with a simple blood glucose check. If unable to obtain a blood glucose measurement and unsure whether the child's behavior is due to hypoglycemia, the parent should treat the infant with a fast-acting sugar source.

Treating the infant's hypoglycemia may be accomplished with glucose water; regular soft drink; fruit juice by bottle; or with 2 teaspoons of honey, jelly, Karo syrup, or cake icing. Parents must have and know how to use injectable glucagon; for children under 3 years old, 0.5 mg (one-half vial) is suggested. If necessary, hypoglycemia may also be treated with an enema of Karo syrup and water.

PARENTAL FOLLOW-UP

Parents need to know that there is always a knowledgeable health professional available for consultation. Frequent phone calls or office visits are reassuring to both parent and professional.

The young child changes frequently: in growth needs, in activity levels, and in temperament. All of these normal childhood changes will affect diabetes control in some way. It is easy for the parents to become frustrated and discouraged with the day-to-day management of their child's diabetes. The professional's listening ear and reassur-

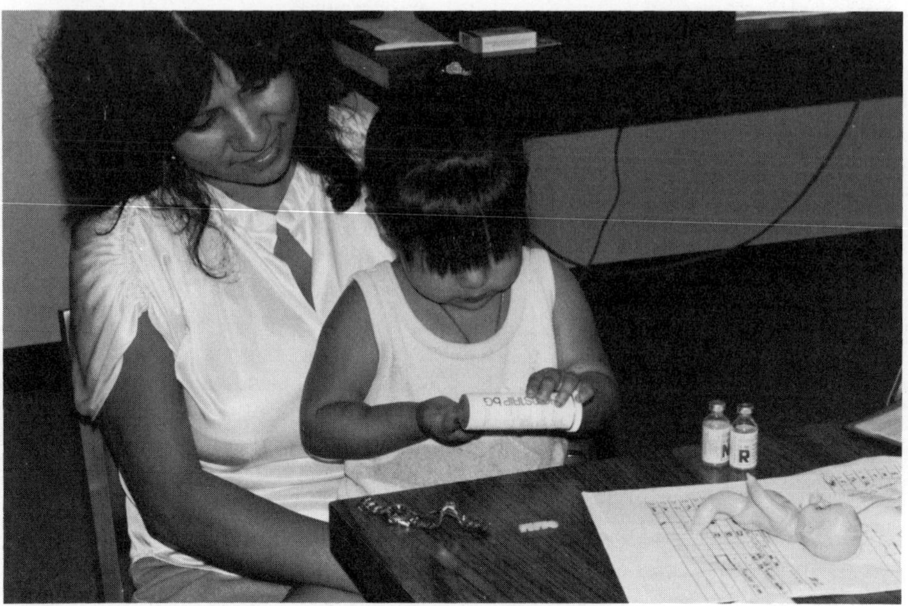

Figure 15–2. The young child's independence is increased by allowing him or her to participate in self-care. Small steps progress to larger steps.

ance become as important as any treatment recommendations.

WELL CHILD ISSUES

The infant with diabetes is still an infant with the same well child needs as all children. Childhood immunizations are to be encouraged, with the implementation of routine immunization schedules. After immunizations, the child's diabetes control may be poor for a few days, with elevated blood glucose levels and occasionally ketones. These alterations are managed as sick days.

It is sometimes difficult for parents to differentiate the child's normal development from effects of the diabetes. Overprotectiveness and overconcern are common. A part of the parent's diabetes education should be a discussion of normal developmental milestones, infant behavior, and normal parenting issues. Anticipatory guidance is more important in the chronically ill child than in the well child.

As the child enters the preschool years, parents must anticipate and plan for relinquishing to the child certain aspects of diabetes care. Such behaviors can and should begin even in the toddler (Fig. 15–2).

SUMMARY

The infant or toddler with diabetes offers a challenge to the health care professional. Manifestations of the young child's diabetes, although metabolically similar to those of the older child, may mimic behaviors of normal development. Monitoring and managing the child's diabetes require a few specialized techniques.

Parents often need frequent reassurance and follow-up care. The occurrence of "a few good days" reinforces the parents' decisions and increases their confidence. As one mother states, "When things are going well, she is just my baby—I almost forget she has diabetes."

16

The Adolescent

The adolescent with diabetes poses certain problems in management that differ from those in the management of the child with diabetes. In order rationally to approach the management of diabetes in the adolescent, it is necessary to understand the developmental tasks and stages of normal adolescence.

There are four basic tasks that adolescents usually address during the transition from childhood to adulthood. These tasks are

1. Emancipation from parents and other significant adults
2. Economic independence
3. Psychosexual differentiation and the adult sexual role
4. Stable adult self-identity in conformity with society

In addition to these tasks, the diabetic adolescent must also accept the diabetic state and adjust to alterations in the pattern of daily activities.

It is helpful to look at the stages of adolescence and their interactions with the specific tasks of normal adolescence and with the additional tasks of diabetic adolescence. Adolescence may be divided into three stages. In *early adolescence*, the primary task involves separation from the parents and from other significant adults. This may take the form of rejection of interaction with family members; rejection of childhood pursuits and interests; reluctance to accept advice, particularly from parents but also from other adults; ambivalence about assuming of independence; appearance of "crushes," often with members of the same sex and sometimes with members of the opposite sex; hero-worship of certain adult models, commonly teachers, coaches, and so forth; wide swings in mood; and the beginning of the physical and hormonal changes associated with puberty. The early adolescent often struggles with the dependent-independent role, sometimes seeking advice from parents while at other times being most reluctant to seek advice or information from anyone. It is essential to understand that it is not possible for the adolescent to be both close to and distant from his or her family simultaneously. This beginning struggle for independence also arouses feelings of ambivalence in parents. Parents often struggle with their upset feelings when their adolescent is no longer willing to come to them for permission or advice.

The *mid-adolescent* is the typical adolescent who is stereotyped in the media. The mid-adolescent has made it through the transition from childhood. By mid-adolescence, most young people have established themselves within a group of friends that is commonly called the peer group. The peer group provides the basis for the mid-adolescent's system of personal support. He or she is rarely willing to turn to parents or other adults for advice, help, or support; the peer group providing the basis for approval of the many behaviors that mid-adolescents engage in. The peer group sets the mid-adolescent apart from everyone else. The mid-adolescent subculture is designed primarily to provide the mid-adolescent with an identity completely separate from every other group. It is at this time that one sees fad behavior, substantial increases in physical activity, and a great deal of behavioral experimentation involving academic achievement, job choices, adult-like sexual behaviors, antisocial group behaviors, substance use and abuse, and increased risk-taking behaviors.

The *late adolescent* is on the verge of assuming the responsibility of the young adult. The late adolescent becomes involved with such issues as physical relocation, economic independence, mature sexual activities, and integration into the general ethical and moral values of society.

INTERACTION OF TASKS OF NORMAL ADOLESCENTS WITH TASKS OF DIABETIC ADOLESCENTS

The Early Adolescent

The primary goal of the early adolescent is to become independent. The early adolescent has been looking forward to this period of increased independence, freedom, and privileges but rarely takes into consideration that along with these desired freedoms he or she is expected to assume a certain amount of responsibility above and beyond that which has been assumed during late childhood. When diabetes has its onset in early adolescence, the adolescent's freedom to act on his or her own and to obtain additional privileges is usually restricted. Adolescents who have been anticipating much less control now find that their parents are exerting much more influence and much more control over their activities.

Many early adolescents will assume some responsibility for the management of their diabetes but exactly how much responsibility they can assume will depend on their past history of accepting responsibilities as a child and on the way they are managing the usual tasks of early adolescence. It would seem to be unwise to ask the early adolescent to assume all of the responsibilities for the management of diabetes. It would seem more sensible to ask the adolescent to assume those responsibilities that the parents, the adolescent, and the physician agree the adolescent may be able to assume. Since ambivalence is a common phenomenon in early adolescence, it is not surprising that adolescents may assume some or all of the tasks of their diabetic management during some periods of time, while they may be neither willing nor able to do so at other times.

In addition to the psychosocial tasks of the early adolescent, the physical and hormonal changes that occur at the onset of puberty have a further influence on the management of diabetes in the adolescent. Both estrogens and androgens may exert significant metabolic effects on the control of diabetes in the early adolescent. In the pubertal early adolescent, it would not be unusual to see a certain amount of lability beyond that encountered during the early months of the diabetic state in preadolescents. In addition to the metabolic changes that are secondary to the sex steroids, the early adolescent is usually emotionally quite labile. There is often some ambivalence and emotional upset about the physical changes that occur in early adolescence, which add to the stresses that early adolescents experience. This lability and stress may result in changes in the secretion of the neurotransmitters, particularly catecholamines, which also may have an effect on control of diabetes. It has been shown that labile diabetic adolescents may gain improved control of their diabetes during administration of beta-adrenergic blockers.

Another characteristic of early adolescents is their inability to think abstractly. Although the ability to engage in formal operations in regard to the thought process begins in early adolescence, a substantial number of teenagers cannot think abstractly. This inability to think abstractly prevents the early adolescent from considering the potentially deleterious long-term effects (complications) that might result from poor management of diabetes. Since the concrete thinking adolescent cannot easily project into the abstract future, discussions in the present of the consequences of poor control in the future are not likely to be regarded as seriously as they might be by a more mature teenager.

The Mid-Adolescent

The mid-adolescent is characterized by membership in a peer group. The mid-adolescent is the adolescent who typically has gone through the process of beginning separation from family and has gained a certain amount of independence. Mid-adolescent behaviors are in many instances dictated by those of the peer group, because this group provides the basis for most of the emotional support and approval that an adolescent receives outside the home. In order to be accepted into the peer group, the mid-adolescent must conform largely to the general behaviors of the group. These behaviors specifically set off the mid-adolescent from the younger adolescent and the child on the one hand and from the older adolescent and the adult on the other. The fad behaviors in which many mid-adolescents participate are often inimical to appropriate management of diabetes. For instance, the eating habits of the mid-adolescent are often quite variable: meals may be skipped or meals may consist of nutrients that are inappropriate for an adolescent with diabetes. However, it is extremely difficult for the mid-adolescent diabetic not to participate in the fad eating behavior of peers. It is therefore helpful to obtain a detailed dietary history of the mid-adolescent's eating behaviors and to devise a nutritional management diet that the adolescent helps plan and to incorporate into that diet as many of his or her eating practices as are consistent with appropriate dietary management.

Another characteristic of the mid-adolescent is the tremendous need for physical activity and the enormous amount of energy that mid-adolescents expend during this activity. This increased physical activity modifies the ultilization of glucose. The adolescent with diabetes who engages in physical activity needs to modify his or her exercise regimen and dietary plan in order to attain optimal homeostasis. This modification is something that other members of the peer group are not doing, so it causes the diabetic mid-adolescent to be different from the peer group. Although many mid-adolescents want to be recognized for their individuality, it seems much more important to them to be similar to rather than different from the peer group, especially in regard to physical activities. The adolescent's peers are often not even aware that their friend has diabetes, because many teenagers are reluctant to reveal their condition to their best friends, probably because having diabetes identifies them as "different." If this is the case, the diabetic adolescent should be encouraged to tell friends about the diabetes and should be given some guidance on how to do this. In most instances, mid-adolescents in the peer group will accept the presence of this disease more easily than will the diabetics themselves,

since it does not affect the members of the peer group personally. Many adolescents can be quite understanding and accepting of the diagnosis and can provide substantial support to their affected friend. However, they can sometimes become overconcerned and overprotective, which occasionally results in strained peer relations.

Mid-adolescence is also a time when behavioral experimentation is very common. This behavioral experimentation seems to be based on the observation that many adolescents feel that they are invulnerable. Elkind has called this phenomenon "the personal fable." The concept that "nothing bad can happen to me" results in risk-taking behavior. The physician needs to be aware that mid-adolescents may therefore find themselves in the position of modifying their diabetic regimen to see if they really need to have insulin every day or to determine if they really need to test their blood or urine glucose as often as the physician suggests. These risk-taking behaviors may result in episodes of diabetic ketoacidosis or in poor general control of diabetes.

In addition to this risk-taking behavior, many adolescents begin to experiment in the use of alcohol and drugs. The ingestion of alcohol by the diabetic causes alterations in carbohydrate metabolism that are not conducive to good control. There are few data about the effect of specific drugs on control of diabetes, but use of sympathomimetic amines, particularly dextroamphetamine, may result in increased blood glucose levels. Heavily sedated adolescents who have taken "downers" or adolescent diabetics who are using a hallucinogenic substance such as marijuana or LSD may find themselves in a clouded state during which time judgment in relationship to the management of diabetes may be quite poor. The adolescent may quite inadvertently miss a meal, not take a dose of insulin, or not perform a blood or urine test while under the influence of drugs or alcohol. It is especially important to discuss this issue in some detail with the mid-adolescent.

The Late Adolescent

The major task of late adolescence is the final separation from the nuclear family and the assumption of complete responsibility for oneself. Many adolescents find this a frightening and somewhat threatening experience.

It is at this time that many adolescents who previously had not paid much attention to appropriate management of their diabetes finally come to grips with the realities of the situation and begin to assume much more responsibility for management. It is at this stage that they no longer have a choice about management of their diabetes, because no one else is going to do it for them. Many adolescents who had management problems during early adolescence and mid-adolescence will continue to have problems during late adolescence and, in some instances, well into adult life. The assumption of responsibility depends to a certain extent on how well the physician, the parent, and the individual adjusted to the diabetic state during early adolescence and mid-adolescence.

There is a great deal of variability in the process of adolescence itself. The adolescent may be working on all of the four major tasks of adolescence in an unequal way. Some of these tasks may be accomplished by the end of adolescence, while others may not be completely resolved. This variability makes it difficult to make very specific statements about the transition from late adolescence to young adulthood. In many instances, adults have never resolved some of the basic issues of adolescence and persist in adolescent-type behaviors throughout their adult life. It is essential to provide additional support to the late adolescent during the separation process, regardless of whether this involves moving out of the home, going away to college, or getting a job.

The late adolescent with diabetes also has to come to grips with the establishment of mature relations with another significant person. Many adolescents are quite worried about revealing to boyfriends or girlfriends the fact that they have diabetes. They are quite worried that their partner will reject them because of their condition. The establishment of mature or permanent social relations occasionally becomes a problem toward the end of mid-adolescence, but it becomes more problematic during late adolescence and early adulthood.

In addition, the diabetic late adolescent woman is often concerned about the effect of her diabetes on childbearing. Most adolescents know that diabetes is a hereditary disorder, and some also know that pregnancy in a diabetic woman is more complicated than is pregnancy in a nondiabetic woman. Therefore, the issue of marriage and childbearing provides the basis for some additional concerns during late adolescence that should be addressed by the physician. Family planning is an issue that particularly needs to be addressed. As mentioned previously, sex steroids may affect glucose homeostasis. Oral contraceptives should be prescribed primarily for those young women with diabetes who have been reasonably compliant and well controlled in the past, since extra supervision is necessary for those who choose this method. However, it is much safer to prescribe some form of barrier-mechanical contraception for those women who have diabetes of over 15 years' duration or who have retinopathy.

Many adolescent diabetics are managed by pediatricians. By the end of late adolescence, the possibility of transfer of care to an internist arises. In many instances, the diabetic will prefer to transfer care, but some late adolescents prefer to remain in the care of the pediatrician who has provided their care for many years. If the physician believes that separation from the nuclear family is causing significant problems for the late adolescent, it might be best to delay separation from the physician until such time as the patient is more comfortable with independent living: too many losses in a short time interval may be too much to manage. It is best to discuss the transfer of care at a time when all other issues seem stable. This should be done over a period of many months before the actual separation takes place in order to allow the adolescent to come to grips with this additional separation.

INTERACTIONS WITH PARENTS AND HEALTH PROFESSIONALS

Understanding Parents' Problems

It is hard to be the parent of a healthy teenager and even harder to be the parent of an adolescent with diabetes. Parents usually try to help their youngster accept the diagnosis and the modifications of activities of daily living that are necessary. Parents themselves may have difficulty accepting diabetes in their child. They may feel guilty, angry, and frustrated when they experience difficulties in trying to help their adolescent manage the problems related to growing up as well as those related to having diabetes. Parents usually feel that they must assume the major responsibility for the management of diabetes in the early adolescent. This would seem to be reasonable and appropriate in many instances, especially at the onset of diabetes, since the young adolescent is often unable to accept responsibilities as parents would like. However, if parents can be helped to realize that the early adolescent is struggling to become independent from the family, it may be easier for them to understand why there may be a great deal of conflict over parental control of the adolescent with diabetes.

It is essential that the physician provide the parents of the adolescent with basic information about the tasks of adolescence and to ensure that the parents understand that many of the resistant behaviors that they will observe are, in fact, based on the normal developmental tasks of adolescence. If parents can understand the tasks that their adolescent is engaged in, it will be much easier for the parent to work out an appropriate management plan in cooperation with both the physician and the adolescent.

Parents and health professionals need to recognize that the management of the behavior of the diabetic adolescent will be easier if there are fewer rather than more rules to follow. The more rules the adolescent has to follow, the more likely he or she is to break rules, at least on some occasions. It is therefore appropriate for the physician and the parents to make clear, unambiguous statements about what rules must absolutely not be violated and about what the consequences of breaking these rules might be. Certainly as a minimum, it is necessary for the adolescent to take injections of insulin as prescribed and to eat appropriately. It is of course highly desirable for the adolescent to perform blood or urine glucose testing and to modify other activities, but the physician, the parent, and the adolescent must decide on how important these other issues are.

The mid-adolescent diabetic is much more likely than the early adolescent diabetic to take chances. It is therefore not surprising that many mid-adolescent diabetics engage in substantial risk-taking behaviors, which may result in moderately to extremely poor control of diabetes. Unfortunately, it is extremely difficult for either the health professional or the parents to prevent behavioral experimentation and the resultant poor or erratic control. Unfortunately, most of us learn by doing ourselves, and the mid-ado-

lescent with diabetes is no exception. The risk-taking behavior should certainly not be condoned either by the parents or by the health professional but should be expected and should be managed in a firm, nonthreatening fashion. The parents should still insist that the basic rules of management be followed, but it is important to keep these rules to the minimum that is consistent with good management. It is essential for the parent to be especially observant, in the most unobtrusive way, for indications that the mid-adolescent is losing control of his or her diabetes. Many adolescents actually welcome a restatement of their parents' commitment to help them manage their diabetes. Parents should not hesitate to discuss poor control of diabetes with their adolescent and with the physician.

The parents of the late adolescent are usually anticipating the freedom that they will experience when their late adolescent finally assumes complete responsibility for the management of diabetes. However, in many instances, parents may be disappointed because the mid-adolescent period may be prolonged in those individuals who have a chronic illness. It is therefore essential that the parents continue to provide as much support as is needed for the late adolescent in the management of his or her diabetes. Parents should be encouraged to understand that the late adolescent with diabetes may need continued parental support well into young adulthood.

Parents themselves are usually under a substantial amount of stress when they have to manage the problems of an adolescent with diabetes. It is important to recognize that there are certain parental needs for support, which, if not identified and managed by the health professional, may complicate the management of the diabetic adolescent. Parents should be given an opportunity to discuss their own feelings of the problems in the management of their teenager's diabetes.

In most families, it is the mother of the child who usually assumes all of the responsibilities for supervision of the child's health. This role may cause the mother to become excessively stressed, especially if she is employed. The physician should be alert to signs of excessive stress in the mother and institute appropriate management. Prevention is best in the case of stress. The husband and wife should attend all patient education sessions, and the diabetes team should discuss sharing responsibilities between spouses. If the wife becomes stressed, the physician and team should discuss this issue with both parents and should arrange for appropriate counseling for both parents. Separate sessions for each parent of a diabetic adolescent may be an effective way for the physician to identify and manage this aspect of diabetes in the adolescent. Some physicians have found that parent groups can be very helpful, and these have been established by the American Diabetes Association and the Juvenile Diabetes Foundation. It may be very helpful to encourage parents to join one of these groups and to participate in their activities, many of which are designed to help alleviate stress in the parents of diabetic adolescents.

Understanding Health Care Professionals' Problems

The health care professionals providing care for diabetic adolescents must understand the developmental tasks and characteristics of adolescents at the three stages of early, middle, and late adolescence. Health care delivery to adolescents with chronic disease that does not take into account these normal development characteristics is not likely to be very successful.

One of the major goals of the health care professional should be to help the adolescent assume responsibility for his or her own health care. Several techniques have been helpful in this respect. It is very important for the physician providing health care to diabetic adolescents to make it clear to the adolescent that the adolescent and not the parent is the patient. One of the best ways to give this message to adolescents in any developmental stage is to treat the adolescent as the patient. This can be accomplished by interviewing and examining the adolescent without the parents present. Most adolescents are perfectly capable of providing the physician with an adequate history and of being examined in the absence of the parents. During the course of the initial interview with the adolescent, it is often very helpful to have a discussion of confidentiality (with the parents present), so that there is no ambiguity about the parents' feelings and the physician's intentions in regard to confidentiality. It is important to remember to make it clear to both parents and adolescents that there

are exceptions to the rules of confidentiality. You must inform both the adolescent and the parents that if the adolescent tells you something that you feel would be very hazardous to the patient's well-being, you will be under an obligation to disclose this information to the parents. It is equally important to stress to the adolescent that you will not disclose confidential information to the parents unless you have discussed it with the adolescent first. In some instances, adolescents will not be paying particular attention to areas that the physician or the parents might be concerned about. Interview the adolescent diabetic's parents alone in order to estimate the reliability of the information that the adolescent provides for you, to hear the parents' viewpoint on the management of a particular problem, and to identify and manage problems that the parents are experiencing. Parents are sometimes reluctant to say things about their children when the children are present during the interview.

Most physicians are placed in a role of authority and tend to become paternalistic when providing care for adolescents with chronic illness. The authoritarian approach is not likely to work well with adolescents. Adolescents are likely to be much more compliant if they feel that they have some control over the situation. It is advisable to discuss in some detail each step of the management plan with the adolescent and to discuss these in very concrete terms. Written instructions should be given so that there is no ambiguity about management.

The physician who takes the psychosocial characteristics of normal adolescence into consideration in his or her management plans for the adolescent with diabetes is not likely to experience anger, frustration, or guilt. These feelings can be minimized if the health provider recognizes that certain types of adolescent behavior that seem very provocative, particularly the risk-taking behaviors, are nothing more than manifestations of the normal developmental tasks. That is not to say that the physician ought to condone risk-taking behaviors such as skipping insulin doses, not adhering to dietary regimens, and so forth. The physician should make it clear to the adolescent that he or she considers these behaviors very risky and not conducive to maintenance of optimal health and functioning. Remember that the fewer the rules that one has to enforce, the easier the job will be.

It is sometimes helpful to discuss the process of decision making with the adolescent. The formal steps in decision making are to

1. Identify *all* the options
2. Examine the potential positive and negative consequences of each option
3. Choose an option based on the balance of the positive and negative consequences
4. Evaluate the results of the option chosen
   a. If results are acceptable, no further action is indicated
   b. If results are inacceptable, return to step 3

Working through this process with adolescents usually gives them the feeling that they have some control over what is planned for their management and tends to increase compliance.

Other methods for increasing compliance include

1. Provide positive reinforcement (that is, compliments, praise) whenever the patient complies, even if it is what you expect and even if it is about a minor issue
2. Send reminder cards about appointments about one week in advance
3. Send birthday, graduation, and other special event cards to show you care
4. Inquire about issues in the patient's life other than diabetes
5. Minimize displays of anger, frustration, and any unhappiness you might feel about the patient's noncompliance

Manipulation

Manipulation is one way in which some people attempt to accomplish a change to their own advantage. Manipulation is usually learned early in life and is a common method of getting what is desired. It may involve a secret or hidden agenda. The person who is doing the manipulation is trying to accomplish something but is not able to state openly and clearly what the objectives and goals are. In diabetic adolescents, manipulation may take the form of refusal to take insulin, test blood, or adhere to diet in order to get more attention, to get more freedom, to get fewer responsibilities, to anger parents, and so forth. Parents and physicians need to be aware of, must recognize, and must deal with these attempts at manipulation by the adolescent. The response to attempts of manipulation must involve the avoidance of giving positive reinforcement for behaviors that one does not want to see, while providing positive reinforcement for desirable behaviors. That is, if the parents or physician reward the adolescent's manipulation attempts, the adolescent will continue to use manipulation as a way to achieve his or her goals and objectives. It is rarely helpful to point out to the adolescent that you recognize these as attempts at manipulation to achieve other goals, because the adolescent usually does not want to hear about it. The best approach is for the parents or the physician to refuse to be manipulated by the adolescent. That means that the physician or parents must not respond positively to attempts at manipulation but rather must ignore them. This may initially result in some adverse consequences for the teenager, who may become sick because of not taking insulin, not adhering to dietary regimens, and so forth; but unfortunately, most people, including most adolescents, learn only by experience. The adolescent who experiences illness because of attempts at manipulation should have that illness managed by the parents or the physician. However, the parents or physician must be very careful not to reward the adolescent for that type of behavior by giving in to their demands. If attempts at manipulation (or risk-taking behaviors) result in poor control, firm action must be instituted. If hospitalization is necessary, the stay should be as short as possible and should not be particularly pleasant. It might be indicated to restrict the adolescent to his or her hospital room rather than to allow him or her to engage in any of the recreational activities that many hospitals have available for teenagers; for if the patient is well enough to play, he or she is probably well enough to be discharged. This suggestion does not apply to those diabetic adolescents who are hospitalized for poor control secondary to infection or other problems.

Parents also can become manipulative. Parents may use the child's diabetes in order to maintain control over the adolescent's behavior and to prevent the adolescent from progressing normally through the tasks of adolescence, particularly that of independence that occurs early in adolescence. The physician must be alert to this possibility and question the adolescent if behaviors emerge that might suggest parental manipulation. The most helpful approach to parental manipulation of the diabetic adolescent is to discuss with the parents the behaviors that they are manifesting and to suggest nonmanipulative methods for obtaining the desired goals.

Physicians can exhibit manipulative behavior too. The use of the hidden agenda in teenagers with diabetes, in an attempt to get them to conform to physicians' ideas about management is not appropriate. Adolescents can usually spot this type of manipulative behavior. As mentioned previously, it is important for the physician to enter into a negotiation process with both parents and adolescents in the management of the diabetic adolescent. This negotiation process is time consuming but usually pays off in the long run and tends to prevent manipulative behaviors.

THE LABILE ADOLESCENT

Some adolescents cannot be helped. The physician who is faced with the adolescent who repeatedly fails to adhere to reasonable regimens, or who repeatedly is hospitalized for diabetic ketoacidosis not related to infections or for other problems poses specific difficulties for management. Every physician should attempt to identify life stresses and other factors that pose problems for the adolescent and that make the management of his or her diabetes more difficult. Adolescents with behavioral problems that contribute significantly to the management of their diabetes should be offered the opportunity to discuss their personal problems either with the primary physician who is managing the diabetes, the patient's primary care physician, or a competent behavioralist. However, some adolescents are not able to accept help in any form from anybody. The best approach to this type of adolescent is to provide whatever episodic care the adolescent requires. This often means making a statement to the adolescent such as, "I think you have a particular problem; I'd like to help you with this particular problem, but if you can't accept the help that I can give you in regard to the things that are really bothering you, that's understandable. I will provide ongoing care for control of your diabetes, will admit you to the hospital whenever you get into difficulty with ketoacidosis, and will always have my door open to you so that if you do want to come and begin to work on some of the basic problems that you are encountering, you can do that at any time." It is not worthwhile for the health professional to expend a substantial amount of time and energy trying to force help on an adolescent who absolutely refuses to be helped. It is, however, important to remind these adolescents that if they do want to have some help for their problems, they can come to you and you can arrange it for them.

In conclusion, management of the diabetic adolescent must be based on an understanding of the basic psychosocial tasks of adolescence and their interaction with the stages of adolescence. Parents and physicians must develop management plans together with the diabetic adolescent. The goals of these plans are to provide for optimal management and to assist the adolescent in assuming complete responsibility of his or her own health care.

17

Management Before and After Surgery

Fifty percent of all patients with diabetes will require surgery at some point during their lives. In the adult, the surgery is often directly related to the diabetes and includes such minor procedures as incision and drainage of abscesses and more complex problems involving compromised vascular supply to an extremity. Infection and complications directly attributable to secondary cardiovascular disease are the most common causes of morbidity and mortality. In contrast, surgery in the child with diabetes usually is unrelated to the disease and includes such procedures as hernia repair, appendectomy, and ear or eye surgery. The overall surgical mortality has been reported at about 3 to 4 percent, with a postoperative complication rate of 17 percent. The child, however, probably has little increased mortality over that of nondiabetic peers, but morbidity from vacillations in blood glucose and infectious postoperative complications remains a problem.

METABOLIC CHANGES

Surgery is a physical stress and is characterized by catabolism, increased metabolic rate, increased protein and fat breakdown, negative nitrogen balance, starvation, and glucose intolerance (see Chapter 11). The degree of metabolic change is related to the surgical procedure, the length of the operation, and the presence of complications such as septicemia or shock. Hormonal changes (that is, increased secretion of catecholamines, ACTH, cortisol, growth hormone, and probably glucagon) during surgery are related to the metabolic disturbances.

In the nondiabetic, there is inhibition of insulin secretion and relative insulin resistance, resulting in increases in blood glucose concentrations during surgery, with persistence for variable lengths of time following surgery. The type of anesthesia also has metabolic effects in the nondiabetic surgical patient, extradural and spinal anesthesia having less effect than general anesthesia. The anesthetic used also plays a role, since ether, chloroform, and cyclopropane are known to cause hyperglycemia, fatty acid mobilization, inhibition of insulin secretion, and increased catecholamine and ACTH release. Newer inhalation anesthetics, premedications, and muscle relaxants have fewer metabolic effects.

All of the metabolic effects of surgery are exaggerated in the diabetic, particularly if there is a virtual absence of endogenous insulin. The pronounced catabolism results in fatty acid production, ketogenesis, hyperglycemia (due to glycogenolysis and gluconeogenesis), and eventually ketosis or ketoacidosis. Therefore, a major aim of therapy during surgery is to prevent metabolic decompensation and at the same time to avoid hypoglycemia. Thus, at least some semblance of good diabetic control is warranted during surgery.

The importance of tight diabetic control during the brief surgical and postsurgical period is not known. Many studies have related short-term control to abnormalities that are important in the surgical and postsurgical periods, particularly as they relate to infectious complications and wound healing. These, therefore, deserve some consideration.

Adherence of polymorphonuclear leukocytes is significantly impaired in diabetics who are poorly controlled, even if they are not acidotic. This defect can be normalized by improved short-term diabetic control. Likewise, abnormalities in random migration, chemotaxis, phagocytosis, and bacterial killing have been noted in leukocytes from diabetics. Some of these abnormalities have been corrected by short-term glucose normalization. Similarly, lymphocyte function may be impaired in diabetics in poor control as seen in certain animal models in which prolonged skin graft survival, decreased phytohemagglutinin response, and decreased mixed lymphocyte culture response is noted. These abnormalities are corrected with treatment of hyperglycemia. Delay in antibody formation has been noted in diabetic children and appears to be correlated with glucose control. These defects of white blood cell function in patients with poorly controlled diabetes may bear some relationship to the increased incidence of infection during the perioperative period.

Abnormalities in erythrocytes and oxygen-carrying capacity have also been noted in patients with poorly controlled diabetes. The concentration of 2,3-diphosphoglycerate is decreased in the presence of ketosis and ketoacidosis, resulting in impaired oxygen unloading to tissues and increased venous oxygen tension. Changes in erythrocyte aggregation and deformability can result in decreased erythrocyte survival, which can be corrected with treatment of hyperglycemia.

Coagulation defects are also noted in persons with diabetes. Although the abnormalities in coagulation are not clear cut, and, although not well defined, any defect in coagulation is obviously important in the surgical patient. Platelet abnormalities are difficult to interpret, but changes in platelet aggregation and adhesion have been noted. Initial hypercoagulability followed by hypocoagulability has been demonstrated in diabetic rats, and these effects are reversed by appropriate insulin administration. Fibrinogen survival is decreased in hyperglycemic patients, and again, euglycemia can reverse this effect.

Wound healing is also of concern in the diabetic surgical patient. Wound healing and strength is impaired in diabetic animals not receiving insulin and is improved with insulin administration.

PREOPERATIVE MANAGEMENT

For elective surgery, the diabetic patient should be admitted to the hospital 36 to 48 hours prior to the surgical procedure. Initial assessment of the metabolic status of the patient should be performed and necessary alterations made. Unless significant abnormalities are discovered, the usual diet and insulin therapy should be continued. It should be noted that the stress attendant to this period precludes this from being an ideal time to attempt tight control. On the other hand, efforts should be made to achieve the best metabolic control possible without making major changes in the patient's usual management. Supplemental doses of Regular insulin may be required.

Each patient should also be assessed for the possibility of any diabetic complication. Most specifically, hypertension and renal functional abnormalities (proteinuria or elevated serum creatinine) should be noted. All members of the patient care team, including diabetologist, pediatrician or family practitioner, anesthesiologist, surgeon, nurse clinician, and dietitian should be involved in assessment and treatment.

INTRAOPERATIVE MANAGEMENT

Numerous methods of glucose control have been used in surgical patients, and, to some extent, these depend on the type of surgery: minor or major, emergency or elective. There is one consistent feature of all these methods: the elective procedure should be performed as early in the day as possible, preferably as the first case. Each method has its proponents, and controversy exists concerning an optimal management program. A significant difficulty in assessing the various proposed methods is that no large-scale, randomized comparative study has been done, and only a few studies report comparisons of even small numbers of patients. Most authors strongly advise intraoperative glucose monitoring.

One early method of management during surgery consisted of withholding both insulin and glucose, with non-glucose-containing intravenous fluids given as needed. Although the original reports appeared favorable, more recent reports demonstrate unacceptable hyperglycemia in some patients and other metabolic derangements, including the presence of increased ketoacids; increased fatty acids; and negative balances of potassium, phosphorus, calcium, and magnesium. Thus, the metabolic status of the diabetic surgical patient was not ideal, and this approach has been largely abandoned.

Another method widely used is the administration of a partial amount of the usual insulin dose as intermediate-acting insulin on the morning of surgery; for example, two thirds of the usual morning NPH or Lente dose without Regular insulin. This is followed by an intravenous infusion containing 5 percent glucose given during the operative procedure, along with serial blood glucose monitoring. Although this represents an improvement over the earlier method, problems still exist, because hyperglycemia occurs in some and in others the glucose infusion does not protect against intraoperative hypoglycemia. Even so, this method is appropriate for many short surgical procedures, especially those in which the child will be receiving oral intake later in the surgical day.

Continuous insulin infusion has become popular in the treatment of diabetic ketoacidosis and recently has emerged as a method of management during surgery. Several variations in technique have been used. One method calls for glucose and insulin to be infused in the same intravenous solution, so that if the infusion is interrupted for some reason, both glucose and insulin are terminated. Another recommendation is for separate glucose and insulin infusions; allowing adjustments to be made in either component separately. In either case, an accurate volumetric infusion pump is necessary, and the ability to monitor blood glucose is essential. Success has been reported in keeping patients euglycemic, in producing euglycemia during surgery in those initially hyperglycemic, and even in maintaining euglycemia in diabetic renal transplant patients with azotemia who are receiving prednisone. Recommendations include intravenous glucose at a rate of 0.1 g/kg/hr and a constant infusion of insulin at a starting rate of 0.05 to 0.1 U/kg/hr. An extension of this method has also been reported wherein a minipump is used to infuse very small amounts of insulin (usually 0.01 to 0.03 U/kg/hr) intravenously in diabetics undergoing minor surgery, when intravenous fluids are not necessary.

The major pitfall in any of these methods of management is undetected hypoglycemia or extreme hyperglycemia during anesthesia. The diabetic may not have the typical reaction to hypoglycemia under anesthesia, and so monitoring of the patient's status becomes critical. Blood glucose determinations must be performed frequently just prior to surgery, intraoperatively, and postoperatively. Most diabetologists recommend that this be done on an hourly basis throughout the surgical procedure and more frequently if the patient is not metabolically stable preoperatively. The method for determining blood glucose must be rapid and accurate. Proper use of glucose-oxidase strips (Chemstrip bG) makes them ideal for intraoperative monitoring. The anesthesiologist must be well acquainted with the method chosen, so that frequent determinations can be accomplished and appropriate decisions made.

Because of the potential problems with hypoglycemia and the need for frequent monitoring, recent reports have assessed the usefulness of an artificial beta cell (Biostator and glucose-controlled insulin-infusion system, or GCIIS) in perioperative management. Using GCIIS it is possible to maintain or achieve euglycemia throughout the perioperative period without the hazard of hypoglycemia. More studies are necessary to assess its cost effectiveness and short-term benefits.

In addition to blood glucose control, fluid and electrolytes must be managed appropriately. Intravenous fluid replacement must be maintained with an appropriate electrolyte composition in addition to the glucose infusion and at a rate determined by the anesthesiologist. An appropriate replacement fluid for children less than 6 years old is one in which the sodium chloride concentration is 0.20 to 0.25 percent. In patients more than six years old, the NaCl concentration should be 0.25 to 0.33 percent. Potassium balance should be maintained with administration of an appropriate amount of potassium. The physician caring for the diabetic surgical patient should choose a method of overall control with which he or she is most familiar and comfortable.

POSTOPERATIVE MANAGEMENT

The aim of postoperative management is the maintenance of good metabolic control until the patient can resume the usual diet and insulin dosage. Again, various regimens have been advocated, including the administration of intermediate-acting insulin in the recovery room and supplements of Regular insulin based on need, as determined by serial blood glucose measurements. A satisfactory level of control can be achieved by continuing the constant intravenous insulin and glucose infusion if begun in surgery. Alternatively, intravenous glucose administration can be continued, and small doses of Regular insulin (0.02 to 0.1 U/kg every two to four hours) can be given intramuscularly or subcutaneously. It does not seem appropriate to use a traditional, retrospective sliding scale for insulin during this time. Such therapy often creates significant problems for the patient. Ideally, blood glucose values should be maintained between 100 mg/dl and 200 mg/dl.

In the severely catabolic patient, total parenteral nutrition (TPN) may be required, and this can be accomplished in the diabetic patient as well as in the nondiabetic. If insulin is not given in sufficient quantities to maintain euglycemia, the large amounts of glucose administered cannot be used for anabolism. Some of the required insulin can be administered in the TPN solution itself and supplemented with constant intravenous insulin infusion, frequent subcutaneous regular insulin, or subcutaneous intermediate-acting insulin. Again, frequent monitoring of blood glucose is required.

Throughout the postoperative period, the diabetic patient should be monitored for complications. Most importantly, infectious complications should be sought; if the patient has had a urinary catheter in place, a urinary tract infection would be a common complication. Additionally, any metabolic derangement such as ketosis, acidosis, or hypoglycemia should be sought and treated appropriately.

EMERGENCY SURGERY

At some time during life, the diabetic, like the nondiabetic, may require emergency surgery. It is worth restating remarks made earlier when considering DKA. Ketoacidosis may closely mimic an acute surgical abdomen, with severe abdominal pain, diffuse guarding and tenderness, nausea and vomiting, and alterations in bowel sounds. The associated leukocytosis may lend further support to the belief that a surgical condition exists. The diabetic care team and the family should be prepared for this eventuality. If the patient is metabolically stable at the time, then management intraoperatively can proceed as for elective surgery. If the patient is in diabetic ketoacidosis or has severe metabolic derangements, treatment should begin immediately for these problems, with surgery postponed as long as possible in order to improve the metabolic status. Treatment of the metabolic problems should continue simultaneously if surgical intervention must proceed immediately. Management with a constant intravenous insulin infusion or with GCIIS is appropriate in emergency surgery.

18

Consequences and Complications

With the increased longevity associated with widespread clinical use of insulin by IDDM patients came the ultimate discovery that certain previously recognized morbid events were occurring with increased frequency, while others were appearing for the first time. Hypertension, retinopathy, glomerulosclerosis, and neuropathy were increasingly recognized, and life-expectancy of patients with these problems did not reach those of nondiabetic peers. Despite 60 years of experience with insulin management, the situation with these patients as compared with the nondiabetic population remains that life expectancy is shortened, perhaps by as much as 20 years; up to 80 percent of children with IDDM develop retinopathy, and about 10 percent become legally blind; renal failure occurs with a fivefold increase in frequency; and a major cardiovascular complication (that is, myocardial infarction, cerebrovascular accident, and so forth) is twice as likely to occur.

As frustrating as our inability to modify these consequences has been, our lack of complete understanding of the pathogenesis of them has been even greater. Even now, there is no unanimity of opinion among diabetes investigators as to the precise cause of these complications. All accept the fact that there is a direct relationship between the insulin-deficient state and the development of degenerative disease, but the specific mechanism(s) remain unexplained. It has become increasingly clear to virtually everyone that microvascular disease is characteristic of diabetes mellitus and that its occurrence and progression is directly or indirectly related to the elevated concentrations of glucose in the blood.

Although it is beyond the scope of this chapter to even consider, much less discuss, the many processes that may lead to the development of a complication, one factor appears undisputed: Hyperglycemia is one element of this multifaceted event. Another factor appears to be almost as important: In general, organ damage occurs in those tissues (cells) in which glucose transport across the cell membrane is not insulin mediated or dependent. Thus, the vascular endothelium, the nerve sheath, the red blood cell, the lens of the eye, and other tissues are suffused with amounts of glucose that are totally dependent on the degree of hyperglycemia and its mass transfer from the extracellular fluid, potentially leading to metabolic and functional alterations within the cell structure. In some instances, it is felt that molecular alterations of cellular proteins (for example, glucosylation) are responsible for physical or functional permutations, or both. In other cases, the accumulation of excess metabolites of glucose (for example, sorbitol and other sugar alcohols) appear as offending agents. In both instances, there are coincident

Table 18–1. **PATHOGENIC FACTORS IN DEVELOPMENT OF CHRONIC COMPLICATIONS OF IDDM**

Possible Responsible Factor	Possible Mechanism or Example
Genetics	Increased predisposition to microvascular disease; ? limited joint mobility
Immunologic injury	Autoimmune disease; disease secondary to exogenous insulin antibodies
Hormonal	
Growth hormone	Increase in microvascular disease after puberty; regression of retinopathy after hypophysectomy
Renin-Angiotensin-aldosterone	—
Hyperlipidemia	Increased atherosclerosis
Platelet abnormalities	Platelet aggregation and adhesiveness Secondary changes
Hyperviscosity state	—
Hyperglycemia	
Glucosylation of proteins	Many proteins
Accumulation of metabolites	Sorbitol accumulation; optic lens, nervous tissue
Metabolic changes in cell	—
RBC abnormalities	Lack of normal RBC deformity
WBC abnormalities	Multiple defects
Hyperfiltration	Increased GFR; sclerosis

Table 18–2. **COMPLICATIONS OF IDDM**

I. Poor Physical or Emotional Health
   A. Symptomatic or asymptomatic hypoglycemia
   B. Symptomatic hyperglycemia
   C. Inadequate coping ability
   D. Others
II. Infectious
III. Metabolic
   A. DKA
   B. Ketosis
   C. Osteomalacia
   D. Others (e.g., limited joint mobility)
IV. Developmental and Statural
   A. Growth retardation
   B. Delayed sexual maturation
   C. Delayed psychologic maturation
   D. Obesity
V. Macrovascular
   A. Atherosclerosis
   B. Hyperlipidemia
   C. Hypertension
VI. Microvascular
   A. Retinopathy
   B. Nephropathy
   C. Cardiomyopathy
   D. Hypertension
VII. Neuropathy
   A. Peripheral
   B. Visceral
   C. Central
   D. Autonomic
VIII. Others

changes in the intracellular environment (for example, electrolytes, minerals, and water) that may contribute to development of structural abnormalities.

Table 18–1 outlines some of the possible factors that are considered operational in the development of the chronic complications of IDDM. Although it was at one time felt that there was a separate genetic defect responsible for the presence of microvascular disease, this is no longer considered a viable theory, tive since similar complications develop in experimental diabetes, regardless of the method of production. Many investigators still believe, however, that there may be some genetic factors that either increase or decrease the vascular response to hyperglycemia.

Table 18–2 categorizes most of the complications associated with the occurrence of IDDM, even though newly recognized ones seem to appear almost daily. The following sections will not attempt to discuss all these complications in any detail but will concentrate on just a few of the most important. Some of the complications noted in Table 18–2 have been discussed in other sections of this book, whereas others will be barely referenced. For these latter instances, the reader is referred to several recent texts dealing with these consequences of the diabetic state.

GROWTH AND GROWTH RETARDATION

Historical Perspective

In 1930, Mauriac published an article that described children in poor diabetic control who developed hepatomegaly, protuberant abdomens, and round facies and who had growth retardation and sexual infantilism. Such children were later found to have fatty livers and hyperlipidemia. This condition, now known as Mauriac's syndrome, has been traditionally attributed to poor carbohydrate control as a consequence of underinsulinization. The periodic reports of this syndrome, even today, all seem to attest to the significance of chronic malnutrition as a causative factor of the growth retardation in children who are maintained in a metabolic state of severe and longstanding underinsulinization. Less clear is the effect of mild to moderately poor carbohydrate control on the growth of children with IDDM.

Literature from early in the insulin era suggested that growth failure was a common association of IDDM but, as the ability to control diabetes improved with better understanding and technology, major disturbances in growth were seen with far less frequency. Still, the debate concerning growth in the average child with diabetes has persisted. Some authors have reported growth disturbances even in patients with well-controlled diabetes, whereas others have maintained that no significant impairment in linear growth occurs in patients in whom carbohydrate control is good. The major difficulty in reconciling these differing reports has, in the past, been the lack of an acceptable standard for determining glucose control, and most of the articles prior to the 1980s do not provide sufficient measurements to allow comparison. Data collected now using glycosylated hemoglobin as a standard should ultimately resolve this controversy.

An interesting and perhaps overcited study is that of Tattersall and Pyke (1973). They looked at 34 identical-twin pairs, in which one or both siblings developed diabetes mellitus before the age of 30. In 12 pairs, one twin developed diabetes before puberty; and in all pairs except one, the affected twin was shorter than the sibling who did not develop diabetes prior to puberty (range of 0.5 to 6.5 inches, mean 2.5 inches). These differences were significantly greater than those observed in six pairs in which both twins developed diabetes before puberty, 10 pairs in which one twin developed diabetes after puberty and the other remained unaffected, and seven pairs in which both twins developed diabetes after puberty. Despite the fact that this study does not provide quantitative data relative to the degree of diabetic control, it does strongly support the argument that something in the diabetic milieu contributes to inadequate growth and that it is not primarily of genetic origin.

As already mentioned, the lack of uniformity in all studies in defining "good control" and the difficulty in differentiating "good" from "not-so-good" control makes comparisons difficult, especially since philosophies of management and goals differ from one locality to another. Additionally, only a few of the reported studies make an effort to look at familial growth patterns and other possible influences. These criticisms notwithstanding, some conclusions about the growth of children with diabetes mellitus appear inescapable:

1. Children with less than optimal carbohydrate control are at significant risk for growth retardation and delayed sexual development.
2. The younger the child at time of onset (that is, the longer the duration of diabetes prior to puberty), the greater the potential for growth retardation.
3. In situations when poor control has led to growth failure, some catch-up growth may be possible if the metabolic state can be adequately controlled.

The suggestion from all studies is that diabetes control does influence rate of growth, but the precise mechanism by which this occurs is by no means clear. What is the optimal degree of carbohydrate control to ensure optimal growth? There is, as yet, no answer to this question. Even more basic to our understanding of this relationship is the elucidation of the pathophysiology of growth failure in those few children who exhibit shortened statures.

Aspects of Growth

A number of interdigitating elements are obviously involved in the process of linear growth. Known factors that have a major influence are genetics, the hormonal milieu, nutrition, and the overall well-being of the individual (physical, emotional, and environmental). The heredity of stature has been termed multifaceted, but, certainly, a major determinant of adult stature is the genetic make-up. However, the "twin" studies and studies on emotionally deprived infants clearly suggest that environment, particularly appropriate nurturing, is important in relation to other factors.

A number of hormones are well known to have significant impact on growth, and many are operational in the diabetic state. In summarizing several studies over the past few years, the following five statements appear appropriate. In the diabetic state:

1. There is a serious deficiency of *insulin* and an associated increase in *glucagon* secretion

2. There is a slight increase in serum levels of *cortisol* with some blunting of the normal diurnal rhythm

3. There are elevated serum levels of *growth hormone* with alterations in the normal diurnal rhythms, marked fluctuations with changes in blood sugar, exaggerated responses to stress and exercise, and lack of suppression with hyperglycemia

4. There is normal (or possibly low) somatomedin activity (*somatomedin C*) even in the face of elevated growth hormone levels

5. There are elevated serum levels of *catecholamines* and increased reactivity of the adrenal medulla

All of these changes are seen from time to time in the majority of Type I diabetics but all are magnified in those with poor carbohydrate control. Additionally, the most striking abnormalities in these hormonal profiles are seen in those patients who are growth retarded, regardless of their degree of poor control. The relationships among these various hormonal factors is uncertain. The effects of elevated cortisol levels on normal growth are well known and can be significant. The importance of such increases in the child with diabetes mellitus is unknown, but the plasma concentrations are often at levels known to inhibit linear growth when steroid analogs are supplied exogenously. At least, a few reports have described a facial feature of Mauriac's syndrome as cushingoid. Less severely compromised metabolic control is often associated with rounded facies, truncal obesity, thickened subcutaneous tissue, and "potbelly."

Adequate nutrition is obviously important for adequate growth. It has a double significance in diabetes, for without appropriate nutritional management, good control is not possible. In inadequately controlled diabetes, heavy glucosuria can result in striking caloric losses with a metabolic shift to alternate energy sources as well as an exaggerated protein catabolism for gluconeogenesis. A few children with IDDM have also been found to have defective gastrointestinal absorption of various nutrients. Additionally, the role of various mineral deficiencies (of zinc, magnesium, and so forth) in overall nutrition and growth is not certain.

Finally, the child's environment and emotional nurturing should not be ignored. Diabetes mellitus carries with it significant stresses and emotional upheaval for children and families alike. This aspect is sometimes ignored by health professionals keyed into insulin, tests, and diet.

Maintenance of Optimal Growth

While it may not be possible to say definitively that mild growth retardation is a totally preventable complication of IDDM, evidence strongly indicates that major alterations in growth rate can be avoided if there is optimal control of carbohydrate metabolism. The concept of optimal diabetic control and its attainment is covered elsewhere in this text (Chapter 4). Suffice it to say here that the definition of good control must include the attainment and maintenance of normal growth and development. To ensure early recognition of problems and successful intervention, the young child with IDDM should be routinely monitored for linear growth, weight, and physical and behavioral development. Heights and weights should be carefully measured at each visit (at three- to six-month intervals) and recorded on growth charts that are appropriate for the sex, race, and genetic background of the patient. Historic information on growth, development, activity, and so forth, also should be routinely obtained, and the examination should include the genitalia (especially during puberty) for documentation and staging of sexual maturation.

The Child with Suboptimal Growth

Even in the best of circumstances, the practitioner caring for children with IDDM will encounter the occasional child who is below the fifth percentile for height or who is demonstrating a deceleration of growth velocity (that is, crossing height percentiles). In order to evaluate such children in a reasonable and efficient manner, the distinction between short stature and true growth failure must be made. Simply stated, short stature refers to an individual who has a length or height greater than two standard deviations below the mean (that is, below the fifth percentile), but whose rate of growth parallels the mean. Growth failure, on the other hand, refers to a person whose rate of growth is below normal and in whom there is a fall-off or decrease in percentile ranking computed over time. A child who is short but who is growing at a normal rate is likely to have a familial or genetic component for short stature, and a family history of this trait should be sought. Alternatively, recognition of a child with a subnormal growth rate should raise the possibility of a pathologic problem, such as a decompensation in carbohydrate control or another endocrinopathology.

In the child with IDDM who has suboptimal growth, it is appropriate to consider the degree of diabetes control as the primary issue. All records of blood and urine glucose results should be carefully reviewed in the presence of the child and parents, with attention being paid to verification of the validity of the recorded results. The level of glycosylated hemoglobin provides objective evidence of such control. A complete history and physical examination should include observation for signs or symptoms suggesting poor control (for example, polyuria, polydipsia, and hepatomegaly), problems with dietary compliance, emotional state and ability to cope with diabetes management, and evidence that would suggest any other coexisting disorder.

Thyroid disease (either hypothyroidism or hyperthyroidism) is the second most common endocrine disorder is childhood and occurs with an increased frequency in individuals with IDDM. Hypothyroidism is associated with decreased growth rate and may be difficult to detect clinically. Often the earliest sign is an apparently asymptomatic goiter; thus, careful inspection and palpation of the thyroid gland should be accomplished. A number of other autoimmune disorders, especially Addison's disease, have been linked to IDDM and thyroid disease, both separately and collectively. Circulating antibodies to various body tissues, such as gastric, thyroid, and adrenal tissues can be demonstrated in some people with IDDM and may be linked to specific histocompatibility antigens.

In the evaluation, other coexisting diseases and chronic illnesses or conditions must be considered and excluded. Among these are conditions in which diabetes is part of another genetic or acquired syndrome, such as gonadal dysgenesis with Turner's syndrome, incomplete rubella syndrome, cystic fibrosis of the pancreas, various neuromuscular disorders, and malabsorption syndromes.

The occurrence of psychosocial deprivation in children with IDDM has not received attention in the medical literature. Emotional and behavioral disturbances often lead to poor compliance, significant control problems, and denial of the condition. Diabetes mellitus is a condition of significant stress and demands on families as well as patients, especially on the youngest ones. It is important that the home environment as well as one that delivers efficient medical and dietary management be a loving, nurturing one.

In the majority of instances of growth failure, diabetes control will be found to be significantly suboptimal. In some, there will be sufficient glycosuria to account for a negative caloric balance, whereas in others, the degree of poor control will be only moderate. In most instances, there is normalization of the growth rate coincident with improved glucose metabolism; and, in some, there is significant catch-up growth when control is maintained over a period of 6 to 12 months.

We have been impressed with intensive insulin therapy (either pump or multiple-dose therapy) in the management of such children. Often, these children will be more compliant than ever before when they understand that improved control will probably lead to accelerated growth. Various investigators have demonstrated an accelerated growth rate that appears to parallel the patient's improved carbohydrate control. Occasionally, the person may almost "explode" into puberty, and this has at times been associated with rapid development of degenerative complications (retinopathy, nephropathy, hypertension). The mechanism for this development is not fully explained, but it is our current practice to ease the control improvement slowly if the growth-retarded child appears to be immediately prepubescent.

THE EYE

The Lens

Transient blurring of vision secondary to acute changes in refraction are not uncommon complaints in people with IDDM, particularly in the first few months after diagnosis. A tendency toward myopic refractive error is observed when blood glucose levels are elevated, while significant reductions in blood glucose levels tend to cause hyperopic errors. Myopia is sometimes described as a presenting symptom. These transient changes in refraction are related to fluctuations in blood glucose and appear most likely due to the osmotic effects of the glucose and of sorbitol. It is for this reason that most ophthalmologists do not prescribe glasses for refractive errors during periods of poor or unstable diabetic control. Transient opacities in the lens have occasionally been seen at onset of IDDM, but these tend to reverse with stabilization of blood glucose.

Of a more serious nature is the development of cataracts, which are not reversible. It is generally accepted that there are two types. *True*, or *juvenile* cataracts are invariably bilateral, develop rapidly, and consist of dense bands of white spots in a subcapsular position, fine needle-shaped opacities of uniform diameter, and posterior subcapsular vacuoles and clefts. These occur in younger patients and are less common than so-called *senile* cataracts. This type is indistinguishable from that seen in the elderly but develops earlier and with greater frequency in diabetic patients. Although the etiology of either form of cataract is still not certain, there is sufficient evidence to implicate hyperglycemia as the predominant force. The lens of the eye is a non-insulin-dependent tissue, and glucose enters by mass transfer; the higher the blood glucose, the higher the intralens concentration of glucose. This ultimately leads to an accumulation of sorbitol (and other polyols) within the lens. As a result of osmotic changes secondary to sorbitol, there are significant fluid and electrolyte shifts, creating a nidus whereby the cataract is formed. Additionally, there may be some glycosylation of lens proteins. Thus, it would appear that the cataract is one complication that should be preventable with successful control of diabetes.

With respect to the frequency of cataracts in those with IDDM, the incidence is said to be about 5 to 10 percent after 10 years' duration and as high as 20 to 30 percent after 20 years' duration. The main indication for extraction of cataracts is impairment of vision below a useful level, and the outcome is usually good if retinopathy is not present.

The Iris

Some reports suggest that as many as one third of diabetics develop pigment deposits along the anterior chamber, usually on the anterior surface of the iris. This is associated with swelling and sponginess of the epithelium, infiltration of the cells with glycogen, and subsequent degeneration. Occasionally, pigment may even be released into the anterior chamber; this process termed *diabetic iridopathy* is of unknown origin.

Pupillary abnormalities can sometimes be found. These include slow reactivity to light, loss of light reflex, excessive miosis in the dark, and nonsyphilitic Argyll Robertson pupil. The pupil may be dilated or miotic. Glycogen deposition is thought to be a possible cause. Recently, electronmicroscopy has revealed ultrastructural abnormalities of the iris musculature and of the adjacent nerve endings.

Rubeosis iridis, a state of neovascularization of the iris, is not specific for diabetes mellitus but is almost always secondary to disease processes elsewhere in the eye. In the case of IDDM, it is generally seen in association with proliferative retinopathy. The rapid growth of new vessels can lead to atrophic changes in the iris and the growth of a fibrovascular membrane. Occlusion of the anterior chamber can result in "neovascular" glaucoma. Panretinal photocoagulation may help arrest or sometimes regress the lesions if vitreous clouding has not occurred. Cryosurgery and sometimes enucleation are required for pain relief if laser coagulation is ineffective.

The Optic Nerve

Retrobulbar neuritis is a rather uncommon entity that has been reported in diabetics, but it is unclear whether there is an increased incidence in this population. One form of optic neuropathy occasionally seen in children is termed pseudopapilledema. Patients may present with no symptoms or with mild or marked visual impairment. Findings consist of optic disc edema with neovascularization, peripapillary hemorrhages, and exudates mimicking true papilledema. Most investigators feel that this is an ischemic manifestation of microangiopathy. Usually the swelling regresses spontaneously with time, but it may lead to atrophy. Primary optic atrophy has also been seen in an occasional child with IDDM. For the most part, this is probably a genetically determined problem and is often associated with diabetes insipidus as well.

The Retina

The reported incidence of retinopathy among diabetic populations shows some similarities and some distinct differences. At the Joslin Clinic, 75.3 percent of 73 patients were found to have retinopathy of some severity after 40 years of diabetes, with about half having proliferative retinopathy. A London study of 92 patients showed 60.8 percent with retinopathy after 40 years of diabetes, but only 17 percent had proliferative changes. A French study of 372 children growing up with IDDM showed a prevalence rate for retinopathy of 53 percent by 20 years' duration and 85 percent by 26 years; the prevalence of proliferative retinopathy was 18 percent by 26 years' duration. In the Oklahoma Indian population, after 18 years of diabetes, the prevalence for all retinopathy is about 65 percent and for proliferative retinopathy about 15 percent. A reasonable summation of this and other data is that approximately 40 to 60 percent of people contracting IDDM in youth will develop some degree of retinopathy by 25 years' duration, and between 5 and 15 percent will have proliferative changes. Rarely are changes seen in the first 10 years of the disease, but the prevalence rapidly increases from that point. The tragedy is that blindness due to retinopathy is 25 times more common in the diabetic population. A patient with proliferative retinopathy has a 50 percent chance of becoming blind within five years.

An interesting note is that in most studies, a significant percentage (15 to 25 percent) of individuals have no retinal changes after 20 to 40 years. What sets these patients apart is not clear. Diabetes control has been considered as one factor, but the variability among populations suggest that genetic predisposition may play a role. Studies of risk factors have consistently shown that the strongest risk factors are the duration of diabetes and young age of onset. Other factors slowly emerging as significant factors are poor carbohydrate control and hypertension. Many have looked at smoking as a potential risk factor, but none of the studies have shown clear differences between the risks of smokers and those of nonsmokers.

The pathogenesis of retinopathy is unclear. Evidence strongly supports the deficiency of insulin as being the initial step and the occurrence of hyperglycemia as the second. At least in animal studies, a lack of control of the hyperglycemia correlates directly with the presence of microvascular changes. Two processes felt to be important in the clinical course of retinopathy are (1) increased vascular permeability leading to retinal edema and exudation, and (2) occlusion of the retinal vessels leading to neovascularization. The list of proposed factors contributing to these processes include lipid thrombi, basement membrane thickening, and swelling of extravascular tissue. More recently increased blood viscosity, red cell aggregation (due to the rigidity of the red cell), and increased platelet adhesiveness have been implicated in the occlusive process.

The most common type of retinopathy seen is called background retinopathy. Usually, the first visible sign is the development of microaneurysms. Other lesions which can be seen are splinter and flame-shaped hemorrhages, "cotton wool" spots representing microinfarctions, and hard yellow-white exudates resulting from extravasation of degenerated cellular material, plasma proteins, and lipids. Other vascular lesions include dilated and hypercellular anterioles, capillaries, and venules. The risk to vision in background retinopathy is small, unless the macula becomes compromised. This can happen by hard exudates extending into the macular region impairing central vision. More serious but less common is macular edema. The prognosis for recovery of central vision is poor; but peripheral vision is usually adequate, and blindness rarely results.

Proliferative retinopathy is the term applied to the proliferation of new, thin-walled vessels in and anterior to the retina. These new vessels are very fragile, and hemorrhages can occur. Massive hemorrhages into the vitreous can severely compromise vision. As the process progresses, proliferation of glial tissue can occur and scar tissue appears. At this point, some regression may occur with partial return of vision. However, contraction of this scar tissue will result in retinal tears and detachment.

Florid retinopathy is a severe, rapidly progressive form of proliferative retinopathy. When it occurs, it is usually seen in younger patients with poor diabetic control. Within months, it can progress to massive neovascularization and vitreous hemorrhages. Blindness is usually the result.

In the opinion of many, the treatment of diabetic retinopathy should begin with the institution of good blood glucose control. Although this is unlikely to result in major improvements and although there may be early worsening, it is hoped that progression of retinopathy will be slowed or delayed. Early results from the Kroc and Steno studies support this concept.

Laser photocoagulation, using a variety of lasers, has been used since the 1960s for the treatment of sight-threatening maculopathy and proliferative retinopathy. The rationale of this treatment is the destruction not so much of new vessels as of ischemic areas. These ischemic areas are thought to produce a substance that stimulates new vessel proliferation. Results of treatment have been improving, and many series are now reporting a 60 to 70 percent reduction in the incidence of blindness.

Pituitary ablation has been advocated in the treatment of proliferative retinopathy based on concerns about the involvement of growth hormone in the pathogenesis of retinopathy. This is rarely performed today, and its effectiveness is unclear. Certainly there are significant consequences to total pituitary ablation. Despite the concerns over this form of therapy, it has been suggested that it be given serious consideration in florid retinopathy, in which laser phototherapy is rarely effective.

In the past, a number of drugs have been suggested in the treatment of retinopathy, such as vitamins, clofibrate, and anabolic steroids; but none have demonstrated convincing effectiveness. Recently, discoveries about the physiology of retinopathy are suggesting other possible approaches. As mentioned earlier, capillary occlusion is a major problem. Abnormalities have been found in the clotting and fibrinolytic systems in diabetes. Platelets are hyperactive and tend to aggregate. At present, drugs that prevent platelet aggregation (such as aspirin) and increase production of prostacyclins (which also inhibit platelet aggregation) are being evaluated. Other cooperative studies are evaluating the role of aldose-reductose inhibitors in some patients. It is hoped that these clinical trials will define the usefulness and safety of these agents. Until more is known, it is probably not advisable to prescribe aspirin or similar agents to patients with proliferative retinopathy who are at risk of retinal bleeding.

Great strides are being made in the understanding and treatment of retinopathy and other microangiopathies allowing for some guarded optimism about the future. The ultimate hope is for the development of preventive measures, so that treatment will no longer be necessary.

THE KIDNEY

Like retinopathy, the development of diabetic nephropathy appears to be directly related to the duration of diabetes. While rarely clinically recognized in the first 10 years of diabetes, the prevalence after that point progressively increases, and over 80 percent of patients with IDDM ultimately demonstrate renal involvement with varying degrees of glomerulosclerosis. Renal failure occurs in almost 50 percent of all patients with IDDM.

Before proceeding to discuss diabetic nephropathy, it is important to recognize that this is not the only renal problem seen in diabetes. Acute urinary tract infections are common in people with diabetes, particularly women, and these can evolve into chronic pyelonephritis. The rate of asymptomatic bacteriuria in the diabetic is also about 10 times that of the general population. The prevalence of urinary tract infections increases significantly in those persons who are inappropriately catheterized.

Pathophysiology of Diabetic Nephropathy

Although there was early evidence that diabetic microvascular disease developed independent of the hyperglycemia of diabetes, extensive investigations in both animals and humans have refuted this concept as a primary factor. There are, however, some investigators who still feel that there is another component, probably genetic, that increases the likelihood in some patients of sustaining damage from longstanding hyperglycemia. Evidence to support this concept is currently lacking.

The development of diabetic glomerulopathy is a complex process involving an intricate interplay of histopathologic and hemodynamic factors, all related in one way or another to the hyperglycemic state. Studies in humans and in animals with diabetes are amazingly similar and herein will be considered together, except when there are differences to be noted.

At onset, in the hyperglycemic state, the whole kidney is enlarged, and the glomerular filtration rate is increased above normal as a direct consequence of the elevated blood glucose levels. Within days of onset (in animals), basement membrane production is shown to be increased, and within two years (in human IDDM), there is a marked increase in basement membrane thickening, both capillary and mesangial. Morphometrically, the glomerular tuft is enlarged and the filtering surface area increased by 50 percent to 100 percent. Glucosylations of basement membrane and mesangial cell proteins can be detected. Most importantly, all of these changes are reversed early in the course of the disease by normalization of the blood glucose level but return anew with further hyperglycemia.

Closely involved in this process are changes in the afferent arteriole with thickening and ultimate decrease in blood flow, owing partly to internal damage but also partly to vasoconstrictive forces, probably secondary to increased levels of thromboxane. Increased platelet aggregation and adherence to vascular endothelium is also in evidence.

The ultimate effect of all these processes is glomerulosclerosis, which is, in most cases, progressive. Evidence in experimental animals that hyperfiltration from various causes will produce progressive glomerulosclerosis and that unilateral nephrectomy in diabetic animals increases the rate of progression toward end-stage sclerosis has led most investigators to favor a primary role for the hemodynamic alterations coincident to hyperglycemia.

From a clinicophysiologic standpoint, microalbuminuria (that is, that detected only by fluorometric techniques or radioimmunoassays; levels less than those usually obtained on standard laboratory tests for proteinuria) is often found initially and disappears as the hyperglycemia is corrected. During the first few years of diabetes, recurrence of microalbuminuria is seen in patients with poor glucose control and may be induced with exercise. Clinical proteinuria (that is, that

detected by usual laboratory methods, including dipsticks) is detected in most persons sometime between the 10th and 15th years of diabetes but is often intermittent. By 20 years' duration, 50 percent of all Type I diabetics will have "fixed," or continuous, proteinuria. These patients generally constitute those who will develop nephrotic proteinuria and those who will progress on to end-stage renal disease, the duration of diabetes for the latter varying from 1 to 10 years.

The clinical manifestations of diabetic glomerulopathy are virtually nonexistent until there is nephrotic-level proteinuria (that is, proteinuria usually greater than 4 $g/m^2/24$ hr) or until there are symptoms of hypertension. It is thus important for the physician routinely to monitor for proteinuria and hypertension during the course of diabetes. By the time the diabetic with glomerulopathy is nephrotic, the patient's glomerular filtration rate (GFR) is usually depressed, and the serum creatinine concentration has risen to levels two or more times the baseline normal for the patient's age. The subsequent decline in renal function is exponential, with end-stage renal disease usually occurring in 1 to 5 years.

As renal failure ensues, the kidneys undergo scarring and contracture, and many of the metabolic functions of the kidney are lost. Periodic hypoglycemia, despite reduced exogenous insulin adminstration, occurs as normal insulin catabolism is reduced. Anemia supervenes as levels of erythropoietin are diminished, and calcium-phosphorus balance is grossly disturbed (manifested by hypocalcemia, hyperphosphatemia, and so forth) as vitamin D hydroxylation becomes less effective. Added to this is the fact that almost 100 percent of such patients will have hypertension, serious retinopathy, and other degenerative complications.

Management of Nephropathy

Prevention of diabetic glomerulopathy is obviously the aim of diabetes management, since a 50 percent renal mortality is totally unacceptable. It is worthy of note that the 50 percent renal mortality figures, although as current as possible, generally relate to those patients who acquired their diabetes 20 to 40 years ago (between 1940 and 1965), in an era when less attention was paid to the adequacy of diabetic control than at present. Thus, if it is the presence of prolonged and significant hyperglycemia that predicts the occurrence of glomerular microvascular disease, then it is conceivable that within the next decade we will begin to see a reduction in prevalence of nephropathy as the era of better-controlled patients reaches the 20-year duration point. The issue then will be whether the degree of control that is clinically possible with standard techniques is sufficient. Experimental data in animals would suggest that the changes may be either delayed or, in some cases, prevented.

Using the sketchy data now available, the practitioner should attempt to keep mean blood glucose levels well under 200 mg/dl, and this generally correlates with the parameters of control noted in Chapters 4 and 5. Obviously, it will be advantageous to keep the GFR normal and to prevent renal enlargement and microalbuminuria, but at present we have insufficient information to warrant a recommendation that additional monitoring in the early stages be made routine. On the other hand, studies are underway that examine routine determinations of microproteinuria and the excretion of beta$_2$-microglobulin (as an index of tubular function).

Reversal of the glomerulopathy would be next best in management of nephropathy if prevention were not possible or if changes had already occurred. In the early stages, hyperglycemia-induced elevations in GFR and microalbuminuria and exercise-induced microproteinuria can be reversed with normalization of blood glucose. Studies suggest that if blood glucose could be maintained in the normal range, progressive glomerulosclerosis could be prevented. However, with the techniques of the mid-1980s and as discussed earlier, complete and persistent normalization of blood glucose is possible in only a few individuals and thus remains only a dream for the majority of patients. The data concerning reversal of clinical proteinuria are conflicting, but most studies suggest that once fixed proteinuria is present, the process cannot be reversed. Whether achieving optimal control after demonstration of fixed proteinuria slows the progress toward end-stage renal disease (ESRD) is uncertain. However, most diabetologists would vigorously push toward optimum control at this time, merely on the chance of delaying the process.

One factor appears certain: uncontrolled hypertension accelerates the progression toward ESRD, and controlling blood pressure seems to retard the progression. Thus, vigorous treatment of hypertension is always indicated. Studies in other forms of progressive renal failure strongly suggest that lowering of the osmolar or solute load that the injured kidney is forced to handle decreases the rate of progression toward ESRD. Thus, a lower protein diet and a smaller sodium load would appear appropriate.

Management of renal failure requires the coordinated efforts of the nephrologist and the diabetologist, occasionally with the close assistance of the transplant team. It is well beyond the scope of this chapter to deal with the problems of transplantation or dialysis or both in this group of patients. To state that they, as a group, represent high-risk patients is a gross simplification. Unlike the situation in most other forms of ESRD, the diabetic patient so involved does not usually have an otherwise normal body. Most of these patients have serious microvascular disease elsewhere, and many will have neuropathy and macrovascular disease. All are more susceptible to infections.

Despite these potential problems, however, most such patients are candidates for either transplantation or dialysis. In our experience, transplantation from living, related donors, if feasible, offers the best long-term results for young persons. However, with the use of some of the newer techniques of immunosuppression, particularly cyclosporine, the success of cadaveric transplantation has shown marked improvement. Although the rate of kidney loss per unit of time is still greater in the diabetic than in the nondiabetic, the prognosis for renal survival has improved greatly in the past few years.

Continuous ambulatory peritoneal dialysis (CAPD) represents a significant improvement in alternative care for the person with ESRD. This has now, in most persons' minds, supplanted hemodialysis as the supportive therapy of choice. When CAPD is used, insulin is usually given also by the peritoneal route and superb glucose control is thus possible.

THE PERIPHERAL NERVOUS SYSTEM

Pathophysiology of Nervous Tissue Changes

Abnormalities in the peripheral nerves can generally be classified into mononeuropathies and symmetric polyneuropathies. Mononeuropathies tend to involve larger nerves singly or multiply but in an asymmetric fashion and are more of a vascular occlusive phenomenon with ischemia than the result of metabolic abnormalities. Metabolic factors appear to be more important in symmetrical polyneuropathies.

Histologically involved nerves can show segmental demyelination and axonal degeneration. A popular concept used to explain nerve changes is the accumulation of sorbitol within certain cells. Schwann cells are easily permeable to glucose even with reduced or absent levels of insulin. Within these cells, there is enzymatic conversion of glucose to its alcohol (sorbitol). Sorbitol accumulates in the cells, causing an osmotic shift of water and electrolytes, with resultant swelling. Other metabolic abnormalities have also been reported, particularly alterations in pyruvate, *myo*-inositol, and lipid metabolism.

Most of the alterations appear intimately linked to the presence of hyperglycemia. Nerve conduction studies have demonstrated a reduction of velocities in both motor and sensory nerves in a large percentage of patients who demonstrate no signs or symptoms of neuropathy. These changes can often be detected at the onset of diagnosis and, at least initially, appear to be reversible with insulin therapy and normalization of blood glucose.

Clinical Manifestations

The incidence and prevalence of neuropathy increases with age and duration of diabetes. Although electrical changes may be present, significant clinical problems are usually not seen early in the disease.

Numbness and paresthesias of the feet or hands or, sometimes, vague back and extremity pain are usually among the first presenting symptoms of distal symmetric polyneuropathy. Often, however, its presence can be detected by careful examination even prior to the development of symptoms. These earliest findings are loss of vibratory sense, loss of ankle jerk reflex, and diminution of sensation to pinprick. With progression, pain in the lower extremity becomes the main complaint, and, when present, the symptoms are usually worse at night. Severe involvement can progress to muscle weakness, joint deformity, ulcerations, and footdrop. Charcot's

joints, or diabetic neuroarthropathy, represents the end stage.

The onset of mononeuropathies is usually acute and variable in presentation, depending on which nerve or nerves are involved. The most common form is that involving cranial nerves, especially those to extraocular muscles. Diplopia and ocular pain can be presenting complaints. Classic third-nerve palsy can occur. If other causes are excluded, resolution usually occurs within a year with only symptomatic treatment.

Radiculopathy is involvement of a single nerve root, causing pain that does not cross the midline. This sensory mononeuropathy is truncal and usually seen in the older patient.

Peripheral mononeuropathies usually involve nerves chronically exposed to pressure and present as entrapment syndromes. Carpal tunnel syndrome, involving the median nerve, is the most common. These are potentially curable and require appropriate treatment and close observation. Surgical intervention is sometimes required.

Autonomic Neuropathy

Dysfunctions of the autonomic nervous system in diabetes mellitus are receiving increasing attention and are said to exist to some degree in up to 70 percent of all diabetics.

As mentioned previously, pupillary response is sometimes diminished and may be due to loss of sympathetic and parasympathetic enervation. Similarly, involvement of sympathetic fibers to secretory glands can result in anhydrosis.

Gastrointestinal involvement can be manifest as esophageal dysfunction, gastric achlorhydria, and gallbladder dysfunction. Intestinal involvement is often manifest as painless, frequent diarrhea with malabsorption. Severe vagal denervation can result in gastroparesis diabeticorum. Treatment usually involves the use of H_2-antagonists such as cimetidine to reduce the volume of gastric secretion and other agents that stimulate gastric and intestinal motility.

Autonomic neuropathy involving the cardiovascular system can be very grave. The first sign of denervation of the heart is a resting tachycardia, unresponsive to the Valsalva maneuver. This denervation increases risk of cardiorespiratory arrest during infection or general anesthesia. Postural hypotension is a result of loss of sympathetic innervation of arterioles in muscles, skin, and splanchnic bed. Other contributory factors may be the lack of cardiac response to hypotension and alterations in renin activity and catecholamine response. The problem can be further aggravated in hypertensive patients on salt restriction and medications.

The urogenital system is almost always involved in autonomic neuropathy. Bladder dysfunction is often insidious, with loss of sensation of the need to void, distention, and hypotonia. This results in problems with micturition and stasis, predisposing to infection and reflux. Instruction on proper bladder care (for example, frequent micturition, double voiding, and abdominal pressure) is important, in an effort to avoid surgical intervention.

Impotence is a well-known sequela in men with longstanding diabetes. It is felt to represent vascular as well as neurologic compromise. Numerous techniques have been developed for the management of this problem.

Management

As with other complications of diabetes, the first recommendation is to institute rigid blood glucose control. Even though electrical studies have indicated that abnormal nerve conduction is not reversible by improved diabetic control, many patients report improvement in symptoms accompanying better control. Analgesics are sometimes needed. Other drugs sometimes used with variable efficacy are phenytoin, phenothiazines, and tricyclic antidepressants. Currently, a combination of amitriptyline (Elavil) and fluphenazine (Prolixin) is recommended. In mononeuropathy, lidocaine and steroids are sometimes injected at the site of entrapment.

THE CARDIOVASCULAR SYSTEM

Microvascular Disease

The microvascular changes seen in diabetes have been alluded to earlier in previous sections on retinopathy and nephropathy, but the capillary basement membrane thickening, altered permeability, and occlusive problems are by no means limited to the eye and kidney. These changes take place throughout the body in every organ system. This is particularly true of the heart, where cardiomyopathy is being recognized with increased frequency. The impact is less noticeable on longevity than are the macrovascular changes, but these changes are present. Often, they contribute to instances of neuropathy with various arrhythmias and probably aggravate large-vessel disease.

Macrovascular Disease

Large-vessel changes seen in patients with diabetes, such as intimal atherosclerosis and medial sclerosis, are identical to those seen in nondiabetics; but they develop earlier and at a more accelerated rate. The coronary arteries, cerebral vessels, and vessels of the legs are the most common sites.

The Framingham study and other studies have borne out the increased risk in diabetics for significant coronary artery, cerebrovascular, and peripheral vascular disease. Coronary artery disease is the major cause of death in the diabetic population. The death rate from myocardial infarction is twice that of the nondiabetic population. There is a threefold to fourfold increased rate of cerebrovascular accidents in diabetics. Peripheral vascular disease is also very common and can lead to circulatory impairment and occlusion.

The search for explanations of this phenomenon continue, but current evidence does not suggest a direct relationship to diabetic control. The mechanisms of atherosclerosis are being examined, and all risk factors of the nondiabetic appear to be operational in the diabetic.

The relative benefits (or detriments) of exercise, lipids, dietary intervention in childhood, and so forth, are still being argued. There seems to be general agreement about smoking, obesity, chronic hyperlipidemia, and chronic hypertension as being significant risk factors in myocardial infarction and stroke.

The ultimate objective of those caring for children with IDDM should be good health maintenance aimed toward a healthy, productive adult life. The most reasonable way of doing that today is the promotion of a lifestyle in which:

1. Optimal diabetic control is achieved through a proper balance of insulin, diet, exercise, and careful monitoring
2. Ideal body weight and regular exercise

are maintained, and potential risk factors, such as smoking are avoided

3. Regular health maintenance visits are provided, with appropriate intervention when risk factors, hypertension, hyperlipidemia, and so forth, are detected.

THE SKIN

Children with IDDM develop cutaneous infections just as do their nondiabetic peers. Cellulitis, furuncles, and mycotic infections have been known to trigger episodes of acute ketoacidosis in the diabetic. It is unlikely in the first decade of diabetes that these infections are more frequent or more difficult to eradicate than they are in nondiabetics. However, as vascular problems occur in the second and subsequent decades, these infections are more bothersome and more prone to complicated courses. The one exception is vulvovaginitis from *Candida* infection, which can be a chronic and recurrent problem in adolescent and older women and is much more difficult to eradicate in diabetics than in nondiabetics.

Necrobiosis lipoidica diabeticorum is a skin disorder that is predominantly seen in diabetes, affecting about 0.1 to 0.3 percent of these patients. It is three times more common in women than in men. Lesions characteristically occur on one or both shins but can be seen also on the abdomen, thighs, back, and arms. The lesions are sharply demarcated plaques with a shiny, atrophic surface. Initially, lesions may be red to reddish brown. The histopathologic condition is that of obliterative endarteritis with secondary necrobiotic changes in the collagen bundles. The pathogenesis is not known. The lesions can even precede the onset of diabetes. Agents that interfere with platelet aggregation, such as aspirin and dipyridamole, have been found useful in the treatment.

Several authors have alluded to differences in the appearance and consistency of the skin in patients with IDDM. It is sometimes pale with a translucent quality and appears thickened and hard or firm to the touch. Most such patients are not in optimal diabetic control, and biopsy samples from affected areas have shown increased glucosylation of collagen.

This skin thickening is often seen in association with limited joint mobility (Fig. 18–1), another condition often associated with suboptimal glucose control. This type of le-

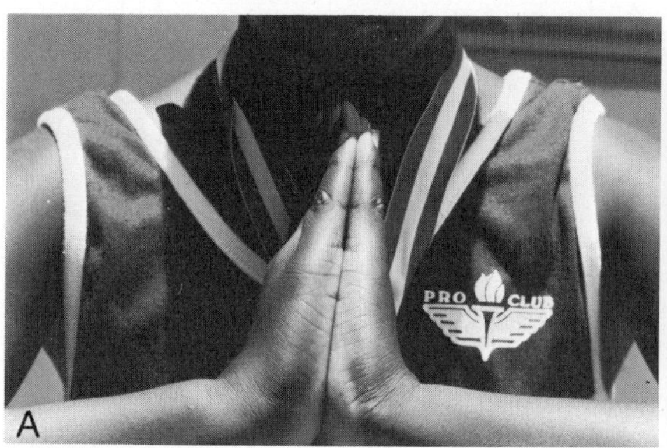

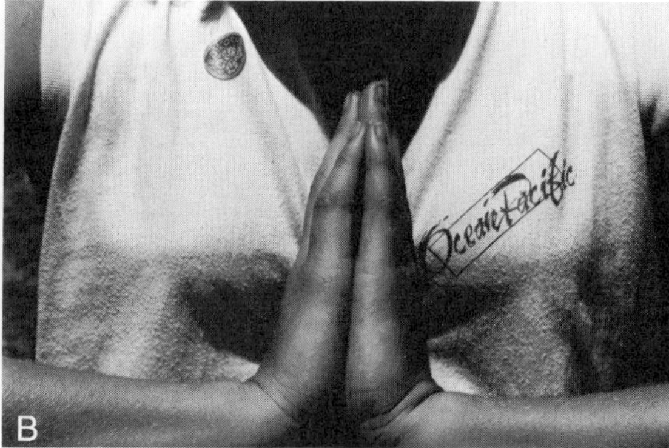

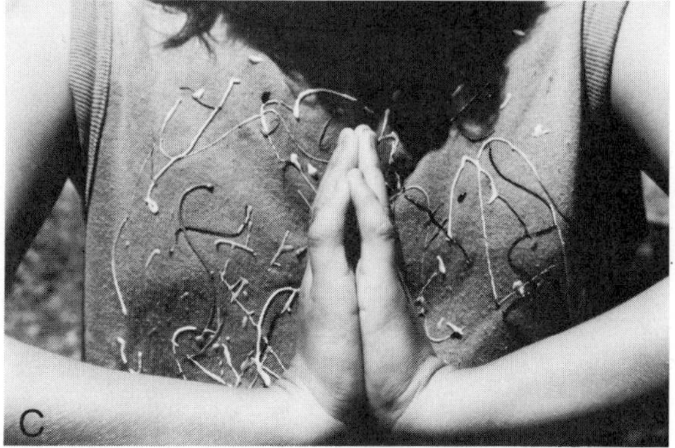

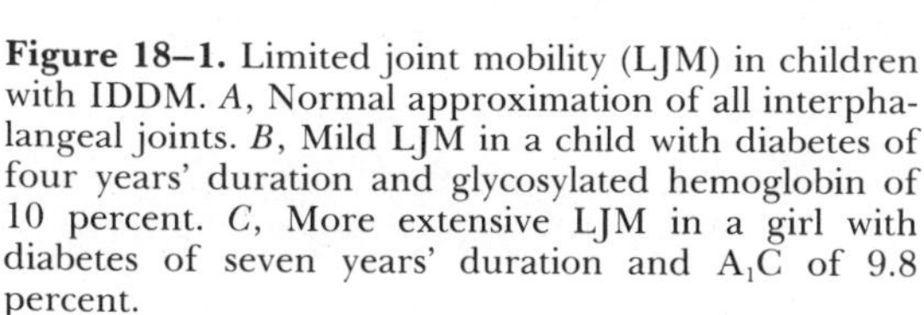

Figure 18–1. Limited joint mobility (LJM) in children with IDDM. *A*, Normal approximation of all interphalangeal joints. *B*, Mild LJM in a child with diabetes of four years' duration and glycosylated hemoglobin of 10 percent. *C*, More extensive LJM in a girl with diabetes of seven years' duration and A_1C of 9.8 percent.

sion, the involvement of which may vary from mild to severe, also appears related to increased tissue glucosylation of collagen around the joints. Why some persons whose diabetes is in terrible control do not develop these findings, while a few whose diabetes is in fair control do, is not yet answerable. One investigator feels that skin thickening serves as a marker for those patients who will ultimately develop microvascular disease.

Other skin lesions not unique to diabetes have also been described with increased frequency. These include vitiligo, granuloma annulare, psoiosiosis, and xanthomas.

OTHER SYSTEMS

As alluded to earlier, a number of abnormalities have been identified in the blood and blood elements of individuals with diabetes. They and their possible role in macro- and microangiopathy are being intensely studied. Some examples of these abnormalities are:

1. Hypersensitivity of platelets to aggregating stimuli
2. Increased platelet prostaglandin and thromboxane synthesis
3. Altered prostacyclin release from vascular epithelium
4. Increased blood viscosity
5. Shortened erythrocyte survival time and altered erythrocyte membranes
6. Shortened fibrinogen survival time
7. Impaired leukocyte adherence and chemotaxis
8. Possibly, altered beta-cell function

Some of these pathologic changes have been shown to be reversible by correction of hyperglycemia and normalization of glycosylated hemoglobin values.

The significance of these changes still requires more refinement. The implications are enormous. If these processes are involved in the vascular changes of diabetes and if they indeed can be reversed or controlled, then the outlook for prevention of severe complications is very promising.

SUMMARY

In this chapter, we have tried to encapsulate the major metabolic alterations and sequelae of diabetes mellitus. The ever-increasing pool of evidence suggests that the initiating factors are insulin deficiency and the subsequent alterations in carbohydrate metabolism. As research continues, the hope is that better ways to control these dysfunctions will be developed. Until then, those caring for children with IDDM should try to optimize care by controlling blood glucose to the best of their ability.

19

Team Approach to Management

As technology and knowledge mushroom, the need for specialized medical care has also increased. Gone are the days of the general family physician providing *all* the care and support to patients and families, especially in the realm of chronic illness. Instead, teams of professionals are now assisting the patient through health and illness. A number of sociologic and technical reasons are responsible for this change.

The focus of health care is shifting from an acute, illness-oriented approach to one of either managing chronic disorders or maintaining health. At the same time, scientific technology has increased the complexity of providing health care. Because no single person can provide the needed breadth and depth of care, allied health professionals have been introduced into the medical care delivery system. It has been projected that during the 1980s, the ratio of physicians to other health professionals will approach 1 to 25.

Not only have health professionals found roles as team members, but the patient also is demanding membership on his or her health care team. The public is becoming increasingly aware of its right in health care—and in its responsibilities as members of health teams.

Comprehensive care is more easily accomplished with a variety of professionals, each lending his or her expertise in a structured, consistent manner. Because of its chronicity and its daily demands on the family, diabetes care lends itself well to the team approach to management.

Probably the earliest diabetes teams were physician-nurse dyads. Models of such teams are described by Joslin as early as 1928. The physician in such teams was responsible for presenting the diagnosis, outlining the medical and educational program, and teaching medical aspects of the disease. The nurse usually taught self-care skills and supported daily activities of preparing meals and hygiene. Dietitians created meal prescriptions and taught nutrition and the use of exchange systems and measuring tools.

Today, specialized multidisciplinary teams may also include psychologists, social workers, physical therapists or exercise specialists, ophthalmologists, podiatrists, pharmacists, dentists, and health educators. Additionally, teams are increasingly including the patient and family as active, responsible members.

CHARACTERISTICS OF TEAMS

A team approach will work best when the group and its members share certain characteristics. A team is a group of people working together for a common purpose. Diabetes teams typically espouse a number of goals: (1) to assist children and families in managing diabetes, (2) to contribute to scientific knowledge about diabetes, and (3) to support team members in their professional growth.

In addition to being goal directed, team members must share a common philosophy of care. Certain aspects of diabetes care are controversial or at best confusing to the child and family. All members of the team must be consistent in their information and interactions with each family.

As in any group, the process of communication is important to that group's effective functioning. Team members must share their treatment plans and collaboratively set management goals. The team that draws on the individual and professional expertise of its members is able to provide comprehensive, quality care for its families. The team members should be able to draw energy from the group, to use other professionals as resources, and to share a sense of comraderie. Periodic meetings and informal interactions strengthen group support and ensure that the team's objectives are being met.

The diabetes team members working with children must share two other characteristics: the joy of communicating with children and the freedom to learn from children and their families. For the professional working with children, patience, empathy, and a positive sense of succeeding are personal characteristics he or she should nurture.

TEAM MEMBERS

The successful team has clear goals, a common philosophy, and distinct, complementary roles for its members. The very nature of teamwork makes this so. Although fringes of the professionals' responsibilities will overlap, there are distinct areas of expertise for each team member.

The Physician

The education or management center physician is the team captain. His or her duties are to determine or verify the child's diagnosis, select the treatment protocol, and initiate the team's interaction with the family. This person is responsible for developing the overall philosophy of care to be followed and ensuring that quality professionals are recruited to the team for defined roles. In this leadership role, the physician also serves as coordinator for the child's overall medical

Table 19–1. DIABETES EDUCATION TOPICS*

Normal blood glucose physiology
What is diabetes?
Relationship of blood or urine glucose
Monitoring techniques
Interpreting test results
Injection technique
Care of insulin
Achieving diabetes control
Hypoglycemia
Hyperglycemia and ketones
Sick-day rules
Pattern control
Social issues
Teenage concerns
Community resources and support
General health measures
Acute and chronic consequences

*These education topics are usually the responsibility of the nurse or health educator.

management. He or she must provide guidance and supervision for team members and for medical students, residents, and others who interact with the child and family. A major role of the team physician is communication with the child's pediatrician or family physician. Diabetes teams, although providing specialized care for the child and family, usually cannot also provide well-child follow-up and care (such as for acute illnesses, immunizations, school physicals, and so on). Hence, the local physician becomes a key link in the child's total health care delivery. Phone communication and written reports to the child's pediatrician or family physician are important duties of the diabetes team physician. The physician's responsibilities to the team include maintaining personal education regarding diabetes research and knowledge and serving as the resource in matters of medical management.

The Professional Nurse

Since the days of Joslin's "wandering nurses," the professional nurse has created a role as a diabetes educator. The team's nurse provides basic education in diabetes care and daily living skills (Table 19–1). The nurse must stay abreast of changes in diabetes care and teaching materials. Furthermore, the diabetes nurse must be aware of improved technology and changes in diabetes supplies. Maintaining his or her own knowledge base is not enough, however. The nurse must be competent also in relaying this information to children and to parents. He or she must

Table 19–2. **DIET EDUCATION TOPICS***

Basic nutrition
Rationale of diet
Exercise and diet
Carbohydrates and blood glucose
The Exchange System
Protein, fat, and blood glucose
Snacks
Hypoglycemia and diet
Dietetic foods
Illness and diet
Special occasions
Restaurant dining
Reading labels
Fiber

*The team dietitian usually coordinates these subjects with the educational program.

continually evaluate not only the results of education but also the methods and techniques of education.

Day-to-day management or care of diabetes is the natural product of an educational program. Thus, it is extremely difficult to separate the two in actual living and practice. Thus, the competent diabetes nurse-educator is also the competent diabetes nurse-clinician. In this aspect, he or she works in a collegial role with the team physician(s).

The nurse's responsibilities to the diabetes team include serving as a resource on teaching materials and techniques and apprising the team of new diabetes equipment and supplies. The university-based nurse may also provide a liaison with nursing programs to train new professionals in diabetes care.

The Dietitian

The role of diet in diabetes management is achieving importance once again, as new knowledge supports the need for normoglycemia. The team's registered dietitian is the group's expert in nutrition, meal planning, and diet education. Even with this expertise, the dietitian must also have an understanding of diabetes—of the disease process and its management. The child's usual pattern of food intake is considered when establishing a meal plan. The dietitian provides classes and information on basic nutrition and other topics relative to diabetes care (Table 19–2).

The dietitian's responsibility to team members include updating the team on changes in diet philosophy and orienting the team to new products, foods, and sweeteners.

The Social Worker

Children and families dealing with chronic illness are also struggling with the emotional and economic aspects of the disease. Through working with the family, the team's social worker assists the family in coping with the diagnosis and with the management needs. Support may come in any number of specific ways: individual or family counseling, social service agency referrals, or support group guidance.

The social worker's intervention with the diabetes team is based on an understanding of child and family dynamics and is guided by knowledge of the effects of chronic illness on family systems. Providing the team with information on the functioning and socioeconomic status of families is an important role of this team member. As the team's liaison with community and state agencies, the social worker ensures continuity of care within the child's community.

The Psychologist

The child development specialist or child psychologist fills a valuable position on the diabetes team. The psychologist offers knowledge in psychoemotional care and behavior management. Families often have difficulty separating the child's normal behavior from the effects of his or her diabetes. Some children also need help in adapting to changes in lifestyle, in coping with family interactions, and in maintaining self-esteem. Counseling, psychologic testing, and therapeutic intervention are services available through the diabetes team's psychologist.

Just as important as the patient-centered responsibilities are the psychologist's services to the diabetes team. The psychologist educates the team in assessing the psychoemotional needs of children and families. He or she may also assist the team in its group process and communication patterns. Furthermore, this person is often a resource for techniques in stress reduction and interviewing skills.

The Physical Therapist or Exercise Specialist

As exercise continues to occupy a place in the diabetic child's treatment plan, services of specialists are increasingly helpful. The physical therapist or exercise specialist provides the child and family with exercise education and fitness testing. The exercise specialist assesses the child's current exercise patterns and works with the family to develop a prescription for daily exercise.

Interfacing with the diabetes team is imperative. The physical therapist must provide consistent information regarding monitoring diabetes and managing exercise-induced hypoglycemia. The physical therapist must have an understanding of the team's dietary philosophy and goals of treatment.

Other Professionals

The diabetes team may be viewed as a nucleus, with surrounding supportive professionals interacting at certain times. In some teams there are two other persons in full-time roles: the health educator and the pharmacist. The health educator is helpful to the team at various stages during its development and practice, particularly in helping establish evaluative programs. The pharmacist is occasionally the professional interface between the team and the patient. In a university-based program, this is sometimes easy to achieve but is much more difficult in the community-based program.

The child and family learn about diabetes from the team and from these other health care professionals. To ensure continuity and consistency, the diabetes team must interact and share pertinent information with hospital nurses, dietitians, medical teams, and health care students. The team makes referrals to members of medical specialities, such as podiatry, ophthalmology, and psychiatry, as needed.

The Child and Family as Team Members

The nature of diabetes places many daily tasks, skills, and judgments in the patient's and family's hands. In addition, the health care consumer (the patient) desires an active role in his or her care. Both of these situations have contributed to the child's and family's roles as diabetes team members. In actuality, the child and family are the most important members of the team and, in the ideal situation, have a partnership role with other members.

To fulfull their role on the team, the child and family have certain responsibilities. They must share certain aspects of their daily life, such as meal and activity schedules, food preferences, and social information. The professional team members collaborate with the child and family to facilitate adherence to the treatment plan.

The family must be knowledgeable about diabetes, in order to share in decision making with other team members. The professional members have the responsibility for providing options and educating the family so that informed choices may be made.

Again, for the diabetes team to perform most effectively, all members must share common goals and philosophies. In this way, the professionals, child, and family become partners in care.

The Pediatrician or Family Physician

This person has an integral role with other members of the diabetes care team. This physician is essential to the success of the whole educational process and to the smooth transition of the child and family from the education center to the real world of everyday living with diabetes. This physician's philosophy of diabetes care obviously must be in concordance with that of the education/management center, and clear lines of communication must always exist between the two. Otherwise, the child and family will be caught between conflicting viewpoints and may become confused, frustrated, and noncompliant. Diabetes control will suffer and long-term health will be jeopardized.

When the education/management center physicians take on the care of a child with diabetes, they also take on the responsibility of continuing medical education for the family physician, who often must initiate treatment for stressful illnesses and who unfortunately may still be required to manage the acute problems of DKA and serious hypoglycemia.

The family physician's additional role as a member of the diabetes team is to keep the team informed regarding problems within the child's family and environment that might affect his or her diabetes care.

Other Hometown Professionals

All persons whose professional roles affect the child with diabetes should be incorporated into the team, at least as far as the incorporation of a single philosophy of care is concerned. Persons who have the greatest impact on children and, thus, on their diabetes include school personnel, particularly teachers, school nurses, and coaches. These persons must be either involved correctly or not involved at all. The center staff, the hometown physician, and the child and family need to identify and define the precise roles that these persons will play in the child's day-to-day living with diabetes.

FUNCTIONS OF A DIABETES TEAM

Thus far, the diabetes team has been defined in terms of its historic development, characteristics of its group function, and roles of its members. But what does a diabetes team do? Is it cost effective? How can the team prevent problems known to happen in groups?

Teams have grown from a need for specialized, comprehensive care. The economics of health care have resulted in delegation of responsibilities to allied health professionals. Theoretically, more patients receive better care from a team of health professionals. Currently, investigators are subjecting this theory to objective study. Deckert and co-workers (1978) found that outpatient supervision in a diabetes clinic benefited patients in a cost-effective manner. They reported that by using a team of professionals, patients who were guided routinely in a clinic received a prognostic benefit of an additional 11.9 years. The authors attributed this benefit to information gained at the clinic visit and to frequent metabolic monitoring by the team.

Further evaluation of the cost-to-benefit ratio of diabetes teams is being conducted by National Diabetes Research and Training Centers (DRTCs). In July 1974, the National Diabetes Mellitus Research and Education Act (PL 93-354) provided for the establishment of the National Commission on Diabetes. This commission set up DRTCs as sources of diabetes research, education, and clinical application. Each DRTC program has established "model demonstration units" and is conducting programs to develop and evaluate innovative methods for diabetes management. Outreach programs and the use of multidisciplinary teams are being studied by selected DRTCs.

Children's diabetes teams have a variety of functions, broadly categorized under education and research.

Education

Each team member is a diabetes educator. Each member has specific responsibility for selected diabetes topics. Even so, all team members must have an overall view of the educational program. Obviously, the team provides diabetes education for children and families; but the team also educates other professionals and the community-at-large.

The team is a resource for diabetes care to these groups. Diabetes professionals reach the medical community through conferences and publications. Providing information to the lay community is accomplished through the team's involvement with support groups, diabetes groups, and the schools. The need for public education is real. It is not uncommon in practice to hear parents describe the misconceptions of school nurses, school principals, and coaches. That some school personnel consider diabetes a handicap and place diabetic children in special education classes says much for the educational need of the public.

Research

The diabetes team has the professional resources to subject clinical questions to scientific scrutiny. This study may take the form of sponsored research or may be an informal problem-solving process. Through formal research, the team gathers data to contribute to scientific knowledge. Through informal study, the team evaluates the outcome of its care and seeks methods for improving those outcomes.

In addition to assessing patient outcomes, the team is obliged to appraise its own functions. The team must assess its effectiveness in terms of the program's cost and goal achievement. The team has a commitment to preventing fragmented care, a potential problem when a group of professionals provides care. By monitoring its communication patterns and its decision making and by keeping these processes open, the team may ensure that the child and family receive quality care.

THE DIABETES TEAM AT UTMB: AN EXAMPLE

The Children's Diabetes Management Center at the University of Texas Medical Branch in Galveston, Texas, currently provides education and follow-up diabetes care for over 400 children and their families. Well over 2000 children and their families have been through one or more aspects of the program. This team has evolved a style of education and a philosophy of care that has been successful for over 20 years. Members of the team now include two faculty member physicians, two master's-prepared nurse specialists, a master's-prepared health educator, a diabetes dietitian, a child development specialist, a physical therapist, and a social worker. The team members are competent child health professionals first, and diabetes experts second.

When a child and family are referred to the UTMB diabetes team, they are either admitted to a nursing unit in the Child Health Center or to a special Care-by-Parent Unit, or, if in close proximity to Galveston, they are seen only in an ambulatory setting. Other patients, who prefer to have the entire family stay in local hotels, are seen daily as outpatients. The Care-by-Parent Unit is managed by a clerk and does not provide skilled nursing care. Families in the Care-by-Parent Unit provide daily care: injections, blood or urine testing, and meal selection. The Unit, closely allied to the outpatient area, has the decor and facilities of a motel rather than a hospital.

Children and parents receive individualized diabetes education planned according to their present knowledge, skills, and attitudes. Educational sessions are generally on a one-to-one basis and are presented by all members of the team. The physicians introduce the family to the team members, the team's philosophy of care, and the teaching plans. The nurse specialist or health educator assesses the child's skills and provides didactic and supervised practice sessions as needed. The child is expected to participate in his or her self-care throughout the program. All children or their families or both are taught methods of self-glucose monitoring and are expected to use these techniques during their

educational program. Children and families are taught to use the information from blood glucose monitoring to make decisions about diet, exercise, and insulin.

The team dietitian completes a diet history with the family and plans meals and snacks with the child's input. She teaches meal planning using the constant carbohydrate diet. Families are encouraged to practice such meal planning throughout their stay.

Most families require a full week-long program of education and evaluation. During that time, the team members interact and plan with each other and with the medical and nursing teams in the Child Health Center.

The team psychologist works with selected families on behavior management and child-rearing skills. As the team's child development expert, she assists the team in interpreting children's responses to diabetes and to education. Team members consult the social worker for help with families needing financial assistance or community support. The team social worker also conducts parent and child support groups during the hospital stay and in clinic programs.

A pediatric physical therapist with knowledge in diabetes works with all inpatients and their parents. She evaluates the child's physical fitness and provides classes on the effects and benefits of exercise. Children are taught techniques of evaluating the effect of exercise on their diabetes.

After discharge, the child is followed closely by phone until the child and his or her family demonstrate ease in managing diabetes. This phone follow-up may be accomplished by any team member but often is the responsibility of the nurse, health educator, and/or dietitian. Families are supported in their accomplishments and appropriate judgments. Their education is reinforced, and their adherence to the treatment plan is assessed. Through this follow-up method, the diabetes team reinforces to the child and family that it is available as a resource and a support.

The UTMB Children's Diabetes Management Team further provides follow-up care in its outpatient clinic. The team believes that education is a lifelong process for the child with diabetes. Traditional clinic appointments do not allow a formal continuing education program or assessment of psychomotor and cognitive skills. To remedy this, the team provides a specialized, half-day

SCHEDULE CARD

TIME	APPOINTMENT	ROOM
8:30-9:00	Data Collection	
9:15-9:30	Diet - Individual	
9:30-10:00	Rap Session	
10:00-10:30	Dr. Travis	
10:30-11:00	Diet Group	
11:00-11:30	Exercise Group	
11:30-12:00	Skills Check	
12:00-12:30	Break	
12:30-1:00	"What's New"	

Figure 19–1. The clinic schedule card given to those who attend the Diabetes Continuing Education Clinic at the Child Health Center, Galveston.

Diabetes Continuing Education Clinic (DCEC). Each child and family is requested to attend one of these half-day sessions each year. For the other one to three routine visits per year, the program is similar to a conventional clinic, the difference being that in these visits all team members participate.

Immediately prior to the DCEC, the team meets to review patient charts, to discuss patient needs, and to plan classes. The children and parents complete data forms (see Appendix), which are used by the team to further individualize the sessions. Children receive a class schedule (Fig. 19–1) listing the continuing education topics for that day.

The DCEC half-day program actually consists of a series of half-hour sessions. Each child, with his or her parents, attends classes or discussion groups on diet, exercise, self-management, behavior management, and skills. The child is assessed by and visits individually with the physician and nurse. He or she also has individual time with the dietitian and other team members, as needed or requested.

At the clinic's end, children and families are asked to evaluate the sessions. Responses have been overwhelmingly positive. Families enjoy the review of information and the renewed feeling of being in control. An additional benefit to families is the interaction among parents and among children in the group sessions. Children and families share with and teach each other.

The team is currently fulfilling its obligation to evaluate this type of continuing education clinic in terms of cost and benefits. There are families who choose not to attend the DCEC, and these are followed in a more traditional setting. The team is assessing the reasons for this decision and is seeking ways of providing ongoing education to these children and families. Another area of study will be the effect of the continuing education programs on children's and parents' diabetes knowledge and adherence.

The diabetes team at UTMB delivers diabetes education in yet another program—summer camps. Team members coordinate two summer camps, which provide diabetes education to an additional 350 to 450 children and families each year. Weekend or teen workshops are another team function.

SUMMARY

In this chapter, we have discussed how interdisciplinary diabetes teams afford children and families specialized care from a variety of professionals. This care is delivered most effectively when team members share their expertise, hold common goals, and deliver diabetes education with consistency and accuracy. Characteristics of teams and of individual team members have been explored. Professional experience with children and knowledge of child development is as important as the team member's diabetes expertise. This chapter has also described components of a children's diabetes team and its clinic program in Galveston, Texas.

20

Camps and Other Similar Programs

In 1925, three years after the introduction of insulin, Dr. Leonard F.C. Wendt began the first diabetic camp near Detroit. Four campers were housed in a cottage owned by another diabetic patient of Dr. Wendt's. Four years later, a second camp for children with diabetes was conducted by Dr. H.J. John near Newburg, Ohio. The outcome from these first programs was so successful that by 1985, there were almost 100 camp programs in North America that were devoted to children with diabetes. In addition, the nature and character of camps have been expanded. Although most "camping programs" are residential locales for children with diabetes, the last few years have seen an unprecedented growth in day camps, family camps, wilderness experiences, weekend retreats, and other variations of a similar theme. Furthermore, no longer are specialty camps (that is, camps for children with chronic illness) almost the exclusive domain of those for diabetes. Similar camping programs are available in many areas for children with such diverse medical problems as orthopedic handicaps, cystic fibrosis, asthma, renal failure and/or dialysis, oncologic diseases, deafness, blindness, cerebral palsy, and seizures.

WHY CAMPS?

Recreational camping programs for children have been part of the American scene almost since our founding as a nation, but until the turn of the 20th century these were primarily reserved for children of the very affluent in our society. Children of the less affluent, particularly from our predominantly rural society, were needed as workers during the summers, and excess leisure time and "summer boredom" were not part of our societal vernacular.

The urbanization of the 20th century, changes in our school systems, and a changed perspective concerning child labor, including such peripheral issues as minimum wages, opened the door to camping programs even for those who were less than affluent. Urban families longed for their children to experience some of the pleasures they had known in the "great outdoors." Such groups as the Boy Scouts, the Girl Scouts, the Campfire Girls, and so on, popularized the theme even further—and the great camp boom was on! Organizations such as the American Camping Association were formed, which set standards for health and safety; and most state governments enacted legislation to aid in the regulation of camps from a health and safety standpoint.

Camping programs are now part of our tradition. We now have "regular" recreational camps, featuring a variety of participatory activities, and "specialized" recreational camps, such as tennis camps, basketball camps, church and Bible camps, arts camps, water-sport camps, wilderness camps, cheerleading camps, soccer camps, and even frisbee camps. Recently, computer camps have become popular.

What do all these camps have in common? They are directed toward what children like to do: have fun. But most are also educational in that they teach skills that may not be learned elsewhere, and their collective strength is the association among peers. Children at camp develop friendships that last throughout life, they learn to interact with others on a live-with basis, and they develop a sense of independence from home and parents that is necessary for their social growth and emotional maturation.

Why "Special Needs" Camps?

Early in this century, camping programs directed toward children with special medical needs began to appear. Initially, the major effort was directed toward those problems that were more visible—the orthopedically disadvantaged, children with a variety of crippling and deforming defects. Such children were not able to participate fully in programs at regular camps and yet they were found to need the same essentials available at such camps. Added impetus was given to such programs in the late 1920s and early 1930s when a popular president ably demonstrated what good supportive recreational programs could do for the residua of poliomyelitis. These camps, thus formed, also took on a rehabilitative task: working with such children in an attempt to assist their full entry into a noncrippled society.

The success of such programs was inspirational to professionals working with other chronic illnesses of children. Empathetic and humanitarian persons and organizations quickly grasped the significance of these programs and fostered their development. Parents of the chronically diseased, groping for ways to support their children and themselves, quickly adopted the concept. All working together brought programs into existence, and the evolution has been gratifying for all to observe.

Why "Diabetic" Camps?

In earlier days, "diabetic" camps were developed primarily because such children were excluded from participating in "regular" camps. Their disease was too frightening to camp directors and parents alike. Additionally, most camps did not have suitable health facilities to care for such "fragile" children. Even today, this is a factor in the continuing growth of camps for the child with diabetes, and well it should be; for many regular camping programs are ill prepared to handle some of the potential problems that are commonplace in the life of a child with diabetes (exercise-induced hypoglycemia, exercise-induced ketosis, stress-induced problems, and so forth).

The major factor leading to the tremendous growth in diabetic camping programs, however, has been the realization of the good that arises through group support and peer interaction. Also contributing to this growth has been the expansion of a dedicated group of professionals interested in the health and well-being of these children. These professionals have appreciated the fact that children with diabetes, more than those with almost any other chronic illness, must make great adjustments in their lifestyle if their diabetes is to be controlled. Such children must develop a degree of self-discipline that is foreign to others of a similar age. They must be strong-willed against day-to-day normal temptations (that is, they must restrict their eating when others eat, they must monitor themselves at inconvenient times, they must give themselves shots regularly, and so forth). Most such children, before camp, do these things in a world alone, knowing no one else with a similar constraint on lifestyle. Camp provides the opportunity for these children to see and know others who have "made it"; to share experiences with others who are similar; to learn how to cope with intrusions into normal living; and to handle being often overprotected by parents, being seen as "brittle" by professionals, and as appearing normal to a unenlightened public.

Affordable, educational camping experiences for the child and adolescent are now available in almost all areas of the United States. The primary purpose of these programs is to aid the child and family in coping with the medical, social, and psychologic problems that diabetes causes. Frequent physician visits, injections, and tests may undermine the child's security and self-concept. The child is at risk of being "different" and isolated. The camping experience combats such isolation. The constraints of medical management may become a constant source of family conflict in even the strongest of families. Camping provides the family with a brief vacation from the constant demands of caring for the child with diabetes: from tests, records, injections, and overall stress. Camps for children with diabetes also provide an opportunity for intense re-education for both child and family and for integration of management of the disease into lifestyle. Whether this is through formal instruction, informal discussion, or example, the camp provides valuable continuing education.

Camp also demonstrates that the child can function without parental supervision and protection, which tends to decrease family anxiety and overprotection. Increased independence and decreased anxiety reduce the potential for behavior disorders induced by chronic disease. There are opportunities for professional education and research in medical and ancillary fields during diabetes camp. Many investigations of metabolic control and psychosocial aspects of diabetes have been conducted during camp.

It is most important that diabetes camps be *fun* for the children, their families, and the health professionals involved. Learning how to deal with a serious illness is obviously important, but one does not necessarily have to be grim or somber in doing so. In fact, learning in a happy atmosphere is easier to accomplish and is longer-lasting.

PURPOSES OF CAMPS

The purposes of camps for children with diabetes are noted in Table 20–1. These objectives are modifications of the ones used over the previous 27 years at the camps operated by the Children's Diabetes Management Center and are similar to objectives that have been approved by the Committee on Camps of the American Diabetes Association.

Fun and Recreation

The primary aim of any camp program should be to provide fun and recreation in a safe, supervised environment. This function is even appropriate for camps for children with diabetes, in which concerns abound. Program staffs must be uniquely qualified to handle young children and teach new recreational and sport skills.

Table 20–1. OBJECTIVES FOR CAMPS FOR CHILDREN WITH DIABETES

All residential camps for children with diabetes should
1. Provide those facilities and personnel necessary to ensure an enjoyable recreational camping experience
2. Provide an appropriate site and program (recreational and medical) necessary to ensure a safe and healthy environment
3. Ensure peer interaction
4. Facilitate the learning of appropriate attitudes, knowledge, and skills that are necessary for effective living with diabetes
5. Promote the development of independence and self-reliance, while increasing self-esteem and self-concept
6. Facilitate a smooth re-entry of the child into the home environment
7. Provide a brief respite for parents from the daily rigors of diabetes care

Some residential camps for children with diabetes will
1. Assist the child in establishing diabetic control, by making appropriate adjustments in medical management
2. Facilitate maturation by fostering programs designed to increase independence, self-reliance, and self-discipline
3. Provide an educational experience for health professionals in management of childhood diabetes
4. Assist children wishing to enter into nondiabetic camping programs
5. Conduct structured observational research or appropriate interventional research designed to benefit the lives of children with diabetes

Adequate supervision by a competent, dedicated staff is essential. In addition, the program should be age-specific and provide a variety of activities to help diminish boredom and homesickness. There is no need to be selective about the type or nature of the activities simply because the camp is for children with diabetes.

Education

Summer camp affords countless opportunities for education about diabetes care, particularly about the day-to-day issues. Many camps provide scheduled group education sessions for the campers. The curriculum for camper education should be age specific and should use creative, attention-keeping approaches. Education sessions are best scheduled after breakfast and before the day's activities begin.

Although campers profit from the group classes and peer sharing, they will likely learn even more during the informal contact with medical staff and other campers. Learning to give a shot can be done in group learning situations. Yet, how much more effective is the peer pressure of a cabin full of self-injectors! Children will readily try new skills, inject new sites, and take on new responsibilities when everyone else (their peers) is doing so.

The close availability and assessibility of competent and compassionate medical staff cannot be overemphasized. These individuals are integral to the campers' learning and to their ability to apply this information about the disease. Older teens and young adults with diabetes are necessary role models for the youngster. These "veterans" are important additions to any camp program for children with diabetes.

Children learn at different stages. The focus of the campers' education should, therefore, be in concert with their developmental level. There are levels or stages in the acquisition of knowledge, attitudes, and behaviors that are necessary for diabetes self-care. The program must incorporate these.

The young camper, 6 to 9 years old, is in a stage of "skills and knowledge acquisition." Children in this age group understand and explain things based on hunches rather than on logic. Consequently, they are not ready to understand relationships. Nor are they equipped to remember rules. Their attention span is limited, and they may still use magical thinking to explain the world around. The educator must focus on skills, with ample time provided for practice and more practice. A few facts may be taught, primarily those related to hypoglycemia and to food exchange groups. A large number of facts, however, brings about confusion and disinterest.

The camper from 9 to 14 years old uses concrete thinking with very little abstract reasoning. Yet, these children are beginning to understand rules and to mentally solve problems. They are beginning to see a cause-effect relationship between aspects of diabetes management. For example, these children understand the effect of diet, insulin, and exercise on blood glucose concentrations. The educator may effectively use games, quizzes, discussion groups, and role playing with this age group.

Older teens are entering a stage of emotional maturation and are able to use cognitive skills of abstract thinking. They are interested in details. They can form theories and can discuss the "possible" as well as the "actual." They learn well in peer groups, in which there is an exchange of ideas. Role playing, debates, and challenging games are tools the educator may find useful in a camp environment. The educator must expand the educational topics to include ones appropriate to teenage issues: alcohol, drugs, sexuality, genetics, careers.

Self-Reliance and Confidence

Another benefit of camp for the child with diabetes is provided through opportunities for the child to achieve self-reliance and confidence, whether on the archery range or in the cabin at "shot time."

Again, experienced and sensitive medical staff members are necessary for the promotion of independence in these children, as they choose the correct method and technique. There is tremendous satisfaction for both child and adult when the first injection is given, the first blood test attempted, or the first collaboration on dosage change made.

A comprehensive camp program will plan strategies to promote continued independence once the child returns home. Often, awards or letters to the home remind the child of personal accomplishments even after camp has ended. The medical staff should make appropriate suggestions to parents and caregivers in order to aid them in maintaining the child's gains in self-care.

Peer Interaction

It is not unusual for a child with diabetes to know no one else who has this disease. Often he or she is the only student at school with diabetes and usually the only child in the community. For a few summer days, the child enters a community where the nondiabetic is in the minority. An amazing realization for the child is that every other child at this place has diabetes—and they all "look normal"! This is an emotionally satisfying event.

Diabetes camp decreases the children's social isolation and offers them peers with whom to share and compare. Friendships are sometimes more easily made during camp. The pressure is off about whether or not to tell a new friend about their diabetes.

Parents sometimes worry that their child

may learn new ways to manipulate or cheat, from more experienced campers. Although this is a real concern, it is one that is readily managed. Medical staff members who are honest with campers about manipulation can often defuse the fantastic plans that some children create mentally. Role playing and talking about decision-making and possible consequences should be a part of an educational curriculum at camp.

Obviously, the camp program is designed to meet the recreational, educational and social needs of the child with diabetes. Yet, there are other people who also benefit from the summer camp experience: parents, siblings, and medical staff, among others.

Parents

For parents of a child with diabetes there truly is no vacation; there is not a day without thinking about meals, insulin, blood glucose levels, and long-term consequences, except for a brief time when the child attends summer camp. This is an important objective of all camps, for these do afford the parent that vacation from the daily demands of diabetes. All parents need the time away from their children to re-energize, gain perspective again, and rest! Parents can and should use this time to be with their spouses and their other children. However, planning and taking major family vacations while the diabetic child is at camp is unfair and hurtful to the child. Most parents want their children to enjoy themselves and learn a few things at camp. Yet, some parents may expect too much from the camp session: excellent control, attitude changes, total self-care—the "perfect diabetic."

Although camp may relieve some day-to-day pressures, it usually does not alleviate the worry. Camp programs must have clear guidelines for parents regarding phone calls and visits. Neither is generally acceptable, as each interferes with the child's program of activities. All parents should have the opportunity to have their questions answered and their anxieties relieved during check-in. Caring and knowledgeable medical staff who take time with families during the checking-in process help tremendously in making the child and parents feel comfortable and secure.

Just as the child has the chance to learn more about diabetes at camp, so should the parents. How difficult for the parent whose child returns home from camp having learned new methods of monitoring and different meal plans! Parents must also have that information. Increasingly, diabetes camps are offering educational sessions for parents. Handouts, check-out conferences, and educational seminars are useful techniques in updating the child's parents.

Siblings

Brothers and sisters of diabetic children carry their own brand of pressures. Amazingly, these siblings have concerns and fears similar to those of the diabetic child and his or her parents. They may worry about their sibling with diabetes, may feel guilty, and may even participate actively in the daily care.

Thus, summer camp for the diabetic child gives siblings a respite as well. If nothing else, they may feel relief from their "parental" concern for a few weeks. For some siblings, it means being able to have a "real" cola drink without feeling guilty.

Metabolic Control

Ideally, summer camp, in providing a fairly consistent environment, should be a place where the child can achieve good metabolic control of diabetes. Yet, although the medical staff may advocate good control, it may not be able to accomplish this goal for every child.

Children arrive at camp from a variety of backgrounds and philosophies of care. Many children come to camp in poor metabolic control. It may take the full camp session just to *approach* reasonable control in such children. Others come to camp in very tight metabolic control, begin a new schedule of meals and exercise, only to find that control begins to slip. Again, it may take the full two to four weeks to stabilize control, only to have the child return home to his or her usual activities and to another period of adjustment.

Parents and referring physicians must be helped to understand this state of flux in the camper's control. Communication with the child's local health care team is important to ensure continuity of care following camp. Such communication should include (1) an overview of the camp experience, including the camp's objectives; (2) a review of the child's health while at camp; (3) an explanation of any changes made in insulin regimen; and (4) suggestions for further education or alterations in care.

MEDICAL STAFF

Summer camp for children with diabetes is a learning experience—but not only for the children. Medical personnel are exposed to aspects of pediatric care only hinted at in textbooks. The medical staff members become surrogate parents, educators, coaches, counselors, family doctors, and confidantes. It is a unique experience for young medical personnel, as they live with, teach, discipline, and supervise children. Superimpose diabetes and its management, and the experience is without equal in its educational value.

The goals for educating the camp medical staff must be considered in planning the program and should include (1) reviewing all aspects of diabetes management; (2) discussing selected issues in child care and management, including homesickness and developmental needs; (3) using first-aid skills; and (4) planning and teaching diabetes care to children.

Medical staff selection must be careful and deliberate, with specific qualities and qualifications in mind. Foremost is the requirement for an ability, willingness, and desire to work with children. Next, experience with diabetes is desirable but certainly should not be requisite. It is highly desirable for members to have a feel for group dynamics and interactions, for, once constituted, the medical team must function together with each member contributing but also supporting. Such a team effort may be a unique experience for some, but each individual's ability to work together cooperatively is imperative. Previous camp experience and past teaching opportunities are helpful. Senior medical staff should meet virtually all of these criteria, but other medical staff members may elect to use the summer camp experience to develop such qualities, under the guidance of those with more experience.

Regardless of whether the medical staff is salaried or voluntary, the success of the summer program rests in large part on the selection, orientation, and guidance of its members.

THE PLACE FOR RESEARCH AT CAMP

Whether to permit selected research studies at diabetes camp is a controversial topic. Camp program planners must decide philosophically the role, benefits, and disadvantages of research at camp. Any research undertaken at camp must be considered and authorized not only by a standard committee for human subjects but also by the camp's medical director.

The obvious advantages to studies conducted at camp are (1) availability of subjects and (2) controllability of the environment. Any research study that interferes with the child's camp experience should be critically evaluated. The camp, after all, is for fun.

OTHER TYPES OF CAMPING PROGRAMS

Camping programs for children with diabetes have traditionally been residential in nature and have directly served only the child with diabetes, but the last decade has seen a tremendous change in such programs. Whereas time and space do not permit an extensive elaboration on all types of programs available, it does appear prudent to mention some of the most important types.

Family Camps

There are many varieties of family camps, but most of the true family camps are residential in nature and are either for brief retreats or full sessions. There are, however, some day programs designed to involve both siblings and parents. Family camps often have a different objective than do conventional residential camps (that is, promotion of family interaction and understanding rather than of peer interaction and self-reliance). Both serve very important functions, but they are not necessarily interchangeable.

Day Camps

These have become extremely popular, particularly in major metropolitan areas, where some children are denied the opportunity to attend residential camps because of either age or expense. Residential camps are costly to operate, and there are not always sufficient campership funds available to serve all who want or need the experience. Day camps, often utilizing city park facilities and volunteer staff, are economical to operate and fun for both the diabetic camper and the community. Furthermore, these are particularly helpful for that group of children (those up to and including age 6 years) considered too young to separate from parents.

Adventure Camps

Wilderness camps, rafting camps, skiing camps, and so forth, are all available to the diabetic camper. Although limited in number, these types of experience, when well supervised by competent medical and program personnel, create a strong sense of self-worth and achievement in the young person. Most persons attending such camps should have previous experience in other residential camps and must possess sufficient knowledge and skills in self-management of diabetes.

Regular Camps

The goal of every diabetic camp should be to prepare its campers for safely attending nondiabetic camps, where the child with diabetes will compete on a par with nondiabetics. It is particularly helpful for children who may be attending cheerleading camp or tennis camp or a similar specialty camp to have previously attended and succeeded at a diabetic camp. This relieves some of the anxiety felt both by the camper and the parent.

21

Social Issues

Sitting around the campfire at diabetes camp, the group of teenage girls shared many concerns and questions: "Can I still have children?" "I heard there's no birth control that's good for a diabetic." "Why haven't my periods started?" "My parents drive me crazy!" "I can't tell anyone about my diabetes—they'd make fun of me."

Some issues in this chapter are basic to all teenagers, some are specific to teenagers with diabetes; but all are of real concern to the young person involved. This chapter will explore some of the major social questions of children and teenagers with diabetes.

THE SCHOOL-AGED CHILD

The school-aged child's social development centers on issues of peer acceptance, role identity, and self-concept. Fitting in and getting along with friends is paramount to the child's social growth.

Telling Friends

The school-aged child risks peer acceptance in telling friends about diabetes. Some children choose to tell friends in a matter-of-fact way. Others anticipate their peers' responses and make light of their disease with such statements as "I have diabetes and take shots, gross, huh?" A few children will boldly tell everyone about their diabetes in fantastic and horrifying details: "I have this disease and I almost died—if I eat sugar I'll go into a coma!"

Often, the child needs help in telling friends. Talking with the child about who to tell, how to tell, and why to tell will assist the child in sharing information with others in a nonthreatening manner.

Social Skills

As with any chronic illness, the child with diabetes will spend time in hospitals, clinics, and at the physician's office. Contact with adults will be increased, as will be exposure to medical jargon. In some ways, this socialization increases the child's ability to relate to adults and health care providers. Yet, this sophistication may hinder or limit the child's interactions with peers.

Although he or she may be fairly sophisticated in knowledge of diabetes and the workings of hospitals, the child with diabetes may have difficulty with "normal" social skills. Social encounters may be limited by poor metabolic control, parental overconcern, or frequent hospitalizations.

Self-Image

Although making a place with peers, the school-aged child is also creating an image of self. Children with diabetes easily see themselves as different, which they often interpret as "not as good" or "inadequate."

Physical health may interfere with sports, school attendance, or social activities. The daily schedule may preclude traveling, sleep-overs, or weekend activities. Parents may be more cautious or concerned with health than are parents of nondiabetic children. The child may feel restricted in activities and burdened by daily requirements of diabetes care.

In an effort to be like others, the young person may disregard overall care, fail to monitor, forget injections, and ignore the meal plan. During these times, parents and professionals may be of most help for understanding the reasons for these behaviors.

Often, giving the child a short "vacation" from diabetes will help to resolve some problems. The parents may take over injections and testing a few days a week or completely for a brief period of time. We often tell children that they may have three or four days per month of "vacation" from a time-consuming task, such as testing. When this technique is used, it is important that the child understand that the responsibility for testing, for example, will shortly return. It may occasionally seem necessary to remind the child of the effect of nonadherence on future health, although frightening the child with threats of future complications is futile. The focus of childhood is, after all, present-oriented, and this fear would be translated into further denial.

School

School attendance and scholastic accomplishment are important tasks of the 8- to 12-year-old. At a time in life when the child is refining beliefs about the world and his or her place in it, the peer contact during school hours is important. For some children with diabetes, however, the peer contact may be too intense and fearful. The child may begin a cycle of school avoidance in response to social anxiety or fear of rejection.

Other children may have physical symptoms as a result of the normal stresses of school demands (for example, tests). Stress in the diabetic child may precipitate hyperglycemia and even ketosis.

In either case, the child may exhibit symptoms such as headache, abdominal pain, lethargy, or other somatic complaints, in addition to elevated blood glucose levels. School avoidance is best handled by assisting the child in the return to school. The child who remains out of school is deprived of social contacts, intellectual stimulation, and structured time. The longer the period of absence, the more apprehensive the child becomes about returning. It is therefore imperative to use all appropriate persons—parents, counselors, physicians, and mental health professionals—to support the child's return to school as soon as possible.

It is helpful for both the team and the child to have an ally in the school nurse. This person is instrumental in helping the child to monitor and treat his or her diabetes during the school day. Figure 21–1 outlines an algorithm we have used with school nurses. Again, the goal is for the child to be at school, even while having to manage diabetes.

Putting Diabetes Into Perspective

From a mother of a 10-year-old: "Please tell the teachers about diabetes. My son's teacher made him stand up in front of everyone and tell about his diabetes. He was devastated!"

From a 12-year-old: "I woke up in the middle of the night; it was dark, and I couldn't see. I screamed and screamed. I thought I was blind."

From an 11-year-old: "My diabetes really is okay. It doesn't bother me—I just wish my parents weren't so sad."

Learning to live with diabetes day-by-day is an added task of the school-aged child. The child has the motor dexterity to perform most care skills and the cognitive abilities to begin to understand the relationships among diet, exercise, and insulin.

Yet, such a child often must integrate diabetes without role models or diabetic peers to assist. It is not unusual for the child with diabetes to know no other child with diabetes. As we have mentioned, this child is often the only one at school with this condition and may be the only one in the entire community. Summer camps and youth groups are invaluable resources for the child and his or her parents. Above all else, these camps address the issue of aloneness.

THE TEENAGER

The teenager's social development focuses on issues of peer relationships, independence, and the future. The teenager with diabetes struggles with the same concerns as

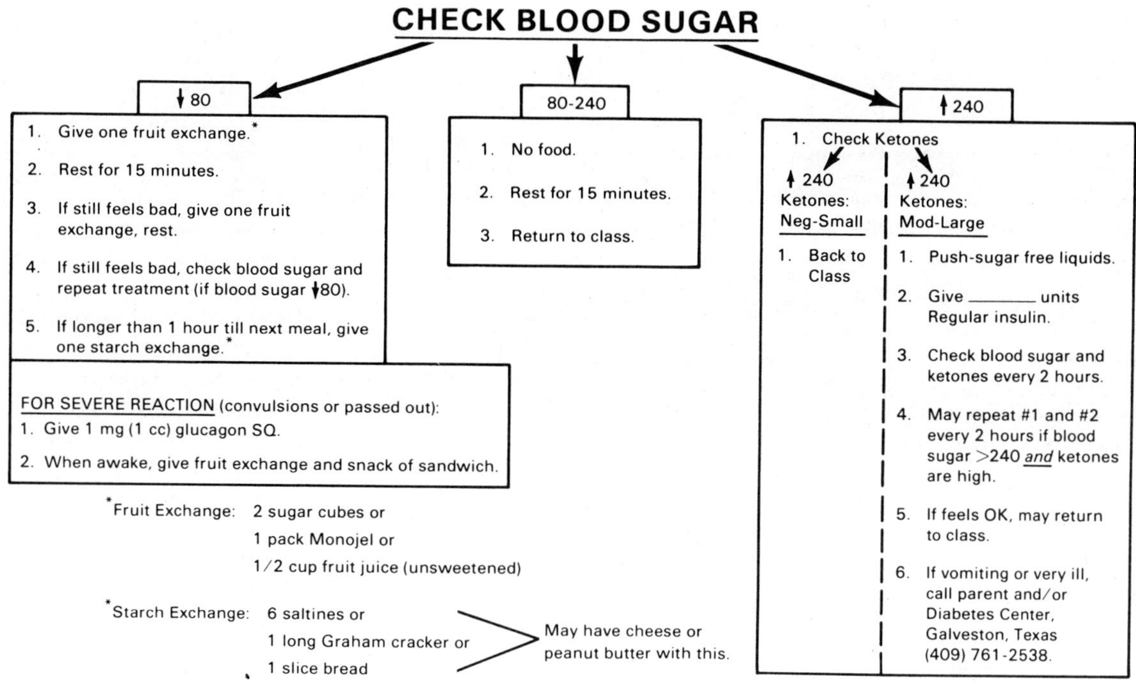

Figure 21–1. Protocols used by Children's Diabetes Management Team for working with children and school nurses during problem times.

any adolescent, but diabetes may place an added strain on the move toward adulthood.

Peer Relationships

As adolescents seek to understand themselves and their proper place within a social group, there may be a fear of rejection from peers. Choosing who and how to tell about diabetes may not be an easy task. In contrast to many other chronic illnesses, diabetes mellitus is hidden; there are usually no outward signs of having diabetes. Thus, the teenager's dilemma is not so much *how* to explain the disease but *whether* to explain it. Such disclosure may readily arouse discomfort in peers already worried about their own physical status. Small wonder that many young persons keep the fact of the disease to themselves.

Telling friends, school teachers, or others about one's diabetes is often difficult or confusing or both. The dilemma may reflect the teenager's attitude about diabetes and its incorporation into everyday life.

The teenager should be helped, often with role playing, to choose appropriate words to relay to others. Obviously, one rationale for informing and alerting friends is to have someone knowledgeable if assistance is needed. Teenagers must weigh this benefit against their need to keep the disease "hidden." A best friend may be the adolescent's only confidante, but even then help may be needed in choosing the best way to disclose various aspects of the disease. Blurting out information at a poorly selected time is an extreme measure that may embarrass or frighten even the closest of friends.

Normal concerns about personal physical adequacy may be amplified if diabetes is interfering with growth and sexual development.

R.P., a 16-year old with diabetes since age 2 years, is retarded in stature (40 kg and 137.2 cm). Depressed and tearful, he has trouble talking about his concerns: his growth, peers, and parents. He wants very badly to grow.

The impact of slowed growth or delayed puberty is devastating for a teenager, but this concern may spark motivation and interest. Such a person usually wants to do or try anything that might stimulate growth. It is at this opportune time that alternative, intensive insulin therapy and education may be accomplished.

On the other hand, thoughts of the future may be overwhelming, pushing further toward disinterest and a sense of defeat. The depression, anger, and guilt must, then, be dealt with in addition (or prior) to a plan for intensive diabetes management.

R.P. is participating in both a program of counseling and a method of intensive insulin therapy: the insulin pump. His depression persists; but he is involved in diabetes management, and his outlook is more favorable.

Various authors have noted that some teenagers with chronic illness are socially immature. The exposure to the medical world may leave the teenager "hospital-wise" but lacking in social skills with peers. In addition, the meal planning may preclude or interfere with the usual foci of teenagers' social lives: parties and eating out. The diabetes professional can help by educating diabetic teenagers about ways to adjust their diet or schedule their meals to permit some flexibility.

S.T. deals with her diet restrictions at parties by sharing food. She regularly bakes cookies for parties and serves as hostess for her friends. To make the cookies less tempting to her, S.T. only bakes flavors she dislikes.

Also, church, school, and civic teen groups may be helpful in increasing the teenager's social outlets.

Most teenagers will experiment with social drinking; some will try drugs. For the teenager with diabetes, both the use of alcohol and the use of drugs may have additional adverse effects. The social or moral questions of using alcohol, drugs, or tobacco are best answered by the teenager and his or her parents. Yet, to choose knowledgeably, the teenager with diabetes must have information, ideally incorporated into the total medical management and education.

Alcohol and Diabetes

Pure alcohol is rapidly absorbed from the intestinal tract. Absorption and resultant blood levels are affected by such factors as type, amount ingested, concentration, frequency of ingestion, and whether taken in the fasted or fed state. Distilled spirits are most rapidly absorbed, followed by wines, then beer. The presence of food in the stomach slows absorption of alcohol.

In the nonfasting state, blood sugar rises with alcohol intake. This seems to be due to glycogenolysis and is therefore dependent on the amount of alcohol and the abundance of glycogen stores. In addition, drinks mixed with regular (nondiet) mixers contribute to the rise in blood glucose.

Alcohol is metabolized by the liver. Although it does not stimulate insulin secretion in the nondiabetic, it does appear to enhance the effect of insulin. In addition, alcohol interferes with gluconeogenesis by inhibiting certain precursors. Because of these actions, blood glucose may fall and the induced hypoglycemia may be refractory to either endogenous glucagon or its administration. Glycogen stores may be rapidly depleted, and severe hypoglycemia may result if alcohol is ingested in the fasting state without the benefit of simultaneous food intake.

Alcohol provides no essential nutrients; yet it is a concentrated source of 7 kilocalories per gram. Distilled alcohol has no carbohydrate content, while beer and wine have variable amounts (Table 21–1). Alcohol is not converted to glucose or amino acids but is used directly for energy or may be converted to fat. Hence, in most exchange diets, alcohol is considered as a fat exchange.

Counseling and educating teens about the effects of alcohol on diabetes should include certain guidelines:

1. Alcohol is more safely consumed in the presence of adequate glycogen stores. Persons with diabetes in poor metabolic control have reduced glycogen stores and are at greater risk of developing severe hypoglycemia.

2. Occasional use of distilled liquor (up to two servings per day) may be regarded as "extra" by those persons with diabetes in good control. Food should not be omitted or exchanged for alcohol in such persons.

3. Consumption of alcohol prior to meals or at peak times of insulin action increases the risk of hypoglycemia.

4. Alcohol should be sipped slowly, allowing the drink to last. Mixed drinks should be selected that are low in carbohydrates, and sugarfree mixers should be used.

5. Alcohol consumption may blur judgment, causing the diabetic person to stray from the meal plan, and may prevent recognition of symptoms of real diabetic problems.

6. The teenager who plans on drinking should wear an identification tag.

7. For weight-conscious teenagers, alcohol

Table 21–1. **COMPOSITION OF ALCOHOLIC BEVERAGES**

	Serving/Size (Ounces)	Alcohol (Grams/ Serving)	Carbohydrate (Grams/ Serving)	Kcal	Exchanges
Beer (regular)	12	13.0	13.7	151	1 starch 2 fats
Beer (light)	12	10.1	6	90	2 fats
Distilled spirits (86 proof)	1.5	15.3	—	105	2 fats
Table wine					
Red or Rosé	4	11.6	1.0	85	2 fats
Dry White	4	11.3	0.4	80	2 fats
Sweet	4	11.8	4.9	102	⅓ starch 2 fats
Light	4	6.4	1–3	48–58	1 fat
Champagne	4	11.9	3.6	98	2 fats
Dessert wines	2	9.4	1.5	73	1½ fats

is best counted as a fat exchange and should be considered in the meal plan.

Tobacco, Drugs, and Diabetes

Comprehensive care for the diabetic teenager should not only include a discussion of alcohol but also provide information about the effects of tobacco and illicit drug use. As before, the choice of whether or not to smoke or use drugs is the teenager's, ideally with guidance from parents.

Studies indicate a definite effect of smoking tobacco on metabolic control. Madsbad and associates (1980) studied 163 adults with IDDM, 114 of whom smoked daily. Those who smoked averaged a 15 to 20 percent greater insulin requirement. In addition, lipid metabolism was affected, with serum triglyceride levels being 15 to 30 percent higher in these individuals. Aside from the effects of smoking on diabetes metabolism, the teenager should be aware also of the general effects of smoking: lung damage and cardiovascular effects.

The use of drugs has a deleterious effect on most teenagers (Table 21–2). The teenager with diabetes is at particular risk when taking mind- and mood-altering drugs. Marijuana, for example, is known to increase appetite and to impair judgment. Both of these effects may lead to dietary indiscretion and a disregard for the diabetic routine.

Stimulants, such as amphetamines and cocaine, increase metabolism and decrease appetite. The person with IDDM is prone to hypoglycemia while using these drugs. Over time, with the use of such drugs, dangerous depletion of glycogen results. Teenage girls are particularly likely to use "legal" amphetamines, or diet pills. Adjustments in diet and insulin therapies are considerably more safe than is the use of diet pills in the diabetic teenager.

Depressants, such as barbiturates and heroin, are used by some to derease anxiety and to enhance a sense of well-being. Use of these drugs produces physical and psychologic dependence. Some depressants, such as heroin, are taken parenterally, and thus the diabetic risks hepatitis as well.

Much is *not* known about the metabolic effects of drugs in the diabetic. It is clear that any substance that alters judgment and appetite will have an effect on the diabetic's daily routine and balance of food, insulin, and exercise.

The teenager should be aware of these general consequences of drug, tobacco, and alcohol use. Appropriate community resources are available for teenagers who become substance abusers. Teenagers with diabetes are not immune to such problems.

Independence

In previous discussions, we have addressed major issues for the teenager: physical adequacy and peer approval. In this section, the teenager's need for increasing independence will be explored.

The adolescent, in the move toward independence, seeks mastery or control of the environment. Diabetes may also have an impact on this mastery. The loss of control imposed by hypoglycemia, for example, is a very real concern for the teenager. Insulin reactions occurring in the presence of peers are frightening and embarrassing and serve to increase the visibility of this usually hidden disease.

Often the teenager will attempt to prevent insulin reactions by purposefully maintaining

Table 21–2. **EFFECT OF DRUGS ON DIABETES CONTROL**

Drugs	How Taken	Personality Type	Desired Effect	Physiologic Actions	Signs and Symptoms	Implications for Diabetes
Marijuana "Reefers" "Pot" "Joints" "Grass" "Weed"	Smoked Rolled cigarettes Pipe Water pipe	High schoolers People of all ages Lonely people	Euphoria Loss of inhibitions Heightened sensitivity Help with unpleasant task Mild hallucinations	Increases appetite Craving for sweets Disorients behaviors Impairs judgment Lack of coordination Sleepiness	Usually none If used recently, red eyes Increase pulse rate Loud talking	Increased appetite and craving for sweets Would raise blood sugar Impaired judgment could disrupt diabetic routine
Cocaine "Coke" "Snow" "Toot" "Stardust" "Speedball" mixed with heroin	Sniffed Spoon Injected Swallowed	Broad thrill-seeker Wealthy junior executive	Confidence Feeling of control Feeling of well-being	CNS stimulant Psychologic dependence Decreases appetite Counteracts sleep Can induce paranoia	Constant sniffing Nostrils numb Energetic appearance Scars on face Dilated pupils (sunglasses) Increased pulse Weight loss	Loss of appetite could lower blood sugar Access to syringes and needles could tempt use and increase popularity with both users and pushers
Amphetamines "Bennies" "Uppers" "Methamphetamine" "Speed" Benzedrine Dexedrine	Pill Capsule Injected intravenously	Students (before exams) Someone under pressure Athletes before competition Overweight person	Intense concentration Self-confidence Assimilate large quantities of alcohol Wakefulness Alertness	CNS stimulant Increases metabolism Depresses appetite Increases breakdown of glycogen in liver Increases stroke volume Increases energy	Talkative Argumentative Serious intent Nervous Dilated pupils Increased pulse Increased blood pressure Arrhythmia	Increased metabolism would burn glucose faster and decrease blood sugar Decreased food intake would decrease blood sugar Increased breakdown of glycogen would increase blood sugar

| *Barbiturates*
"Downers"
"Goofballs"
"Nembutal"
"Yellow Jackets"
"Seconal"
"Reds" | Pill
Capsule
Injected intravenously | Person who is depressed
Speed freak | Decrease anxiety
Combat insomnia
Counteract "speed"
Dull reality
Shut out world | CNS depressant
Physical and psychologic dependence
Stimulant of hepatic enzymes so drugs metabolize faster and are less effective | Slow movements
Thick, slurred speed
Uncoordinated
Sleepy
Pupils dilated (sunglasses) | Increased activity of hepatic enzyme would alter the effectiveness of oral agents
Drowsiness could disrupt routine of meals and treatment |
| *Heroin*
"Junk"
"Joy powder"
"White stuff"
"H" | Injected intravenously; subcutaneously
Mouth | Thrill-seeker
Addict | Rush of well-being
Absence of tension | CNS depressant
Severe physical and psychologic addiction
Depresses appetite
Decreases gastrointestinal motility, so could increase cardohydrate absorption | Itching-scratching
Confused
Staggering
Drowsy
Nausea
Constipation
Needle marks or tracks (arms covered)
Pupils constricted (sunglasses) | Access to syringes and needle could be influential
Diabetics would be more susceptible from infections from needles
Hepatitis from dirty needles could impair glycogen storage
Decreased GI motility could increase absorption of carbohydrate from the gut and elevate blood sugar
Loss of appetite would decrease blood sugar |

From Holyoke A: Drug abuse assessment guide. Diabetes Educ 5:24, 1979.

hyperglycemia. Such comments as "Normal blood sugars for *me* are 120 to 180; I feel bad around 80" are clues that the adolescent may have worries about hypoglycemia. There are other measures the teenager may take to prevent hypoglycemia or to treat it inconspicuously. Learning to adjust insulin or diet, monitoring frequently, carrying a carbohydrate source, and treating symptoms early are all measures the teenager may employ.

Parents

"My parents are always nagging." This lament is echoed by many teenagers as they attempt to gain control over their lives and their diabetes. The teenager may begin to feel that his or her judgments are not trusted, that personal abilities are not respected. The teenager whose parents make all diabetes care decisions and who are overprotective often worries about his or her own health excessively. After all, if parents are constantly worried, maybe the diabetic, too, should be anxious.

The adolescent must be given the opportunity to take gradual responsibility for diabetes care. Counseling parents and negotiating contracts with the teenager are both interventions that will aid this emerging independence. Although the teenager needs this increased control, there is usually ambivalence about assuming total responsibility. There is a continuing need of the parents to support and provide guidance. What may be helpful is for the teenager to assume care and to "meet" with parents on a scheduled basis to discuss diabetes control.

Problems with Self-Care

Most adolescents will pass through phases of denial or disregard for their care. The following two vignettes are typical:

T.K., a 16-year-old with diabetes for 18 months, called her dietitian to report that she had just returned from the bakery with her friends where she had eaten "one of everything." Her blood glucose level was high, and she was feeling badly. But she really wanted to talk about how she had ignored her diabetes and that it probably was not "worth doing it again."

S.R., a 15-year-old with a two-year duration of diabetes, had reported at his clinic visit blood glucose levels of 80 to 180 "all the time." Yet his glycosylated hemoglobin at that visit was 15.6 percent (less than 10 percent being acceptable).

Long, thoughtful discussion with S.R. revealed that he had skipped his evening injections numerous times during the summer months. He was recording false readings to appease his parents. When sharing his feelings of guilt and shame, S.R. was visibly relieved to learn that he could achieve control again and feel better. Weekly phone calls and monthly visits helped maintain that motivation. Within three months, the glycosylated hemoglobin was 10.4 percent; his health and emotional outlook had also improved.

Such testing of limits is not unusual in the teenager. It is painful for parents and professionals to watch as mistakes are made; yet such errors in judgment are often necessary for growth and maturity. The wise parent and caring professional will be available when the adolescent needs and wants supervision and guidance to regain control. Threats and scare tactics are generally ineffective tools in helping such a teen.

Planning for the Future

The third major focus of social development for the adolescent is planning for the future. As with all teenagers, diabetic teenagers think about sexuality, marriage, and family, and about further education and career. He or she may think about all of these in reference to future health and wonder what influence diabetes will have on this future.

Birth Control and the Teenager with Diabetes. Risks during pregnancy are four to five times greater in the woman with diabetes. The risks are compounded when that person is also a teenager. All sexually active teenagers need information about contraceptives; sexually active teenagers with diabetes may need additional help in choosing a safe method.

Efficacy rates for the current methods of birth control for nondiabetics are presented in Table 21–3. As we shall see, some of these rates do not hold true for the diabetic woman. The following is a discussion of three of the more common and effective contraceptive methods.

Oral contraceptives are of two varieties: the combination pill and the mini-pill. The combination pill contains both estrogen and progesterone; the mini-pill contains progesterone only.

Studies of diabetic women who have used the combination pill suggest there is consid-

Table 21–3. EFFECTIVENESS OF BIRTH CONTROL MEASURES WHEN USED PROPERLY

Method	Effectiveness
Combination pill	99.3%
Mini-pill	97–98%
IUD	96–98%
Diaphragm	96–98%
Condoms and foam	96%
Rhythm	76%
Vaginal mucus	76%
Vaginal sponge	80–90%

erable risk of thromboembolic disease, including cerebral ischemia and myocardial infarction. In addition, these oral contraceptives mimic the hormonal changes of pregnancy and may put diabetic women at risk for the rapid progression of retinopathy occasionally seen in the pregnant, insulin-dependent, diabetic woman. Thus, this method of contraception is generally not recommended for the teenager with diabetes.

The mini-pill, on the other hand, may be a good choice for teenagers. The reports of use of this method are encouraging: little to no risk of cardiovascular disease, and retinopathy and insulin requirements are unaffected. The recognized disadvantages include a reduced reliability and erratic menstrual cycle. Other side effects include increased appetite with weight gain.

Intramuscular injections of progesterone are occasionally advocated for the sexually active teenager who is noncompliant in the use of other methods. This is generally successful if the dose is repeated at intervals.

Intrauterine devices (IUD) were, at one time, discouraged in diabetic women because of a hypothesized increased risk for intrauterine infections. However, Gosden and co-workers (1982) reported disturbing data about the failure rate of these devices in their diabetic patient population. Eleven of 30 diabetic patients became pregnant within the first year after insertion of an IUD. This finding led the investigators to examine the IUDs from women with diabetes, which revealed that the IUDs contained high deposits of sulfur and chloride and that the coils had eroded. Neither these deposits nor such erosion occurs in IUDs in nondiabetic women. These differences may be connected in some way to a difference in the endometrium of diabetic women. Hence, the use of intrauterine devices is discouraged in light of its higher failure rate in diabetic women.

Mechanical methods such as condoms, diaphragms, foams, and creams are generally effective contraceptive methods when used properly. Unfortunately, most teenagers do not find these methods as acceptable as others. Both partners must be responsible, mature, and willing to plan for and to use the devices. The woman must have a diaphragm that fits properly, and she must know how to insert it correctly. The efficacy of any such barrier devices is increased when spermicidal jelly or foam is used in combination.

A new device, the vaginal sponge, may offer added advantages to the teenager. These sponges are easier to insert and have spermicide already in place. The sponge is inexpensive and may be inserted well before sexual contact.

Any teenager choosing to become sexually active needs accurate contraceptive information. This is particularly true for the diabetic teenager who is at even greater risk during pregnancy. The teenager needs to be supplied with information about contraceptive methods and pregnancy in a nonjudgmental, straightforward manner.

Marriage and Pregnancy. The adolescent's look to the future includes thoughts about marrying and starting a family. It is not uncommon for the diabetic teenager to have self-doubts and real concerns about having children. There is always the worry, "What are the chances of my children getting diabetes?"

Since this is a difficult question, the physician may choose to consult genetic counselors* for help in providing information to the adolescent or young adult. Basically, diabetes is a disorder with hereditary overtones, multifactorial in etiology and polygenic in nature. Some authors have recommended the use of HLA typing in counseling couples in family planning, but current population studies would suggest that the risk of a Type I diabetic having a child with diabetes is about 10 percent.

In any event, the teenager wants and needs information about what differences and risks she must consider as a diabetic in planning pregnancies. Teen "rap" groups are good vehicles for relaying such information.

Employment. Although strides have been made in reducing barriers to employment

---

*Genetic counseling services are generally available through local chapters of the National Foundation of the March of Dimes.

for persons with diabetes, the teenager must be aware of problems that still exist. Both federal and state statutes have attempted to uphold the rights of persons with diabetes. Such laws as Public Law 93-113, the Rehabilitation Act of 1973, seek to prevent job discrimination of handicapped persons; persons with diabetes are included in this category as well.

Persons who are insulin-dependent diabetics generally do not qualify for jobs in which it would be difficult or dangerous to stop work in order to treat hypoglycemia. Such jobs include piloting commercial airlines and serving in the military and possibly also jobs involving heavy equipment operation.

Work involving frequent shift rotations, odd shift work, or split shifts are generally undesirable in terms of the person maintaining good metabolic control. Such jobs include driving commercial buses or trucks in interstate commerce.

Employers voice concern over potential increased absenteeism among persons with diabetes; yet studies demonstrate that the majority of diabetic employees present (70 to 73 percent) have no more absenteeism than do their nondiabetic counterparts. When such studies have eliminated a few frequently ill, diabetic employees, the remaining diabetic workers have been found to have fewer sickness absentee days than nondiabetics.

The majority of diabetic teenagers will likely maintain good attendance records, and each worker should be evaluated on an individual basis. Whether diabetic teenagers should inform their employer or potential employer of their diabetes is an issue to be addressed in vocational counseling. Teenagers should be aware of the laws that protect them from discrimination. These laws do not mandate disclosure of the diabetes. If teenagers choose to discuss their diabetes with the employer, they should state clearly that the diabetes is in good control, if indeed it is; and that they are under close medical supervision, if in fact they are.

Employers are generally uninformed about diabetes, particularly about IDDM. If the mature teenager so chooses, he or she may use this opportunity to educate the employer. The worker should be ready to discuss diabetes with the employer, specifically the effects of diabetes on work performance. Table 21–4 outlines guidelines for the teenager seeking work.

In working with teenagers, the health care professional should have resources to help with job counseling and placement. Most areas have vocational rehabilitation programs, located in state agencies, employment offices, or high schools. In addition, the American Diabetes Association provides excellent literature for workers and employers regarding diabetes.

Insurance. Although not an immediate concern for the teenager, the parents often have questions about the diabetic teenager's insurability. Generally, life insurance standards have been modified to account for the improved mortality statistics for persons with diabetes. Insurance carriers now consider not only the type of diabetes but also its duration, the degree of control, the severity of the disease (often measured by the amount of insulin required), and the presence of complications. As insurance companies become more specific in their criteria, more diabetics are being insured at lower risk levels. A list of such progressive insurance carriers is available from the American Diabetes Association.

Health insurance is also a concern for parents and teenagers. Because the morbidity for diabetics is higher than that for nondiabetics, health insurance is generally more

Table 21–4. GUIDELINES FOR THE TEENAGER SEEKING EMPLOYMENT

Be honest with the employer about diabetes.
Use the opportunity to educate the employer about diabetes.
Maintain diabetes in good control so that it will not interfere with work performance.
Find a job with regular work hours.
Ensure that someone at work can help with hypoglycemia.
Wear identification.
Be a good employee and worker.

Table 21–5. FINANCIAL IMPACT OF DIABETES: SUPPLIES

Disposable syringes	$0.15 each
Insulin	$8–$15/bottle (1000 units)
Puncture devices	$8–$30 each
Lancets	$8–$10/box of 200
Chemstrip bG	$12.50–$16.50/ bottle of 25
Dextrostix	$40–$50/bottle of 100
Blood glucose meters	$150–$200
Clinitest tablets	$0.05 each
Acetest tablets	$0.09 each
Glucagon	$12–$14/each bottle
Insulin infusion pumps	$1900–$2500
Infusion sets	$2–$3 each
Pump syringes	$0.33–$0.66 each

costly or more difficult to obtain. Usually, the diabetic teen can obtain only limited coverage if he or she seeks insurance individually.

Group health and life insurance, however, offers the diabetic employee an opportunity for affordable premiums and adequate coverage. Generally, group insurance coverage is based on the overall claim experience of the employer. Diabetes usually figures into an overall claim experience in only a minor way. Hence, the teenager is wise to choose employment that offers such benefits. It is important for the worker to sign up for such coverage shortly after employment to be considered in the group plan rather than as an individual policy holder.

Financial Impact of Diabetes. As the teenager plans for the future, one concern will likely be the ability to afford diabetes. Insulin, syringes, and monitoring materials are costly, necessary items for self-care. Table 21–5 offers broad ranges of the cost of some of these materials. It has been estimated that the six million Americans with diabetes last year spent $9.7 billion on hospital costs, physician visits, medication, supplies, and lost time at work. Unfortunately, there are few financial resources for the person with diabetes. National diabetes organizations primarily direct their funds to research and not to individuals. The diabetic may, however, find assistance from local church and civic groups. In addition, the person may employ such cost-saving practices as reusing syringes and lancets and cutting blood testing strips in half.

Driving. Certainly a major milestone for the adolescent is obtaining a driving license. In most states, application for a license requires a physician's statement of health for the person with diabetes. Obviously, the main danger in operating a motor vehicle is the possibility of hypoglycemia for the insulin-dependent diabetic driver. Teenagers should be aware of this danger and determine plans to prevent insulin reactions or to identify and treat them early.

SUMMARY

This chapter has explored the major social developmental tasks of children and adolescents in relation to their diabetes. The child or adolescent may need additional guidance and problem-solving skills to handle the social situations involved in growing up.

22

Pregnancy

CLASSIFICATION

As proposed by the National Diabetes Data Group, diabetes during pregnancy may be divided into two subgroups: (1) those women who develop diabetes during pregnancy and (2) those women who have diabetes before becoming pregnant. The former are known as gestational diabetics and thus at the end of pregnancy must be reclassified into the category of either diabetes mellitus or impaired glucose tolerance (if the postpartum blood glucose levels meet the criteria) or into the category of previous abnormality of glucose tolerance (if the postpartum blood glucose values are normal). Identification of the category gestational diabetes is important because (1) such patients are still at increased risk for perinatal morbidity and mortality; (2) there is an increased risk of fetal loss; and (3) these women are at higher risk of developing diabetes 5 to 10 years later.

It has been estimated that gestational diabetes will develop in approximately 1 percent to 2 percent of all pregnancies. Indications for performing an oral glucose tolerance test (OGTT) during pregnancy include (1) presence of glycosuria, (2) history of diabetes in a first-degree relative, (3) history of an earlier stillbirth or spontaneous abortion, (4) presence of a fetal malformation in a previous pregnancy, (5) previous large-for-gestational-age baby, (6) pregestational obesity in the mother, (7) high maternal age, and (8) parity of five or more. The presence of more than one of these factors further increases the risk of having an abnormal glucose tolerance test

(GTT). The criteria for an abnormal OGTT during pregnancy originally taken from studies of O'Sullivan and Mahan (1964) are given in Table 22–1. The criteria for an abnormal glucose tolerance are defined as two or more blood glucose values greater than two standard deviations above the mean. Women who meet or exceed these criteria have about a 30 percent chance of becoming diabetic during the following eight-year period.

If the patient is a known diabetic and becomes pregnant, another classification has been proposed and widely accepted. This grouping relates conditions existing before pregnancy to perinatal outcome (Hare and White, 1977). The most recent revision is given in Table 22–2. Although perinatal mortality figures are changing, it is clear that classes A through C have much better rates of fetal survival than do classes D through T. A second classification, proposed by Pedersen and associates in 1974, is based on factors that arise during pregnancy (Table 22–3). The more signs present, the worse the fetal prognosis. In fact, a better estimate of mortality may be obtained when the two classifications are combined for use.

METABOLISM

Normal Pregnancy

In the fasting state, the effects of pregnancy on carbohydrate metabolism are primarily secondary to transfer of glucose and

Table 22–1. CRITERIA FOR ORAL GLUCOSE TOLERANCE TEST DURING PREGNANCY

Time	Plasma (mg/dl)	Whole Blood* (mg/dl)
Fasting	105	90
1 hr	190	170
2 hr	165	145
3 hr	145	125

*Two or more of these values are necessary (following a 100 g oral glucose challenge). Modified from the National Diabetes Data Group, Diabetes 28:1039, 1979.

amino acids from the maternal to the fetal circulation. The glucose transferred is utilized for energy (that is, for protein and fat synthesis and for the formation of glycogen). The glucose utilization rate in such a state has been estimated to be 6 mg/kg/minute, compared with normal adult values of 2 to 3 mg/kg/minute. Since the fetal blood glucose level is 10 to 20 mg/dl lower than that of maternal circulation, simple diffusion cannot explain glucose transport; thus the process is described as one of "facilitated diffusion." Unlike glucose, insulin is not transported across the placenta. Insulin production can be measured in the fetus at 12 weeks' gestation, and its secretion is stimulated by both amino acids and glucose. Besides being utilized for protein synthesis, amino acids are also used as an energy-yielding fuel, as suggested by fetal lamb studies. This passage of amino acids from mother to fetus results in maternal hypoaminoacidemia, notably a decrease in alanine, which is a key precursor to

Table 22–2. CLASSIFICATION OF DIABETES IN PREGNANCY (WHITE)

Class A: Glucose tolerance test abnormal; no symptoms; treatment with diet and without insulin

Class B: Onset after age 20 and duration less than 10 years

Class C: Onset between ages 10 and 20 or duration between 10 and 19 years

Class D: Onset before age 10 or duration greater than 20 years or evidence of minimal vascular disease (e.g., background retinopathy)

Class E: Pelvic vascular disease

Class F: Renal disease

Class G: Multiple failures in pregnancy

Class H: Arteriosclerotic heart disease

Class R: Proliferative retinopathy

Class RF: Both renal disease and proliferative retinopathy

Class T: Pregnancy after renal transplantation

Adapted from Hare JW, White P: Pregnancy in diabetes complicated by vascular disease. Diabetes 26:953, 1977.

Table 22–3. PROGNOSTIC BAD SIGNS OF PREGNANCY (PEDERSEN'S)

A. Clinical pyelonephritis
B. Precoma or severe acidosis
C. Pregnancy-induced hypertension
D. Neglecters—women present themselves in labor or are within 60 days before birth at first presentation

From Pedersen J, Molsted-Pedersen L, Andersen B: Assessment of fetal perinatal mortality in diabetic pregnancy. Diabetes 23:302, 1974.

glucose production. Thus, in the fasting state, the fetus causes hypoglycemia, hypoaminoacidemia, and hyperketonemia in the mother. In association with maternal ketonemia, ketone bodies may be found in amniotic fluid and are probably available to the fetus for use as energy. The major factor determining ketone use by the fetus is substrate delivery. Thus, in situations of limited glucose availability, ketones may serve as an alternative fuel to meet fetal energy requirements.

In the fed state, the metabolic response in the nondiabetic pregnant female is one of hyperinsulinemia, hyperglycemia, hypertriglyceridemia, and diminished sensitivity to insulin. The hyperinsulinism is most marked in the third trimester and is demonstrable in response to either glucose or amino acid administration. Despite the hyperinsulinemia, however, the blood glucose response to a glucose load is decreased tissue sensitivity to insulin. Nevertheless, blood glucose excursion still remains in a narrow range, indicating that homeostasis is achieved by the compensatory increase in plasma insulin. This decrease in tissue responsiveness plus the unmasking of diabetes during pregnancy and the increase in insulin requirements form the basis for characterizing pregnancy as a diabetogenic state. Various hormones have been implicated in this diabetogenic response: human placental lactogen (HPL), progesterone, and estrogen. HPL, a polypeptide hormone produced by the syncytiotrophoblast, is similar to the growth hormone; and a mild but definite impairment in glucose has been noted after acute infusions of this hormone. Like the growth hormone, HPL alters glucose metabolism by diminishing the effectiveness of insulin. However, at term, HPL circulates at a concentration 1000 times that of the growth hormone.

Following the luteal phase of pregnancy, the placental phase is characterized by increasing placental secretion of estrogen and progesterone. These hormones cause glucose intolerance, with an increase in plasma insulin secretion. This suggests that these hormones act as insulin antagonists rather than as inhibitors of insulin secretion.

Indeed, the mechanism of insulin resistance induced by these hormones appears to be due to a postreceptor event. Studies indicate that insulin receptors on circulating monocytes or erythrocytes do not decrease during human pregnancy, despite an increase in plasma insulin. Values for insulin binding have been the same or slightly greater than those for nonpregnant females.

The changes of significance during normal pregnancy may be summarized as follows: fasting levels of glucose are reduced and postprandial increments are increased in late pregnancy; levels for most amino acids are lower in the fed as well as in the fasting state; plasma cholesterol is increased in late pregnancy and unaffected by dietary excursions; and plasma triglycerides are increased.

Diabetic Pregnancy

The effect of pregnancy on the clinical course of diabetes is variable, and it is useful to divide the pregnancy into two parts rather than the usual three (Fig. 22–1). During the early months of pregnancy, the major factor contributing to altered glucose homeostasis is the transfer of glucose to the fetus. This effect results in hypoglycemia, with a subsequent necessity to lower the insulin dose. This need for less insulin does not indicate a change in tissue sensitivity but is a consequence of decreased availability of circulating carbohydrate. In the second half of pregnancy, the diabetogenic action of HPL, estrogens, and progesterone outweighs the glucose-transfer effect. Thus, insulin requirements increase by as much as two thirds. At this time, there is also an increased tendency for ketosis and ketoacidosis. After delivery, with the rapid fall in concentrations of the diabetogenic placental hormones, insulin requirements decrease dramatically, frequently to less than prepregnancy levels. A gradual increase to usual levels occurs over the ensuing 3 to 6 weeks.

MANAGEMENT OF DIABETIC PREGNANCY

Diet

The energy cost of pregnancy has been estimated to be about 75,000 kcal. This figure is derived from the energy expenditure required to accommodate the normal compositional changes of pregnancy, which vary

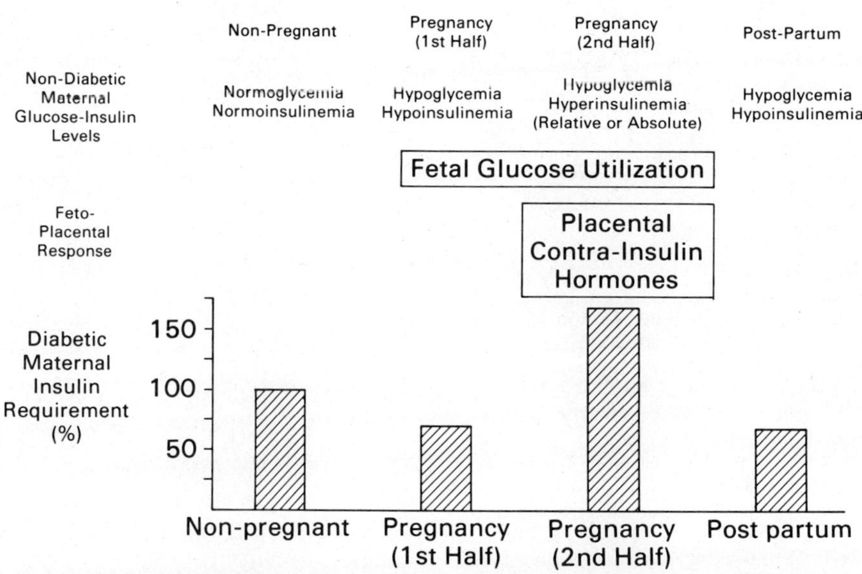

Figure 22–1. The diabetic pregnancy. Multiple changes occur during the normal pregnancy in the handling of glucose. This is easier to understand if the pregnancy is divided into two parts and contrasted with both the nonpregnant and postpartum states. See text for discussion. (From Tyson JE, Felig P: Medical aspects of diabetes in pregnancy and the diabetogenic effects of oral contraceptives. Med Clin North Am 55:953, 1971.)

from 38 to 50 kcal/kg. In clinical terms, an increment of 300 kcal/day above basal requirements should provide calories sufficient to meet the nutritional needs of pregnancy. Approximately 45 percent of these calories should be in the form of carbohydrate, but supplements are required if there is excessive renal glycosuria. The total accumulation of protein during pregnancy, calculated from known sites of protein deposition in mother and fetus, averages 925 g. Thus about 1.3 g/kg body weight will satisfy the extra protein requirement. The remainder of the calories are provided as fat (40 to 60 g). Adequate vitamins and minerals should be provided.

Sodium restriction beyond maintenance requirements should not be imposed. Pregnancy is normally associated with increased renin-substrate and subsequently angiotensin I and II and aldosterone. Teleologically, this may be to preserve the increase in effective circulating blood volume associated with pregnancy. Thus, the increase in aldosterone and sodium retention associated with pregnancy are normal events and do not necessarily warrant sodium restriction. The Committee on Maternal Nutrition of the National Research Council recommends a weight gain of approximately 24 pounds. The presence of diabetes should not influence this anticipated weight gain. There should be minimal weight gain the first trimester followed by a progressive linear rate of weight gain of 350 to 400 grams per week for the last two trimesters.

For the diabetic or nondiabetic, pregnancy is not the time for dieting. If successful, dieting results in fat breakdown, with resultant ketosis. Several investigations suggest that ketonemia may have adverse central nervous system effects on the fetus.

Insulin

Since blood glucose levels normally tend to be lower during early pregnancy, insulin therapy should be altered accordingly. Thus, fasting levels around 70 mg/dl and postprandial levels around 90 mg/dl should be a goal. Rarely should whole blood glucose exceed 100 mg/dl. Several regimens have been used to attain this goal. Clearly, it cannot be achieved with one injection of insulin per day. At least two, and perhaps three or four, injections per day are required. One injection of intermediate-acting insulin with Regular insulin at breakfast and a second injection of this mixture before the evening meal are recommended. Some authors prefer a long-acting insulin (ultralente) plus shots of Regular insulin at mealtimes. Such therapy can mimic the glycemic control of the subcutaneous insulin infusion pump. The doses of insulin must be sufficient to maintain euglycemia without frequent or severe hypoglycemia. Mild hypoglycemia is unavoidable. Home blood glucose monitoring is mandatory.

Monitoring

Blood glucose levels should be checked at least twice a day; while fasting and at another time, which may be at peak insulin action or two hours postprandial. Most experts recommend more frequent blood glucose monitoring, and this is particularly desirable if there are a significant number of fluctuations outside the desired range. Glycosylated hemoglobin concentrations should be monitored at least every two months and perhaps as often as monthly.

After delivery of the placenta, the patient becomes very sensitive to insulin for several days. Since the patient is fasting during labor and delivery, frequent blood glucose monitoring, with a dextrose infusion and either frequent subcutaneous insulin or intravenous insulin injections, is recommended. It is important to attempt to maintain euglycemia during labor and delivery, since it has been shown that the incidence of respiratory distress syndrome among a group of premature babies was significantly lower in mothers who became neither ketotic nor acidotic during labor. At the time of delivery, insulin can usually be stopped while the glucose infusion is maintained, until stable blood glucose levels in the range of 90 to 120 mg/dl are obtained.

Fetal glucose levels are a direct function of maternal glucose levels. However, the fetus does not have a compensatory capacity to protect against maternal hypoglycemia. Thus, decreased blood glucose levels are experienced by both mother and fetus. Although it appears that the fetus has the ability to withstand such insults, this may reflect our inability to detect subtle damage rather than its actual absence.

MATERNAL MORBIDITY AND MORTALITY

With careful monitoring of blood glucose during pregnancy, the morbidity and mortality for the pregnant diabetic has improved greatly. In the preinsulin era, few pregnant diabetics were seen; among 1300 diabetics followed by Joslin, only 10 pregnancies were noted. Today, with the exception of those in class H (see Table 22–2), maternal morbidity should be completely eliminated. Of four class H mothers seen at the Joslin Clinic, only one was alive for four weeks following pregnancy, and she had undergone a coronary artery bypass operation.

Retinopathy in pregnancy can follow an unpredictable course for any individual patient. Prepregnancy background retinopathy or background retinopathy acquired during pregnancy is often a benign process. However, such retinopathy may take any of three courses during pregnancy: remit, remain stationary, or progress to proliferative retinopathy. Background retinopathy should be initially evaluated with fluorescein retinography during the first trimester and then followed with ophthalmoscopic examinations at each visit. If progression to proliferation occurs, treatment with argon laser therapy is initiated. Data indicate that such therapy can usually halt the progression of proliferative lesions appearing during pregnancy and preserve vision. Patients with prepregnancy, laser-treated, proliferative retinopathy must be carefully observed during pregnancy.

The course of patients with diabetic nephropathy is more difficult and demanding. These diabetics require intense attention in order to control blood glucose and hypertension and to maintain fluid and electrolyte balance. Even patients with kidney transplants may maintain a successful pregnancy despite the need for extensive monitoring in addition to the continual administration of immunosuppressive therapy.

FETAL MORTALITY AND MORBIDITY

Fetal mortality and morbidity in all cases has improved remarkably in the last years. Mortality figures range from 0 to 21 percent in reported series, with a continual decline over the last 10 years. Congenital malformations are reported to occur in 5 to 18 percent of cases; cerebral dysfunction in 20 to 36 percent; macrosomia in 16 to 40 percent; hypoglycemia in 16 to 76 percent; erythremia in 10 to 45 percent; hyperbilirubinemia in 19 to 35 percent; and respiratory distress in 2 to 9 percent of cases studied. Improvement in recent years is due to better monitoring of the fetus during pregnancy and better control of maternal blood glucose levels. Procedures for fetal monitoring include ultrasonography, urinary estriol determination, amniotic fluid phospholipid assay, and intrapartum fetal monitoring. Ultrasonography permits the gathering of information concerning the size of the fetus: gestational age can be assessed from crown-rump measurements in the first trimester and from serial measurements of biparietal diameter in later pregnancy. Ultrasound can also be used for placental localization before amniocentesis and to detect fetal malformation. Plotting the infant on the intrauterine growth curve will determine whether the fetus is macrosomic, indicating maternal, and hence fetal, hyperglycemia; or whether it is small for gestational age, indicating perhaps placental insufficiency. Furthermore, reduced or slowed fetal growth can also alert the perinatologist to additional problems that may occur in a small-for-gestational-date infant.

Another measure of fetal and placental well-being is the 24-hour urinary excretion of estriol. This test is based on the property of the fetal adrenal glands to secrete dehydroepiandrosterone, which is converted by the fetal liver to 16-OH dehydroepiandrosterone; this in turn is converted by the fetal liver to 16-OH dehydroepiandrosterone sulfate. Placental enzymes remove the sulfate molecule and aromatize the compound to produce estriol, which, after conjugation in the maternal liver, is excreted in the urine. It has been pointed out that although estriol determinations may be extremely valuable, certain precautions in interpretation must be observed. First, urinary estriol excretion is highly correlated with birth weight and, thus, is also correlated with findings on ultrasonography. Second, urinary estriol excretion in patients with diabetes mellitus is more variable than that in the nondiabetic. Third, there is marked day-to-day variability in estriol determinations. Thus, if a fall in estriol excretion is to be judged significant (greater than 35 percent), comparison with previous stable excretion values is required. Last, owing to the variability, it has been recommended that such excretions be measured daily.

An important advance in the care of the newborn has been the determination of the lecithin to sphingomyelin (L/S) ratio in amniotic fluid. This ratio provides an assessment of functional lung maturity. In past years, in order to prevent intrauterine fetal death, preterm delivery (33rd to 37th week of gestation) of patients with complicated diabetes mellitus was performed. Such early delivery often produced a live fetus but one with immature lungs who required ventilatory assistance after birth. These infants often succumbed in the neonatal period.

Respiratory distress syndrome (RDS) is related to inadequate surfactant production, and the increasing concentrations of lecithin in the amniotic fluid indicate the completion of lung maturation. An L/S ratio of greater than 2.0 usually indicates that the infant's lungs are sufficiently mature to sustain normal pulmonary function and that the risk of RDS is slight. The origin of the increased incidence of RDS in infants of diabetic mothers remains controversial. Possible explanations include increased incidence of prematurity, cesarean-section delivery, and birth asphyxia. Studies in glucose-intolerant Rhesus monkeys suggest that the polyhydramnios often associated with diabetic pregnancy may result in more rapid removal of lecithin after its production in the lung, resulting in lower concentrations in tissues and higher amounts in the amniotic fluid, with a higher incidence of RDS in neonates of affected pregnancies.

Fetal heart monitoring, particularly during stress testing, is another method of testing placental sufficiency. During uterine contractions, blood flow can transiently decrease, thus producing transient ischemia to the fetus. If uteroplacental blood flow is compromised, the transient fetal hypoxia may produce delayed slowing of the heart rate. This is considered a positive stress test, suggesting fetal compromise. Other indicators of uteroplacental insufficiency are absence of beat-to-beat variability or acceleration of heart beat with fetal movements or both. Such monitoring should be performed from the 32nd week of gestation. A positive test serves to prompt other examinations, which will aid in the decision as to when to deliver the fetus. If positive, urinary estriol levels and amniotic L/S ratio should be determined. If urinary estriol is unchanged and L/S ratio is less than 2.0, the patient may be followed with daily estriols and frequent monitoring of fetal heart rate. If the L/S ratio is greater than 2.0, the pregnancy may be terminated. Also, if the stress test is positive, with low levels of estriol, the pregnancy may be terminated. In fact, if the stress test is positive, with low levels of estriol, the pregnancy should be terminated regardless of L/S ratio. If termination is elected and if vaginal delivery is decided upon, scalp electrode monitoring plus measurements of pH is highly desirable. These measures more closely reflect the metabolic state of the fetus than do such indirect measures as heart rate status.

Infants of diabetic mothers have an increased incidence of hypoglycemia, hypocalcemia, and hyperbilirubinemia, as well as RDS. These are often a result only of immaturity and not of the diabetic condition of the mother.

Neonatal hypoglycemia is related to the persistence of fetal hyperinsulinemia. The fetus of a diabetic woman has an abundance not only of glucose but also of insulin. This hyperinsulinism results in rapid utilization of the glucose available, and profound hypoglycemia may result within minutes to hours after birth. Although there are ample supplies of glycogen in the liver and adipose tissue triglycerides, the hyperinsulinism results in an inability to mobilize glucose from these sources. Infants subjected to hypoglycemia early in the neonatal period (<30 mg/dl for the term infant; <20 mg/dl for the preterm infant) are at risk for neurologic damage whether or not they are asymptomatic.

All neonates born to diabetic mothers of any class or any macrosomic infant should be carefully monitored with serial blood glucose analyses. Symptoms of hypoglycemia can range from jitteriness and poor feeding to cyanosis, seizures, pallor, apnea, and bradycardia. Intramuscular injection of glucagon (200 μg/kg) will aid in mobilizing glucose from the liver; but hypertonic dextrose intravenously with a constant infusion rate of 4 to 10 mg/kg/min may also be necessary to maintain euglycemia.

The cause of the increased incidence of hypocalcemia is not clear. Symptoms of hypocalcemia include seizures, apnea, neuromuscular irritability and jitteriness, vomiting, poor feeding and other nonspecific symptoms. A hypocalcemic infant (ionized calcium <3 mg/dl or serum total calcium level <7 mg/dl in a term infant) should be treated by an intravenous infusion of calcium gluconate, 200 mg/kg over 20 minutes, with cardiac monitoring. If constant infusions are desired, 500 mg/kg/24 hr of calcium gluconate can be used.

Classes A, B, and perhaps C are frequently associated with macrosomia as well as with the other biochemical alterations noted. In contrast to the large babies seen in these classes, patients with vascular disease often have babies that are small for gestational age, which is presumably due to secondary complications of compromised placental function. Congenital malformations are also increased in infants of diabetic mothers. Skeletal defects and congenital heart disease are the most common. Infants of diabetic mothers have an incidence of congenital heart defects five times the incidence in the nondiabetic population. These infants are also more susceptible to persistence of the fetal circulation. Major malformations are noted in White's classifications D and F, in women with complications during pregnancy, and in infants with low birth weight. Pedersen has suggested that malformations were more common also in women with higher blood glucose levels in the first trimester.

RESULTS FROM METABOLIC CONTROL

Since neonatal hypoglycemia and macrosomia appear related to maternal hyperglycemia, attempts have been made to assess the influences of maternal tight metabolic control on fetal morbidity. In two studies, Jovanovic and coworkers (1980, 1981) have found significantly decreased neonatal complications

Table 22–4. **A DIABETIC PREGNANCY: ACTUAL 1981 EXPENSES***

Hospital charges (mother for 11 days)	$4151.65
Hospital charges (infant for 6 days)	$ 733.00
Physician charges	
a. Obstetrician	$1267.20
b. Anesthesiologist	$ 250.00
c. Endocrinologist	$ 175.00
d. Pediatrician	$ 120.00
Miscellaneous	
a. Stress tests (8)	$ 588.00
b. Laboratory tests	$ 267.80
c. Nondiabetic medications	$ 19.00
TOTAL	**$7571.65**

*These are actual expenses incurred by a pregnant woman with diabetes (in 1981 dollars). The patient was in good health, had superb diabetes control throughout pregnancy, and incurred no perinatal complications.

after introducing rigid blood glucose control. In their initial project, these investigators followed 10 patients who were less than eight weeks pregnant and had had diabetes for a mean of eight years (range, 1 to 23 years). Control of blood glucose levels was achieved through education concerning diabetes and pregnancy, three injections of insulin per day, home blood glucose monitoring, and a diet to provide 30 kilocalories per kilogram per day. Blood glucose values were maintained between 60 and 70 mg/dl in the fasting state, with postprandial values of around 140 mg/dl. Normal plasma glucose levels were achieved after one week of the program and were maintained throughout pregnancy. Bimonthly HbA_{1C} levels, which were initially elevated in all patients (9.4 $\pm$ 1.6 percent), fell to normal (<5 percent) five weeks after the blood glucose values normalized. Serum estradiol, prolactin, and serum human chorionic gonadotropin, although elevated initially, normalized after glucose control was achieved. All patients were delivered at 37 to 40 weeks, and none of the infants showed signs of macrosomia, hypoglycemia, hyperbilirubinemia, hypocalcemia, erythremia, or RDS. In a later comparative study, 52 diabetic women were followed by using the same measurements and were compared with 42 nondiabetic control subjects. There was no fetal mortality in the diabetic group; infants of diabetic mothers of classes D, R, and F had somewhat smaller babies. There was one blood glucose level less than 45 mg/dl in a single infant, but none showed a bilirubin level above 12 mg/dl, a calcium level below 7.0 mg/dl, a hematocrit above 65 percent, or RDS. Furthermore, there were no major or minor congenital malformations. These studies emphasize that euglycemia is achievable with clinically available tools in a motivated population. Additionally, if euglycemia can be maintained throughout gestation, outcome may be more dependent on antenatal care than on diabetes per se. Nonetheless, mothers with vascular complications did tend to have smaller babies.

The presence of congenital malformations may also be related to preconception blood glucose control. Evaluation of 200 pregnancies in which blood glucose was well controlled before conception demonstrated no congenital anomalies. In a retrospective study of 116 insulin-dependent diabetic pregnant women who were studied in the first trimester, 15 infants had major congenital anomalies. The mean HbA_{1C} level was significantly higher in the group of mothers who delivered infants with major anomalies than in the group who delivered normal infants. There was no relation of high or low initial HbA_{1C} to White's classes. Furthermore, there was no evidence that diabetic women with microangiopathy had more hyperglycemia in early pregnancy than did diabetic women without microangiopathy. The overall incidence of major anomalies has been reported to be 6 percent to 9 percent in several larger series, a figure some three to four times that in the general neonatal population. Since fetal malformations occur before eight weeks' gestation, improved biochemical control should begin before conception.

Children of diabetic mothers have also been found to have lower intelligence quotients later in life. Factors contributing to such decreased IQ include maternal acetonuria; birthweight less than 3000 g; and White's classifications C, D, and F. Both Churchill and Stehbens and their coworkers found maternal acetonuria to significantly lower scores on the Bayley and Stanford-Benet scales, at eight months and four to five years, respectively. Interestingly, Churchill and associates also noted that maternal hypoglycemic episodes had no demonstrable impact on later neuropsychiatric status. Yessing found that cerebral dysfunction was more common in White's classes C, D, and F. This dysfunction also increased with low birth weight and low gestational age. Although early studies showed impairment of neuropsychologic development in infants of diabetics, particularly those who had pregnancies complicated by ketonuria, more recent data suggest no adverse effects of diabetes on subsequent neurologic development. Advances in control of diabetes during pregnancy, decisions concerning time for delivery, neonatal resuscitation, and care of the neonate will result in excellent prognosis for neurologic development in infants of diabetic mothers.

Although the child of a diabetic mother is more likely to have congenital malformations, decreased cerebral function, and diabetes mellitus, the first two can be minimized or eliminated by careful metabolic control of glucose metabolism, careful perinatal monitoring, and the use of well-equipped and staffed delivery and neonatal intensive care units. It is also important to remember that pregnancy in the diabetic should be a well-planned event, for it is costly (Table 22–4).

23

Insulin Delivery Systems

It has been less than 10 years since the first reports appeared on the clinical use of external insulin infusion devices, giving rise to a therapy now collectively known as continuous subcutaneous insulin infusion (CSII), or insulin pump therapy (IPT). To appreciate even superficially the rapid advances that have been made in this field, one needs only to look at Figure 23–1. The device on the left (Fig. 23–1A) was the first pump used by our group in Galveston in 1978. It was this instrument (by Autosyringe) that, as much as any other, gave diabetologists the experience necessary to evaluate this new modality of management. Despite its many undesirable features (that is, weight over 1 pound, external knobs, inability to separate effectively bolus from basal doses, sealed battery that required recharging while being worn, and so forth), therapy delivered by this pump altered the lives of many in a very positive manner. Figure 23–1B depicts a pump (circa 1984) that has become the major one used by the Children's Diabetic Management Center (CDMC) but that is similar to approximately a dozen other "new" microprocessor units currently being marketed. The differences in patient appeal are obvious. Less obvious, but of more importance, are processing and safety features now common to virtually all third-generation pumps.

Closed Versus Open-Loop Pumps

The ideal pump would have the characteristics depicted in Figure 23–2. The major feature of such a device would be an effective and continuous monitor of blood glucose (that is, the glucose sensor). A computer interface between the sensor and an insulin pump would facilitate precise delivery of insulin (and, perhaps, of other glucoregulatory hormones) to the body. As the sensor detected lowering of glucose, delivery of insulin would cease until such time as blood glucose again rose to some predetermined level. This feedback-controlled device would thus be similar to an artificial beta cell. Such an instrument does, in fact, exist (Fig. 23–3) and is widely used in research laboratories, as seen here in the diabetes control unit of our center. Technical problems have thus far prevented prolonged ambulatory use of such instruments in patients. On the other hand, technologic advances predicted over the next few years may provide such a device for clinical use.

Insulin pumps today, however, are all open-loop devices (Fig. 23–4). The pumps are preprogrammed to deliver a basal insulin infusion at a relatively constant rate during the 24-hour period and are supplemented by premeal boluses or pulse infusions that are

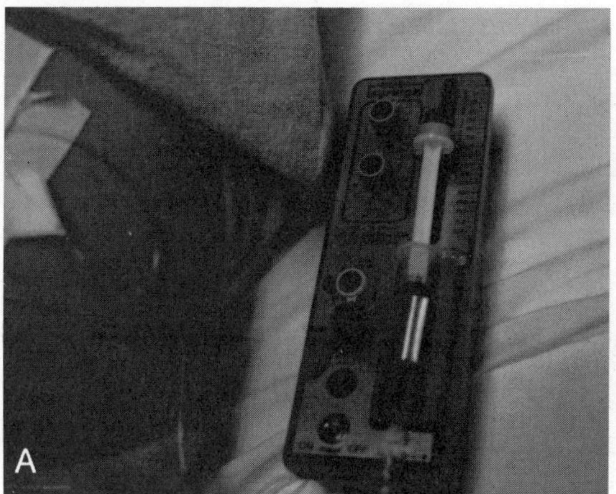
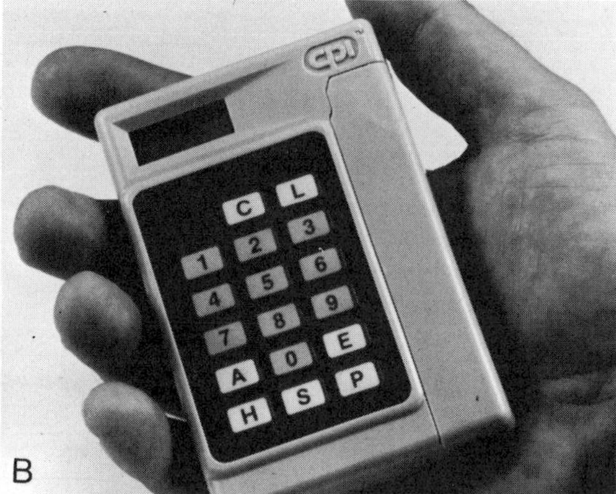

Figure 23–1. *A*, CSII delivery by one of the first devices (by Autosyringe) in 1978. *B*, One of the more popular infusion devices in our unit (CPI-Betatron II) in the mid-1980s.

specific for each meal. Blood glucose excursions are then measured in the traditional manner (usually preprandial and postprandial levels) with subsequent adjustments being made in either basal or bolus amounts. Open-loop pumps are, thus, just that—sophisticated and programmable pumps without the internal feedback loop. Multiple fingerstick determinations of blood glucose are thus part of the package that is bought when CSII is instituted. Additionally, someone (the patient, it is hoped) must make decisions external to the pump about the appropriateness of doses and must have the necessary judgmental skills to alter these doses when indicated.

ARTIFICIAL DEVICES

CLOSED LOOP SYSTEM (Artificial Beta Cell)

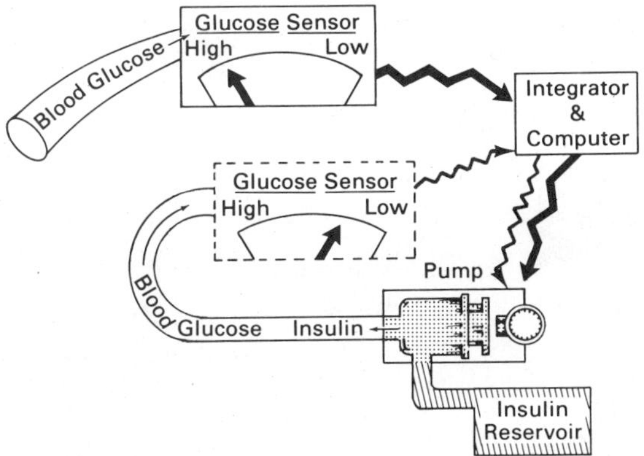

Figure 23–2. Closed-loop delivery system (see text).

CONTINUOUS SUBCUTANEOUS INSULIN INFUSION (CSII)

As the name implies, in CSII insulin is delivered from the pump reservoir into a subcutaneous site, usually via a microinfusion set (that is, a small-bore, flexible, polyethylene catheter with needle attached). Regular or crystalline insulin is used exclusively, and most investigators have found that Velosulin (pure pork insulin by Nordisk) is the best. Other crystalline insulins are more prone to crystallize in the microtubing and thus potentially to interrupt smooth and continuous insulin delivery.

M.B., a 12.5-year-old boy, was referred to the Children's Diabetic Management Center because of hyperlabile diabetes. He had onset of IDDM at age 11 years, and, almost from the beginning, the diabetes had been difficult to control. He had multiple eipsodes of both hypoglycemia and ketosis—DKA. Multiple therapies and interventions had been used without success. About three months prior to his referral, he had been started on CSII, using biosynthetic human insulin (Regular). His diabetes control was dramatically improved for two to three weeks but then returned to its previous unstable state.

At the time of referral, he was receiving over 1.8 units per kilogram body weight per day but was still quite hyperglycemic and intermittently ketotic. His glycosylated hemoglobin was 9.8 per cent (normal 3 to 6 per cent). Although both child and parent denied having noted any crystallization of insulin in the tubing or any noticeable change in daily delivery rate, we switched his insulin to Velosulin and made no other changes.

He quickly became hypoglycemic and, over five days, his dosage decreased to 0.92 U/kg/day. Five

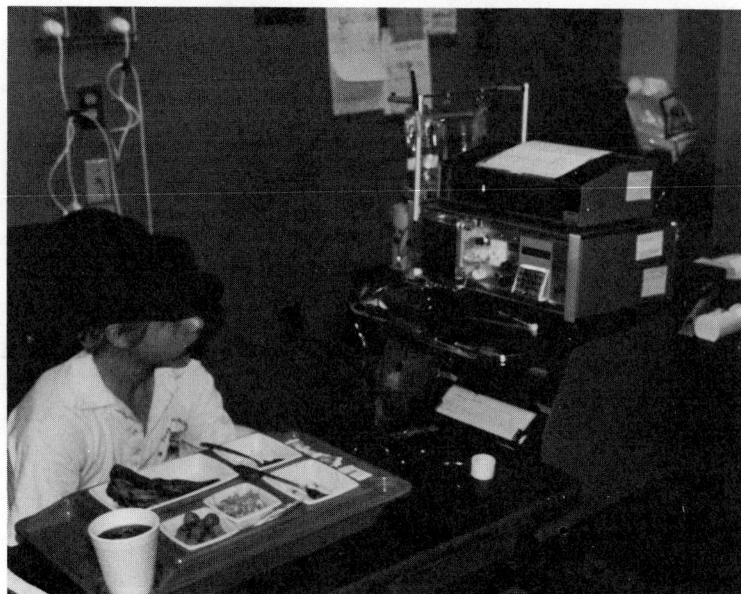

Figure 23–3. A glucose-controlled insulin-delivery system (GCIDS), the Biostator (Miles Laboratories), a closed-loop system. This one is in use in the Diabetes Control Unit of the Clinical Research Center, Children's Diabetes Management Center, Galveston.

months later, his dosage has remained around about 1.0 U/kg/day, and his glycosylated hemoglobin has fallen to 6.1 per cent. No other episodes of DKA have occurred.

PHYSIOLOGIC CONTROL

Generally, it might be said simply that the advantage of pump therapy is that normal glucose-insulin relations may be best simulated by this means. Figure 23–5 describes the simplest example of an insulin pump program. It consists of a constant *basal level* (long arrow) given continuously throughout the day, usually at a constant rate per hour; *pulse doses* (inverted triangles) given prior to meals; and a *basal supplement* (or alternate) to blunt the predawn hyperglycemic surge (open arrow). Some of the newer devices have the capacity for several "alternate" basal rates per day, which may be preprogrammed in such a manner that appropriate individualization of insulin need is met.

Total Insulin Requirements

It is impossible to predict precisely the amount of insulin that will be required by CSII when moving from usual or conventional therapy. In our experience and in those of most others, the daily dosage of insulin required to obtain control of blood glucose initially increases (from baseline depot insulin doses) and subsequently (days to weeks later) declines below prepump levels. It is usually our practice to start pump doses either at the patient's current dosage or at 1.0 U/kg/day, whichever amount is larger, and then carefully to monitor, making changes as indicated by the blood glucose excursions.

ARTIFICIAL DEVICES

<u>OPEN LOOP SYSTEM (Insulin Dose)</u>

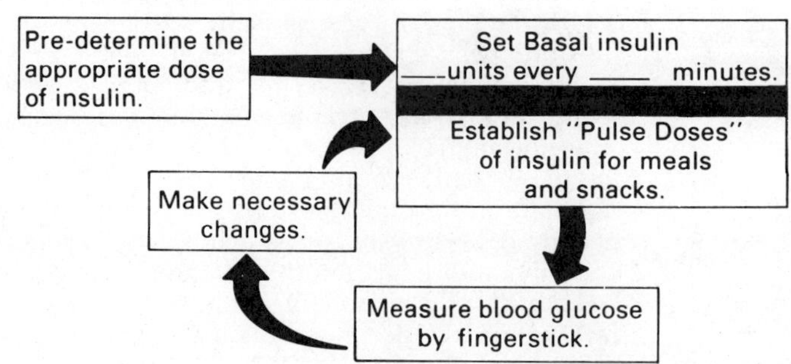

Figure 23–4. Schematic of the open-loop system (see text).

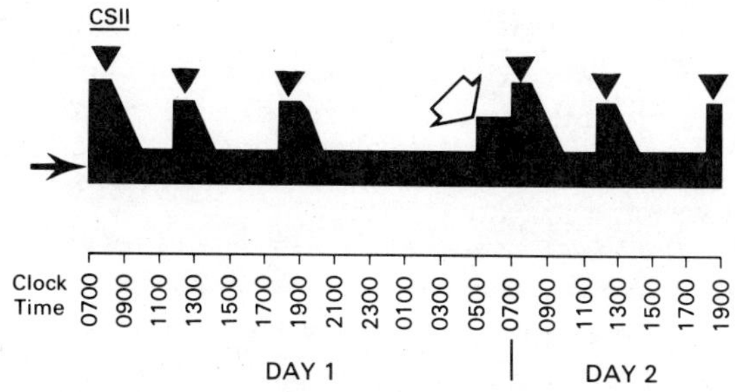

Figure 23–5. The plasma insulin profile in a pump patient (see text for description).

Basal Level or Rate

This must be individualized. We have noted that some patients do best on as little as 20 per cent of total dosage, whereas others have seemed to require 40 percent to 60 percent of total in the basal mode. Our general program is designed to start with a basal dosage of about 35 to 40 percent of total dosage and to be adjusted accordingly. An occasional patient seems to do better on a variable basal rate alone, without pulse dosing.

Basal Supplement

In our experience, the "dawn phenomenon" is variable in time of onset, length, and degree of need for extra insulin. In most patients, the period of extra need occurs between 3:00 and 7:00 AM, and we usually double the hourly basal rate as a starting point. Some patients do not appear to have a predawn surge of counter-regulatory hormones, while others begin this as early as between midnight and 1:00 AM. It has been noted by us as well as by others that the usual circadian rhythm of counter-regulatory hormone secretion is altered by poor control of diabetes.

Premeal Boluses

Premeal bolus doses are usually recommended 30 to 45 minutes prior to the meal, with the size depending both on the premeal glucose and on the glycemic response to the meal. Usually, the prebreakfast dose is greater in amount than the other two, but the only way really to determine the "usual" or "best" dose is through the monitoring of premeal/postmeal glucose values, following

administration of varying amounts of insulin. We have not routinely given presnack doses, but these may be required in some.

SUMMATION OF LITERATURE AND CDMC RESULTS

Control of Diabetes

A number of studies have demonstrated an improved glycemic control in those patients placed on insulin pump therapy. The mean amplitude of glycemic excursion can be reduced and glycosylated hemoglobin concentrations returned to normal. In patients who are well selected and properly motivated and followed, prolonged euglycemia can be achieved.

Prevention or Reversal of Complications

Some studies have demonstrated a reversal of microalbuminuria, but most studies have not demonstrated significant reduction in clinical (fixed) proteinuria once it has appeared. However, this is not always the case, as is demonstrated by the following example:

K.B. had onset of IDDM at age 1.8 years and had no real problems with diabetes until age 16, when she was discovered to have proteinuria. In retrospect, her diabetes control was probably only fair, but, except for two hospitalizations for hypoglycemia, she had never been ill. She had, during most of this time, taken two injections of insulin daily.

Upon referral at age 16.5 years, her glycosylated hemoglobin was 8 percent (normal 3 to 6 percent). She had mild increases in blood pressure for age (130 to 140/88 to 94) and persistent proteinuria measured at 400 mg/24 hours. Her glomerular filtration rate was 92 ml/min/m^2 (normal 60 to 80 ml/min/m^2).

In December 1979, she was placed on CSII and, except for a few days, has remained on such continuously, now for almost six years. Her Hb A$_1$C values have ranged between 5.6 percent and 8.0 percent. Her BP has not required treatment, and after two years of CSII therapy, her proteinuria has cleared and has never returned. Her GFR has ranged between 78 and 84 ml/m^2/min.

In two controlled studies of CSII patients, there has been some regression of previously noted retinal (that is, nonproliferative) changes after one to two years of improved control. Likewise, there have been documented reports of improvement in diabetic neuropathy. In all such studies, there is obviously a point in the progression of the degenerative complication at which improved diabetic control will not significantly alter disease progression. The greatest benefit appears to be in those patients who have not yet developed clinical evidence of sequelae.

Growth

Various studies have demonstrated that poorly controlled diabetes can lead to a falloff in growth rate. Improved control, whether secondary to CSII or to other interventions, may reverse this process. Figure 23–6 demonstrates this in one child.

P.A. had onset of IDDM at age 6.4 years. He did well for about two years but then developed marked hyperlability associated with severe social and environmental stresses. He had multiple hospitalizations for DKA. His height, previously in the 25th percentile, fell to below the 5th percentile. Multiple interventions were unsuccessful, and CSII was finally instituted at age 12.5 years. Control dramatically improved, and after about 6 to 9 months accelerated growth occurred, allowing P.A.'s height to return to about the 10th percentile.

Hyperlabile Diabetes

As indicated in earlier chapters, hyperlabile diabetes may have multiple causes, but psychologic and social problems are among the most common. In many instances, it is difficult to tell which came first, however, for they become so intertwined. It is always appropriate to attempt to identify the specific cause of the hyperlability and to eradicate it, but this is often almost impossible to accomplish without some dramatic intervention. Restoring diabetes control may lessen the stress on the child and family, leading to less hyperlability. Often, psychologic interventions take a long time before being effective. We feel that we can hasten the return to good physical and psychologic health by attacking both problems simultaneously.

At other times, the cause for the hyperlability may be difficult to uncover. A trial of CSII may be a worthwhile consideration as demonstrated in Figure 23–7. This patient had onset of diabetes at age 10 years, and hyperlability was apparent from that point on with multiple hospitalizations owing to

DKA. Even while on multiple dose insulin therapy (MDIT), or three shots per day, she did not do well; neither was psychologic intervention helpful. However, when placed on CSII, she showed improvement in control, and her hospitalizations stopped. For a short time in 1984, her pump was discontinued with a return to an ultralente/Regular regimens (MDIT). She quickly decompensated with two bouts of DKA before returning to pump management.

CDMC EXPERIENCE WITH CSII

The primary indication for institution of pump therapy in our first 29 children is seen on Table 23–1. This does not include the additional persons we have treated by use of the pump during management of pregnancy. Our total number of pump patient is now almost 50, but the proportions are approximately the same as seen here. The patients have ranged in age from 8.1 to 18 years, with a mean of 13.8 years. Of the first 29, 18 were female and 11 male.

Failure to grow at a normal rate for a period of greater than 18 months was the primary indication for use in our center (12 children). For the group as a whole, the average growth rate was 1.7 cm per six months in the 18-month period prior to CSII. Over the 18 months following institution of CSII, the average rate of growth was 4.3 cm per six months, with every child increasing the six-month rate by 50 percent or more. Whereas we had been unable to motivate these children to control their diabetes, each was highly motivated to grow.

Hyperlability was the initial indication for CSII in seven children. These seven were selected from a much larger group of hyperlabile children referred to our institution. Excluded were persons with obvious causes for their hyperlability (that is, another unassociated disease, recurrent and intentional noncompliance, overtreatment syndromes, or serious psychopathology). In addition, all seven of those chosen had failed to be helped by MDIT. Significant improvement occurred in four of the seven; one discontinued the pump after only two months; while the other two had no significant improvement in diabetes control.

A desire for better control of diabetes was the primary reason for pump use in four children, and three of the four have continued

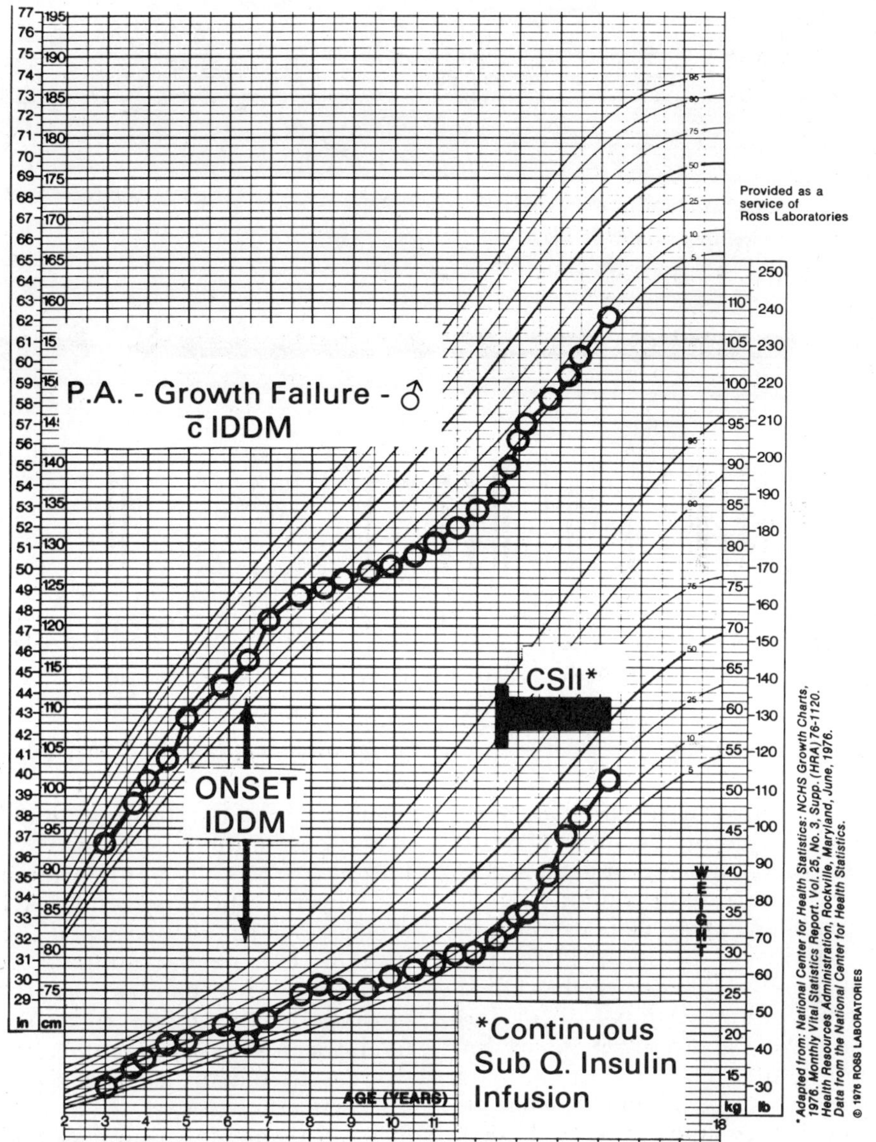

Figure 23–6. Growth failure, due to poorly controlled IDDM, which was corrected with CSII (see evidence of "catch-up" growth). (Adapted from National Center for Health Statistics: NCHC Growth Charts, 1976. Monthly Vital Statistics Report. Vol. 25, No. 3, Suppl. (HRA) 76–1120. Rockville, MD: Health Resources Administration, June 1976.)

using the pump for periods exceeding 18 months; the other child, a 12-year-old, discontinued use of the pump after two months. For every child who wanted better control and was started on CSII, there were 16 other children who wanted CSII but were not started, because they each "failed" our preinstitution test. We require that all persons who desire a pump qualify before being started on CSII. To qualify for pump installation, they must (1) perform HBGM three to four times per day for three to six months, (2) keep accurate records and mail them to the CDMC twice monthly, (3) maintain weekly phone contact with a team member, and (4) demonstrate seriousness of resolve by altering insulin dosage sufficiently to lower glycosylated hemoglobin by more than 1 percent. Most persons fail this test and remain on their conventional management. All three children who remained on the pump program improved their glucose control.

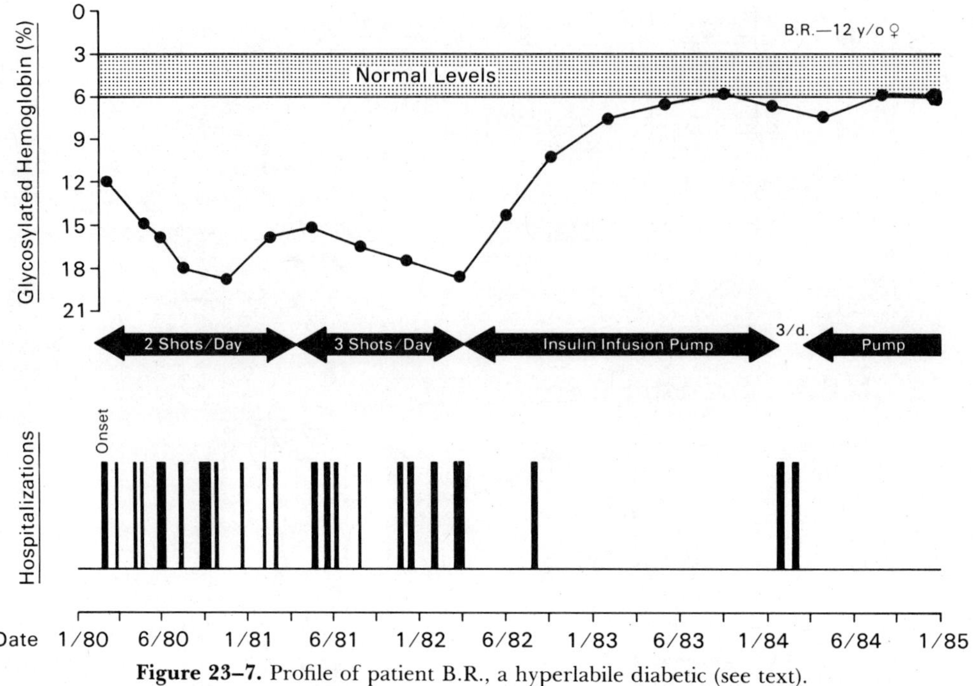

Figure 23–7. Profile of patient B.R., a hyperlabile diabetic (see text).

COMPLICATIONS OF CSII

Overall, our complication rate has been relatively small. Three of the 29 had more than one site infection, and in one it was serious enough to warrant discontinuation of pump therapy. This experience is similar to that in the literature. In most cases, the person who acquires a site infection has failed to use meticulous preinsertion care or has attempted to leave the needle in place for longer than 48 hours.

DKA is reported to be a common complication, and there were nine episodes of DKA in our 29 patients. In five, there was evidence of either pump malfunction or cannula clotting; in one the needle had come out of the subcutaneous site, and in the other three the cause was not apparent. Patients must be continually cautioned about the rapid onset of hyperglycemia and ketosis once insulin

Table 23–1. PRIMARY INDICATIONS FOR CSII IN 29 CHILDREN

Failure to grow normally	12
Hyperlability	7
Desire for better control	4
Proteinuria (<1 g/day)	2
Nephropathy/Hypertension/Retinopathy	2
Seizure disorder	1
Painful neuropathy	1

administration is interrupted, particularly in the presence of stress. Since the Regular insulin is rapidly absorbed and has a short action curve, the patient is virtually uninsulinized two to four hours after interruption of delivery. The onset of DKA is therefore much more rapid than when there is depot insulin. The newer pumps have pressure-sensitive alarms that are able to detect most obstructions in the line; thus, the prevalence of this as a causative factor appears to have decreased. When the hyperglycemia-ketonemia syndrome occurs, it is our practice to give supplemental insulin (see earlier), and we prefer not to give this through the pump.

Serious hypoglycemia with seizures, coma, and potentially death is a real concern as glucose control becomes tighter. In the presence of excessive insulin, the liver may be unable to release glycogen or promote gluconeogenesis even if the stimulus (that is, hypoglycemia and glucoregulatory hormone secretion) is present. This concern is potentially greater in the pump patient, in whom Regular insulin delivery continues even in the presence of hypoglycemia and inactivity.

Pump "runaway" has been reported and documented, but considering the large number of pumps being used this appears rare. On the other hand, some potentially disturbing events have happened. Two of our patients (unknown to one another) have reported the unexpected (and unprogrammed) delivery of "boluses" upon turning on a large, unshielded, fluorescent light. One of these patients also had several other spontaneous discharges of bolus doses, some observed by others. We have learned of several patients in other centers who have occasionally experienced similar occurrences. Since pump technology is so new and the pumps so small as to make proper shielding from electromagnetic fields difficult, it is surprising that more such episodes have not occurred. The practitioner must be ever alert to such possibilities.

RECOMMENDATIONS FOR USE

The Candidate

Not everyone who wants the pump should have it, and only a few can and will use it to its full advantage. Many adolescents, young adults, and parents are seriously misinformed about what a pump is or does. They consider it a way to solve all problems and lessen the time and attention they are required to spend on control of diabetes. It is often not sufficient merely to tell them of the additional attention required. It is for this reason that we established the "compliance test" alluded to earlier. It makes information become a reality.

Extremely careful selection is required for the group of patients who will use the pump. There are few children below the age of 10 years who can or should use the pump. Generally, the family should be actively involved in the care, and a degree of home stability appears important, although not absolutely essential.

The Program

Pump management can actually be dangerous to the person's health! Pumps should not be prescribed by any physician or diabetes team without the addition of two essential features: (1) a detailed educational program for the patient, coupled with close supervision and follow-up, and (2) 24-hour availability of one or more members of the team. It is not sufficient to rely on the pump manufacturer to give the instruction and to provide the toll-free phone number. It is also not sufficient for a practitioner, regardless of his or her level of expertise, to sign out to an inexperienced partner or colleague who may have little knowledge of CSII. Thus, at this stage, CSII should probably be reserved for those teams operating from diabetes centers who have both the expertise and the time to commit to such a program.

Patient Selection

Patients with hyperlabile diabetes, those with growth problems, those with early proteinuria, and those who wish to become (or are) pregnant constitute, in our minds, those with prime indications for pump usage. But, as the pumps are further improved and as our quest for good control continues, more who merely wish to obtain the best control will become viable candidates.

Alternatives

Several studies have demonstrated that MDIT (see Chapter 6), when properly used, is comparable to CSII in the ability to obtain glucose control. Thus, MDIT is a suitable option and is certainly less expensive. Additionally, all patients receiving CSII must have a back-up MDIT program that can be initiated in the event of pump malfunction or if they wish to be "off" the pump for a while.

24

Pancreas and Islet Transplantation

As noted in Chapter 18, microvascular complications are the major cause of morbidity and mortality in the insulin-dependent diabetic. Between 40 percent and 60 percent of patients who have onset of IDDM before age 15 years will ultimately develop renal failure. Evidence strongly suggests that blood glucose control directly influences development of these secondary complications. The advent and success of renal transplantation in relieving illness has fostered the concept of pancreas or islet cell transplantation to correct the disordered diabetes metabolism and thus to prevent or reverse complications. The first attempts at pancreas transplantation were made in the 1960s. Although the endocrine pancreas eliminated the need for exogenous insulin, technical complications related to the exocrine secretions were frequent. For that reason, interest in islet cell transplantation evolved; however, difficulties in isolating islets from human pancreata and in overcoming the immune barrier have made this procedure equally difficult. Nonetheless, recent technical advances and more effective immune suppression offer hope that these methods of curing the metabolic abnormality of diabetes will be feasible in the future.

WHOLE PANCREAS TRANSPLANTATION

Technical Considerations

The first pancreas transplant was reported by Lillehi and coworkers from the University of Minnesota in 1970. With these first grafts, it became apparent that, although the endocrine secretions could obviate the need for exogenous insulin, the technical problems in handling the exocrine secretions were difficult to manage. The initial procedure drained the digestive enzymes into a section of duodenum, which was transplanted with the pancreas. Drainage into the bowel, although the most physiologic way to handle the exocrine secretions, is also the most hazardous in cadaveric grafts. Exposure of the proenzymes to gut enterokinase activates these enzymes, which can lead to anastomotic breakdown, with subsequent leakage of enzymes, tissue destruction, and infection. This is particularly bothersome in the presence of the relatively large doses of immunosuppressive medications required to prevent graft rejection. The members of the group at the University of Minnesota, who have the largest experience with pancreas transplantation, currently use this method for their living-related donor transplants, since the need for immunosuppression is less in these patients than in those with cadaveric donors. Other methods of draining the exocrine secretions have included anastomosing the Wirsung duct to the ureter or to a retroperitoneal Roux-en-Y loop; however, fistulas and leaks with pancreatic enzyme activation have occurred in some of these cases also. Free drainage of the pancreatic duct into the peritoneum has also been used with success; with this approach, activation of proenzymes does not occur. In this technique, the pancreas is placed in the peritoneum, as opposed to the iliac fossa; and thus, only vessel anastomosis is required. The peritoneal absorption of pancreatic secretions results in elevation of serum amylase and lipase, but this is usually without sequelae. However, one patient developed areas of subcutaneous fat necrosis, which may have been related to the increase in serum lipase. Ascites necessitating graft removal has also been reported.

Ductal injection has also been widely used to eliminate exocrine secretion. The material injected into the duct is neoprene, a synthetic rubber that is liquid in its natural state and made up of an aqueous suspension of chloroprene, which has the chemical characteristic of flocculation when its pH is modified by pancreatic juice. In early animal studies, neoprene injection appeared to be a simple, efficient way to suppress exocrine function of the pancreas. However, it has been noted to cause fibrous atrophy around the islets, which may continue for up to 20 months. The experience with this technique in humans has been satisfactory, although some grafts have failed because of islet fibrosis induced by the injected agent. For cadaveric grafts, this injection technique may be the method of choice for eliminating exocrine secretions. Other polymers have also been used; these include prolamine, polyisoprene, silicone rubber, and cyanoacrylate.

Patient Selection

Since prevention of secondary complications of diabetes is the ultimate goal of pancreas or islet transplantation or both, the transplant ideally should occur before the onset of complications. However, owing to the uncertainty of a successful outcome and the need for immunosuppression, most pa-

tients already have advanced microvascular disease before transplantation is considered. Of 56 patients who had transplants before 1977, 29 (52 percent) either had a transplant-related death or died soon after transplant; 14 of these patients (25 percent) were alive in 1981. Of 424 patients worldwide receiving 130 transplants between July 1977 and November 1981, only 25 (20 percent) died with transplant or perioperative complications, and 82 (66 percent) were alive in 1984. Since not all patients develop life-threatening complications of diabetes and because the hazards of immunosuppression and surgery are significant, such surgery is generally limited to patients already receiving immunosuppression for renal transplantation. Although the order of transplantation has varied slightly, the success rate has been highest when transplanting the pancreas after a successful kidney transplant. The most widely used immunosuppression consists of prednisone and azathioprine, and this is often supplemented with antilymphocyte globulin or cyclosporine A or both. Although prednisone can have an adverse effect on carbohydrate metabolism, most recipients of pancreas transplants have had normal or nearly normal metabolic profiles during glucose tolerance tests. This demonstrates that steroids do not preclude or diminish the effect of a functioning pancreatic transplant (Fig. 24–1).

Results

The University of Minnesota group performed the first human pancreas transplant in December 1966. During the next 6 years, a total of 14 such transplants were performed simultaneously with kidney transplants. Only 1 of the 14 pancreas grafts functioned for more than a year. From 1978 to May 1982, 49 pancreas transplants were performed in 43 patients. Eighteen patients received a living-related segmental pancreas transplant. As of June 1982, of 45 patients undergoing transplants, 13 had functioning grafts and were insulin dependent 1 to 46 months after transplant. Nineteen patients lost graft function between 1 and 7 months, 16 for technical reasons. Eight patients died between 1 and 21 months, 3 with functioning grafts. Graft survival at 1 year was 25 percent, with patient survival being 84 percent. Metabolic studies after transplantation have shown normal glu-

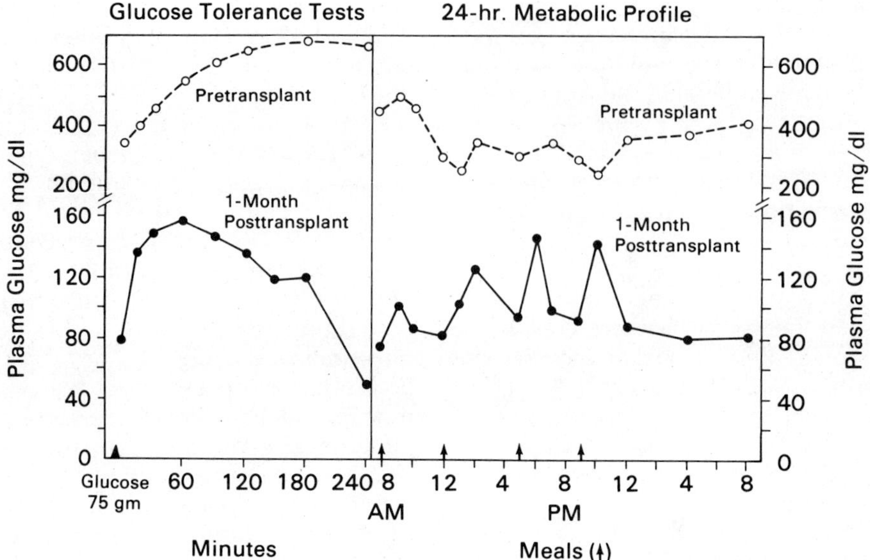

Figure 24–1. Results of glucose tolerance tests and 24-hour metabolic profiles in patients prepancreatic and six months postpancreatic transplant. (Adapted from Rynasiewiez JJ, et al: Diabetes 31(Suppl 4):92 1982.)

cose tolerance tests with normal values for serum and urinary C-peptide levels.

The group at Lyon have performed a similarly large number of pancreas transplants, 21 grafts in 20 patients. Five patients died with functioning grafts, 11 died secondary to rejection or from sclerosis secondary to neoprene injection. Figure 24–2 demonstrates the cumulative data on survival.

The American College of Surgeons/National Institutes of Health maintained an Organ Transplant Registry until June 30, 1977. Since July 1, 1977, information on pancreas transplants has been recorded by the International Human Pancreas and Islet Transplant Registry. The two registries compiled information on 190 pancreas transplants performed in 178 patients at various institutions. As of December 1981, there were 19 patients (of those 178) who had functioning grafts. Of grafts not functioning, approximately one fourth failed for technical reasons, one fourth functioned until the patient died, and one half were apparently rejected after an initial period of good graft function.

Those grafts lost to rejection are notable in that this process appears to differ markedly from renal allograft rejection, which

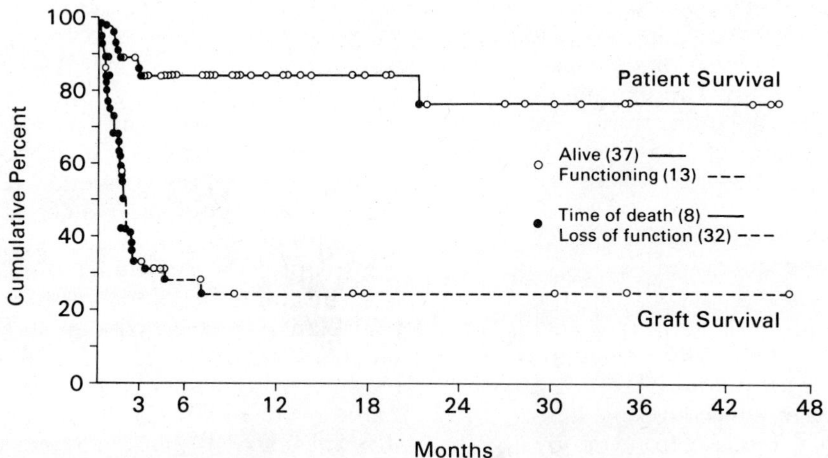

Figure 24–2. Graft and patient survival following pancreas transplantation. (From Sutherland DE, Goetz FC, Elick BA, Najarian JS: Experience with 49 segmental pancreas transplants in 45 diabetic patients. Transplantation 34:330–338, © by Williams & Wilkins, 1982.)

may be accompanied by fever, malaise, hypertension, and local tenderness and swelling. Pancreas graft loss has been accompanied by no systemic or local signs or symptoms. It has also been noted that although the pancreas undergoes rejection, this does not necessarily indicate that the same will happen to the renal allograft.

At the time of this writing, the group from Minnesota offer the option of pancreas transplants to diabetic patients who have previously received renal allografts and who are well more than one year after that transplant. Pancreatic grafts are also offered to patients whose complications of diabetes are judged to be more severe than the side effects of immunosuppression. For patients receiving cadaveric grafts, the whole pancreas is transplanted after silicone rubber injection. For living-related donor transplants, the pancreaticojejunostomy technique is used. As more experience is gained, undoubtedly recipient-selection criteria, surgical technique, and immunosuppression methods will change also.

ISLET TRANSPLANTATION

Because of the initial problems associated with whole or segmental pancreas transplants, isolated islet cell transplants were investigated. Early studies demonstrated that pancreatic fragments could be dispersed onto the peritoneum of diabetic and nondiabetic rats, and, although graft survival was demonstrated, no effect on blood glucose was noted. Later studies showed that islet cells could indeed reduce glucosuria, decrease plasma glucose, and enhance weight gain. In 1973, two groups of investigators used highly in-bred strains of rats such that there was no rejection of the islet tissue. After the islets were obtained, they were injected into the peritoneal cavity of the experimental animal. At sacrifice seven weeks later, the peritoneal cavity was dotted with normal-appearing islets with insulin-containing beta cells. Mauer and associates confirmed and extended these data to show that reversal of early diabetic nephropathy could also take place with islet transplantation. Rats with streptozocin-induced diabetes develop renal changes characteristic of diabetic nephropathy within six to eight months after becoming diabetic. When the animals received transplants of pancreatic islet cells, not only did their blood glucose return to normal but their diabetic

glomerular changes were also reduced or normalized. Thus, islet tissue itself can be used to reverse the acute metabolic abnormality as well as to prevent microvascular sequelae. However, obtaining sufficient numbers of islets and protecting against rejection of the islets remain problems.

Technical Considerations

Many of the problems in isolating islet cells are associated with the difficulty in obtaining enough human pancreatic tissue with minimal warm ischemia time, inadequate distention of the pancreas to provide sufficient disruption for animal enzymatic reaction to release intact islets, inefficient chopping methods, use of collagenase of variable composition (and thus effectiveness), and inefficient methods for separating and purifying the islets from the ductal, acinar, and fibrous components. Islets are prepared by mincing the pancreas and then incubating the tissue with collagenase. The tissue is then subjected to Ficoll gradient sedimentation. Although the product is a pure one, the numbers of islets obtained are relatively small—certainly not enough to correct diabetic hyperglycemia without exogenous insulin. Isolated islets are capable of producing insulin in greater or lesser amounts in response to varying glucose concentrations in the medium.

Many methods have been sought to maximize islet isolation. Najarian and associates (1977) used a tissue culture method, which enabled them to destroy more acinar tissue while at the same time preserving islet tissue, thus increasing the number of islets recovered per pancreas. Andersson and associates (1976) isolated up to 400 hand-picked islets from the body and tail of pancreata obtained within six hours after death of nine patients between 23 and 45 years of age. In contrast, they could not isolate islets from the more fibrotic pancreata of five patients between 46 and 65 years of age. Yasunami and co-workers (1981) demonstrated that separation of islet and acinar tissue could be accomplished by culturing in vitro fragments of collagenase-digested but unseparated pancreas. Data suggest that 20 percent of the islet cell mass of the adult pancreas is needed to maintain normoglycemia. The total mass of islet tissue in a fetus is 24 per cent that of the adult; thus, if all islet tissue could be extracted from the fetal pancreas, it should be sufficient to maintain normoglycemia without exogenous insulin. Furthermore, the separation of islet and acinar tissue is somewhat easier in the infant than in the adult. Methods to improve retrieval of viable islets are being pursued.

Clinical Experience

The Minnesota group has reported 15 patients who have undergone islet cell transplantation. The first group of seven was given a total of 10 islet cell transplants. All had normally functioning renal allografts. The pancreata were obtained from cadaver donors; six donors were infants, and four were adults. The tissue was injected into three sites: five intraperitoneally, four into the portal vein, and one into a muscle pocket in the groin. All patients continued to require exogenous insulin, although the dosage required decreased. Furthermore, transplantation into the portal vein caused no increase in portal vein pressure or measurable hepatic dysfunction.

The feasibility of islet transplantation has been difficult to determine for a number of reasons. In an attempt to eliminate one source of failure (that is, rejection), the group at the University of Minnesota evaluated the potential of autotransplantation of islet cells in patients with chronic pancreatitis. Such patients underwent near-total pancreatectomy, the pancreas was then chopped, digested with collagenase, washed, and infused into the portal vein within 2½ hours after pancreatectomy. Such a procedure has been performed in 10 patients, only three of whom required exogenous insulin but who remain ketosis-resistant. These patients demonstrate the technical feasibility of islet transplantation in humans. According to published cases and those submitted to the International Human Pancreas Transplant Registry, 76 islet allotransplant procedures were performed in 71 diabetics between 1970 and December 1981. Most attempts failed; only four patients were reported to be insulin independent for sustained periods of time after islet transplantation. Although the procedure is not uniformly successful, it is a safe procedure with no patient mortality. Thus, rejection remains the most significant problem of islet transplantation.

Experimental Approaches

Pure islets are antigenic in and of themselves. This is demonstrated when allogenic islets are transplanted into diabetic rats across strong histocompatibility barriers. This antigenicity remains whether fetal, neonatal, or adult islets are transplanted, although well-established fetal allografts may be less susceptible to immune destruction. In nonimmunosuppressed recipients, fetal pancreatic islet allografts are almost always rejected before they have matured sufficiently to reverse diabetes. The site of transplantation may also be a factor; islets dispersed to liver or lung tend to survive longer than islets in the peritoneal cavity.

In experimental studies, several agents have been used to prolong islet graft survival; azathioprine, cyclophosphamide, erthyro-9-2-hydrox-3nony adenine (an adenosine deaminase inhibitor), and cyclosporine A have been used. Clinically these drugs are used in combination with prednisone. The immunosuppressive agent that has been most effective in delaying rejection of islet allografts is antilymphocyte serum. The fact that such sera can prevent rejection has given rise to the concept that leukocytes physically associated with the islets may play a major role in sensitizing the host. Lacey and associates (1980) have shown that survival of islet allograft transplanted across a major histocompatibility barrier could be enhanced when the islets were cultured in vitro at 24°C for seven days before transplantation and the recipients were given a single injection of rabbit antiserum to rat lymphocytes before transplantation. Low temperature per se did not markedly prolong graft survival. Transplantation of islets from rats to streptozocin-induced diabetic mice rendered the mice normoglycemic when the islets were cultured for seven days at 24° and the mice given one shot each of rat antilymphocyte serum and of mouse antilymphocyte serum. From these studies it would appear that passenger leukocytes may be integral to the rejection process of islets and that culturing at low temperatures also aids in prolonging islet survival.

Several attempts have been made at preventing rejection by placement of a physical barrier between recipient antibodies or lymphocytes and functioning, transplanted islet cells. In this technique, islets are separated from the host by a semipermeable membrane that excludes passage of cells or large molecules but allows free passage of glucose and insulin. Theoretically, the islets will not be rejected, owing to the barrier to cells or molecules; however, there have been multiple technical problems with this method, and although initially encouraging, long-term results have not been satisfactory.

If islet transplantation proves effective and immunologic problems can be overcome, better methods of obtaining sufficient islets will need to be improved. One such method involves various procedures for islet preservation. Long-term preservation could allow islets to be accumulated from several donors, and thus a sufficient number to reverse the carbohydrate disorder could be transplanted at one time. Culture of islets at 37°C is one means of preservation; such islets remain effective for up to one week before transplantation. Although cultured fetal and neonatal pancreatic tissue will differentiate into islets, no long-term pure islet cell cultures have been established to provide a continuous source of insulin-producing tissue. Storage of islets at 4°C has also been tried; successful transplantation has been demonstrated after cold storage from 24 hours to four days.

Cryopreservation, storage of cells or tissues or both at −196°C for variable periods of time, has been applied to white blood cells, red blood cells, and sperm without loss of viability. Critical cryobiologic factors affecting cell survival include cooling and warming rates, the concentration and extent to which agents used to protect against intracellular ice crystal formation penetrate the cells, and the osmotic changes that occur in attempts to remove the cryoprotectants. Transplantation of cryoprotected islets has been successfully performed in rats; there have been no reports in larger animals or humans. However, this approach has the potential to assist in the solution of the problems of obtaining sufficient material for transplantation and of decreasing the likelihood of rejection.

Clinical pancreas and islet transplantation are technically feasible procedures. Both rodent and large-animal studies are numerous. Pancreas transplant ensures metabolic correction, and pancreas grafts may be less susceptible to rejection than are islet grafts. As experience increases, more patients should become suitable recipients of transplanted pancreata, from either cadaver or living-related donors. As improvements are made in harvesting, preserving, and preventing rejection of islets, islet cell transplants will also be realized as a potential cure for diabetes.

25

Diabetes in the Year 2000

Contemporary treatment of total insulin deficiency is frustrating for the patient, family, and physician. Insulin injection is given into the wrong place (the subcutaneous tissue) from whence it is absorbed at the wrong times (unrelated to feeding and fasting) and in the wrong amounts. The wonder is that people with diabetes are able to achieve the level of metabolic balance that they generally do.

Thus, our basic limitation in the management of insulin-dependent diabetes in the 1980s is the inability to reproduce physiologic insulin responses. All else is commentary to this fundamental constraint. The need for frequent monitoring to attain good to excellent control, the vagaries of exercise and emotional state with only partly predictable metabolic effects, and the need to assume a lifestyle few can achieve to maintain excellent diabetic control reflect an attempt to adjust to an unphysiologic diurnal insulin level in the circulation and tissues. If therapeutic insulin were administered into the portal circulation for delivery first to the liver and if the dose were adjustable to variations in physical activity, stress, and nutrition, this book would be largely irrelevant.

If we really had such a physiologic means of delivering insulin, the patient with diabetes would need as much education about energy metabolism and its regulation as the recipient of a cardiac pacemaker needs about cardiac physiology. Both the reasons for and the secondary effects from failure to adhere to the treatment regimen would shrink, and a whole generation of therapists could virtually abandon the labor-intensive tasks of attempting to deal with the psychosocial issues of diabetes. The means to these ends are imminent.

A SYSTEM FOR PHYSIOLOGIC DELIVERY OF INSULIN

Small portable pumps preprogrammed for administration of frequent pulses of insulin by the subcutaneous route have become highly sophisticated since introduction of the concept in the mid-1970s. However, these so-called open-loop systems require enormous patient diligence in closing the loop (that is, monitoring control). Most importantly, improved control is achieved only by chronic overinsulinization of peripheral tissues. Insulin is still delivered in the wrong place (subcutaneously), and the absorption from the injection site, particularly of bolus doses, is not precisely correlated to the food intake. Intravenous administration of insulin using a mechanical pump, even if connected to a continuous-monitoring, glucose-controlled system, also results in hyperinsulinemia. The simple explanation for this is that insulin is being delivered to the peripheral circulation and must reach unphysiologic levels in the

266

circulation to bathe the liver adequately. The intact pancreatic beta cell, on the other hand, delivers its insulin into the portal vein, thence to the liver, where 80 percent of the secreted insulin is extracted to do its work at the primary site of insulin activity.

Injection of insulin into the peritoneal space is the next best choice to direct infusion of insulin into the portal vein. The peritoneal space is nonreactive; for example, a shunt tube draining cerebral spinal fluid can be tolerated indefinitely by patients with obstructive hydrocephaly. Most important, the drainage of the peritoneal space is largely to the liver. Intraperitoneal insulin administration could be accomplished by one of two methods currently under investigation. A small button with a self-sealing diaphragm can be placed in the anterior wall of the abdomen, and through this a needle can be inserted, which, in turn, is connected by tubing to a small pump worn at the waist. Alternatively, a telemeter-adjusted pump can be implanted in the abdominal wall.

All that remains is to establish control of the insulin release by the level of glycemia. In contrast to the advanced state of development of delivery systems, continuous monitoring of glycemia has remained a perplexity. The computer technology to translate glycemia information to insulin release is the simpler of the two aspects of this problem. Rather, the limitation has been the development of a glucose sensor that is reliable, durable, and small. Blood withdrawal at frequent intervals, as with glucose-controlled intravenous infusion systems (automatic pancreas), such as the Biostator, is only practical for short-term use. Long-term placement of a sensor in the circulation would convey risks of thrombosis, infection, and embolization. Thus, a sensor is needed that is completely inert and does not require blood withdrawal or that can be implanted in a nonvascular location.

By 1990, four competitive systems should be available; choice will depend on cost, compatibility with the telemeter-computer-pump system, and features such as recycling time, correction of drift, and speed of transmission of readings. Electrochemical glucose sensors are of two types, electroenzymatic or electrocatalytic. The enzyme electrode measures oxygen concentration change or hydrogen peroxide production from glucose oxidation using immobilized glucose oxidase enzymes. Short-term use of this system has demonstrated that subcutaneous tissue glucose concentration corresponds to circulating levels. This approach to glucose sensing is, however, limited by the inactivation of the enzyme, making this a useful device for the patient to insert as a needle but impractical for long-term implantation.

The electrocatalytic sensor measures electron transport when glucose is oxidized on a platinum electrode. This method consumes no reagent and is practical for long-term implantation. However, physiologic co-reactants (aminoacids, urea) can interfere with readings, and the electrodes eventually need replacement. These problems can be diminished by manipulation of recharging current and method of data analysis.

Another method of glucose monitoring is by affinity sensing. Fluorescein-labeled dextran is bound to the protein lectin, concanavilin A (Con A), which has specific binding sites for glucose. The Con A is immobilized on the inner surface of a hollow dialysis fiber and sealed by a membrane freely permeable to glucose but retentive of the larger molecular-weight dextran. A single optical fiber in the lumen of the dialysis fiber measures unbound fluorescein-labeled dextran-displaced from binding sites in proportion to glucose concentration. This system is renewable and selective, thus suitable for implantation.

A problem with all implantable systems is the fibroblast and giant cell reaction that produces an avascular encapsulation of the sensor implant, isolating it from extracellular fluid. Surface design will need to obviate anchor points for encapsulating cells. The best prospect is a filamentous structure of diameter less than 2 mm, which will stimulate minimal scar formation.

One available sensor will be unaffected by the problem of encapsulation, because it will be noninvasive. Optical rotation of the aqueous humor, determined by using polarized light, reflects glucose concentration in that area, a value that corresponds to extracellular levels elsewhere. A contact lens covering cornea and sclera will incorporate a polarizer, detector, telemetry transmitter, and power source.

The 1990 model glucose-controlled intraperitoneal insulin infusion system, then, will consist of sensor-transmitter, either placed permanently or temporarily in the subcutaneous tissue or worn as a corneal-scleral contact lens, informing the implanted or externally worn computer-controlled pump. The system will have a 24-hour memory, which can be removed and stored for subsequent review. This will be necessary to permit adjustments of insulin administration algorithms in response to glycemic changes. Since insulin is being delivered more or less directly to the liver, there will not be a need for separate infusion of glucagon or glucose to prevent hypoglycemia, as there is in intravenous glucose-controlled systems which must achieve hyperinsulinism in peripheral tissues to insulize the liver adequately.

Although the system described would be near-perfect treatment, it is not a cure for diabetes. It is a stop-gap measure. Patient compliance will still be required, since the glucose probe will need changing periodically, and the patient will need to report to the physician for a telemeter equipment check and verification that the computer is making appropriate changes in insulin administration on a day-to-day basis. Children and adolescents will find the probe obtrusive to their physical activities and may have to resort to a preprogrammed regimen based on probe data gathered on weekends.

As outlined earlier, the present decade is the era of the biomedical engineers, as well as of the biochemical geneticists, who will ensure an unlimited supply of insulin chemically identical to our own insulin molecule. However, the last decade of this century will see the conquest of diabetes by the immunobiologists and the immunogeneticists.

DIABETES DETECTION AND PREVENTION

There is no point in detecting diabetes before the development of clinical disease unless one has a means of preventing it. By the year 2000, we will have such a means.

Most of the at-risk individuals will be identified through neonatal screening, which will provide a capillary tube of heparinized blood to be analyzed for specific subtypes of HLA-DR 3 and 4 antigens or for specific DNA sequences associated with these HLA genes and having specific disease associations. This screening test will have a specificity of approximately 40 percent (60 percent false-positive results) and a sensitivity of nearly 100 percent, imperfect because a few individuals will have insulin-dependent diabetes on a non-HLA-related basis.

Those individuals designated as high risk because they carry specific HLA-DR–related genes for insulin-dependent diabetes will have annual blood specimens obtained to test for islet cell antibodies, islet cell surface antibodies, and activated (killer) T cells directed against beta cells (determined by monoclonal antibodies to HLA-DR, transferrin, and other determinants). If any of these are positive, nuclear magnetic resonance (NMR) scan of the pancreas will detect edema if autoimmune insulitis is present.

The pathologic process that will be detected by NMR has also been demonstrated by abdominal computed tomograph (CT) scans, showing migration to the pancreas of peripheral lymphocytes labeled with indium or iodine isotopes and reinjected into newly diagnosed patients. Thus, in vivo demonstration has confirmed the pathologic process (insulitis) implied by in vitro studies of autoimmunity and activated lymphocytes. This insulitis, with reduction in beta cell mass to less than 10 percent of normal, is seen in most recently diagnosed IDDM patients. Regeneration occurs as the formation of new pure alpha-cell (glucagon-producing) or pure beta-cell islets, but the latter undergo further inflammatory destruction while the former survive; the old islets regenerate pancreatic-polypeptide–producing and alpha cells only. This process of ongoing regeneration and recurrent insulitis is reflected in the clinical remission and invites intervention.

In the BB strain of rats with spontaneous insulin-dependent diabetes, immunosuppression with antithymocyte globulin reduces the frequency and severity of diabetes and can reverse the process even after clinical onset. Long-term immunosuppression is, however, a more complex issue in human diabetes. Nevertheless, within the next few years the first successful reversals of insulin-dependent diabetes will be accomplished using general immunosuppressive agents such as cyclosporine A, which can completely prevent the development of diabetes in BB rats. More specific therapy will ultimately be necessary for intervention in all newly diagnosed patients.

This therapy will come in the form of monoclonal anti-idiotypic antibodies directed at surface antibodies on T lymphocytes, which will be administered to those with edema on NMR scan and with the disappearance of the specific killer T cells monitored. In addition, should antibody-dependent beta-cell lysis be found important, antisera directed against B lymphocytes and plasma cells expressing islet cell–reactive idiotypes will be used. Patients undergoing these forms of therapy will require long-term monitoring and occasional repeat therapy, since they are likely to remain susceptible to a variety of environmental triggers of autoimmune insulitis and will thus be subject to relapses.

Because of the high frequency of autoimmune disease of the thyroid (chronic lymphocytic thyroiditis) and gastric parietal cells (pernicious anemia) among first-degree relatives of persons with Type I diabetes, the finding of islet cell antibodies in the proband will require testing family members for thyrogastric autoimmunity. Particularly at risk are mothers (27 percent thyroid autoimmunity, 15 percent gastric) and sisters (20 percent thyroid) of diabetic persons.

CURE

Several approaches to the cure of diabetes will be available before the year 2000. For the newly diagnosed patient born before the screening era, the presence of autoantibodies against the islet cells and of specific killer T cells, with evidence of edema on NMR scan, will confirm autoimmune pathogenesis. Immunosuppressive therapy will be important to reverse these processes. Anti-idiotype antibodies will be curative and relatively safe.

This approach will not help two groups of patients: those with diabetes dating from the era before the development of monoclonal anti-idiotypic antibody and those with non-autoimmune diabetes (for example, diabetes due to pancreatic hypoplasia). For these individuals, improved techniques of separating porcine islets from passenger macrophages and lymphocytes will permit transplantation of these islets across species lines (xenogeneic transplantation).

This will be possible to accomplish, because the islet cells themselves do not express HLA-DR antigens and, thus, will not initiate the rejection process. Pretransplantation recipient whole blood transfusions or other techniques to minimize the sensitization process will enhance graft activity. Isolation of the islets can be achieved by in vitro incubation adjusting temperature (low) and oxygen (high) to permit only islet survival while the passenger cells wither. A technique that may obviate the need for in vitro preparation is the use of specific antiserum against HLA-DR (immune response antigens) of the non-islet cells from the donor pancreas.

The preferred sites of transplantation will be either injection into the portal vein or direct implantation in the spleen. Injections into the portal vein will embolize the portal triads and establish neo-islets. Seeding the peritoneal space may be equally effective and considerably easier, with insulin being discharged into the space or through capillary channels developed from the peritoneal surface.

For Moslems or Orthodox Jews, a limited supply of ovine, bovine, or even human islets will be available. Jehovah's Witnesses and doctrinaire vegetarians will remain users of the glucose-controlled insulin infusion system.

CONCLUSION

The children's diabetes team of 1986 consists of general pediatrician, pediatric endocrinologist, nurse clinician, psychologist, social worker, dietitian, and others as needed in the specialties of ophthalmology, nephrology, cardiology, neurology, gastroenterology, and urology. In the year 2000, the core team, along with the pediatrician, will be the clinical immunologist and the immunopathologist. The rest of the team, including the specialists in diabetes complications, can then apply their skills in the adult clinic, since people with Type II diabetes will continue to resist efforts at weight reduction and since these non–insulin-dependent patients will be at increased risk for the development of vascular complications.

Selected References

A. Texts, Symposia, Books

Ahmed PI, Ahmed N: Coping with Juvenile Diabetes. Springfield, IL: Charles C Thomas, 1985.

American Diabetes Association: Curriculum for Youth Education. New York: American Diabetes Association, 1983.

Bille DA: Practical Approaches to Patient Teaching. Boston: Little, Brown, & Company, 1981.

Bleicher SJ: Symposium on home blood glucose monitoring. Diabetes Care 3:57, 1980.

Brownlee M: Handbook of Diabetes Mellitus. New York: Garland STPM Press, 1981.

Burrish T, Bradley L: Coping with Chronic Disease. New York: Academic Press, 1983.

Castells S: Symposia on juvenile diabetes. Pediatr Clin North Am, 31, 1984.

Committee on Dietary Allowances: Recommended Dietary Allowances. 9th ed. Washington, DC: National Academy of Sciences, 1980.

Craig O: Childhood Diabetes and Its Management. 2nd ed. London: Butterworth, 1981.

Creatzfeldt J, Kobberling J, Neel JW: The Genetics of Diabetes. Berlin: Springer-Verlag, 1976.

Eaton P: Symposium on insulin delivering systems. Diabetes Care 3:257, 1980.

Ellenberg M, Rifkin, H: Diabetes Mellitus: Theory and Practice. 3rd ed. New York: Medical Examination Publishing Company, 1983.

Erikson EH: Childhood and Society. 2nd ed. New York: Norton, 1963.

Friedman EA, L'Esperance FA: Diabetic Renal-Retinal Syndrome. New York: Grune & Stratton, 1980.

Havighurst FJ: Developmental Tasks and Education. 3rd ed. New York: Longman, 1972.

Katzen HM, Mahler RJ: Advances in Modern Nutrition. Vol. 2. Washington, DC: Hemisphere Publishing, 1978.

Kozak GP: Clinical Diabetes Mellitus. Philadelphia: WB Saunders, 1982.

Laron Z: Diabetes in Juveniles: Medical and Rehabilitation Aspects. Vol. 12: Modern Problems in Pediatrics. New York: Karger, 1975.

Lazarus RS: Psychological Stress and the Coping Process. New York: McGraw-Hill, 1966.

Martin JM, Ehrlich RM, Holland FH: Etiology and Pathogenesis of Insulin Dependent Diabetes Mellitus. New York: Raven Press, 1981.

Mansolf FA: The Eye and Systemic Disease. St. Louis: CV Mosby, 1980.

Minuchin S, Rosman B, Baker L: Psychosomatic Families. Cambridge: Harvard University Press, 1978.

Peterson CM: Diabetes Management in the 1980s. Philadelphia: Praeger Scientific, 1982.

Piaget J: The Origins of Intelligence in Children. New York: International Universities Press, 1952.

Podolsky S: Clinical Diabetes: Modern Management. New York: Appleton-Century-Crofts, 1979.

Redman BK: The Process of Patient Teaching in Nursing. 4th ed. St. Louis: CV Mosby, 1980.

Schnatz JD: Diabetes Mellitus: Problems in Management. Reading, MA: Addison-Wesley, 1982.

Seligman M: Helplessness: On Depression, Development, and Death. San Francisco: WH Freeman, 1975.

Selye H: The Stress of Life. New York: McGraw-Hill, 1976.

Shade DS, Santiago JV, Skyler JS, Rizza RA: Intensive Insulin Therapy. Princeton, NJ: Excerpta Medica, 1983.

Skyler JS, Cahill GF: Diabetes Mellitus. New York: Yorke Medical Books, 1981.

Symposium on Optimal Insulin Delivery. Diabetes Care 5:1, 1982.

Symposium on Potentially Implantable Glucose Sensors. Diabetes Care 5:147, 1982.

Travis LB: An Instructional Aid on Insulin-Dependent Diabetes Mellitus. Austin: American Diabetes Association, Texas Affiliate, 1985.

B. Etiology, Pathogenesis, Classification

Cahill GF Jr, McDevitt HO: Insulin-dependent diabetes mellitus: The initial lesion. N Engl J Med 304:1454, 1981.

Champsour HF, Battazzo GF, Bertrams J., et al.: Virologic, immunologic, and genetic factors in insulin-dependent diabetes mellitus. J Pediatr 100:15, 1982.

Cudworth AG, Woodrow JC: Genetic susceptibility in diabetes mellitus: Analysis of the HLA association. Br Med J 2:846, 1976.

Fajans SS, Cloutier MC, Crowther RL: Clinical and etiologic heterogeneity of idopathic diabetes mellitus. Diabetes 27:1112, 1978.

Fleegler FM, Rogers KD, Drash A, et al.: Age, sex and season of onset of juvenile diabetes in different geographic areas. Pediatrics 63:374, 1979.

Gorsuch AN, Spencer KM, Lister J, et al.: Can future type I diabetes be predicted? A study in families of affected children. Diabetes 31:862, 1982.

Lebovitz HE: Etiology and pathogenesis of diabetes mellitus. Pediatr Clin North Am 31:521, 1984.

Ludvigsson J, Safwenberg K, Heding LG: HLA-types, C-peptide and insulin antibodies in juvenile diabetes. Diabetologia 13:13, 1977.

National Diabetes Data Group: Classification and diagnosis of diabetes mellitus and other categories of glucose intolerance. Diabetes 28:1039, 1979.

Pincus G, White P: On the inheritance of diabetes mellitus. I. An analysis of 675 family histories. Am J Med Sci 1:186, 1933.

Pyke DA, Nelson PG: Diabetes mellitus in identical twins.

In Creutzfeldt W, Kobberling J, Neel JV (eds): The Genetics of Diabetes. Berlin: Springer-Verlag, 1976, pp. 194–205.

Rabenowe SL, Eisenbarth GS: Type I diabetes mellitus: A chronic autoimmune disease. Pediatr Clin North Am 31:531, 1984.

Rayfield EJ, Seto Y: Viruses. *In* Brownlee M (ed): Handbook of Diabetes. New York: Garland STPM Press, 1982, pp. 95–120.

Rimoin DL: Genetics of diabetes mellitus. Diabetes 16:346, 1967.

Rosenbloom AL, Kohrman A, Sperling M: Classification and diagnosis of diabetes mellitus in children and adolescents. J Pediatr 98:320, 1981.

Rosenbloom AL, Hunt AS: Prognosis of impaired glucose tolerance in children with stress hyperglycemia, symptoms of hypoglycemia or asymptomatic glycosuria. J Pediatr 101:340, 1982.

Rotter JI, Rimoin DL: Etiology. *In* Brownlee M (ed): Handbook of Diabetes Mellitus. New York: Garland STPM Press, 1981, pp. 1–93.

Unger RN, Orci L: Glucagon and the A cell: Physiology and pathophysiology. N Engl J Med 304:1518, 1575, 1981.

Yoon JW, Austin M, Anodera T, Notkins P: Virus-induced diabetes mellitus: Isolation of a virus from the pancreas of a child with diabetic ketoacidosis. N Engl J Med 300:1173, 1979.

C. Clinical Disease and Management

Aleyassine H, Gardiner RI, Tonks DB, Koch P: Glycosylated hemoglobin in diabetes mellitus: Correlations with fasting plasma glucose, serum lipids and glycosuria. Diabetes Care 3:508, 1980.

Bleicher SJ: Symposium on home blood glucose monitoring. Diabetes Care 3:57, 1980.

Brouhard BH: Control and monitoring for the child with insulin-dependent diabetes mellitus. Am J Dis Child 137:787, 1983.

Bunn HF: Evaluation of glycosylated hemoglobin in diabetic patient. Diabetes 30:613, 1981.

Clements RS, Keane NA, Kirk KA, Boshell BR: Comparison of various methods for rapid glycose estimation. Diabetes Care 4:392, 1981.

Drash A: Diabetes mellitus in childhood: A review. J Pediatr 78:919, 1971.

Galloway JA, deShazo RD: The clinical use of insulin and the complications of insulin therapy. *In* Ellenberg M, Rifkin H (eds): Diabetes Mellitus: Theory and Practice. 3rd ed. New York: Medical Examination Publishing Company, 1984, p. 519.

Gonen B, Rochman H, Rubenstein AH, et al.: Haemoglobin A: An indicator of the metabolic control of diabetic patients. Lancet 2:734, 1977.

Jovanovic L, Peterson CM: The clinical utility of glycosylated hemoglobin. Am J Med 70:331, 1981.

Langdon DR, James FD, Sperling MA: Comparison of single- and split-dose insulin regimens with 24-hour monitoring. J Pediatr 99:854, 1981.

Laron Z, Volovitz B, Karp M: Linear growth and insulin dose as indices of control in children with diabetes mellitus. *In* Laron Z (ed): Medical Aspects of Balance of Diabetes in Juveniles. New York: S Karger, 1977.

Morris LR, McGee, JA, Kitabchi AE: Correlation between plasma and urine glucose in diabetes. Ann Intern Med 94:469, 1981.

Reeves M, Forhan S, Skyler J, Peterson C: Comparison of methods of blood glucose monitoring. Diabetes Care 4:404, 1984.

Rizza RA, Gerech JE, Jaymond MW, et al.: Control of blood sugar in insulin-dependent diabetes: Comparison of an artificial endocrine pancreas, continuous subcutaneous insulin infusion, and intensified conventional insulin therapy. N Engl J Med 303:1313, 1980.

Rudolf MCJ, Sherwin RS, Markowitz R, et al.: Effect of intensive insulin treatment on linear growth in the young diabetic patient. J Pediatr 101:333, 1982.

Schiffrin A, Belmonte MD: Comparison between continuous subcutaneous insulin infusion and multiple injections of insulin: A one year prospect study. Diabetes 31:255, 1982.

Schmidt MI, Hadji-Georgopoulos A, Rendell M: The dawn phenomenon, an early morning glucose rise: Implication for diabetic intraday blood glycose variation. Diabetes Care 4:579, 1981.

Shade D, Eaton R, Friedman N, Spencer W: Prolonged peritoneal insulin infusion in a diabetic man. Diabetes Care 3:314, 1980.

Skyler JS: Selection and management of the patient receiving intensive insulin therapy. *In* Shade DS, Santiago JV, Skyler JS, Rizza RA (eds): Intensive Insulin Therapy. Vol. 10 Princeton, NJ: Excerpta Medica, 1983, p. 144.

Skyler JS, Siegler DE, Reeves ML: A comparison of insulin regimens in insulin-dependent diabetes mellitus. Diabetes Care 5:11, 1982.

Skyler JS, Skyler DL, Siegler DE: Algorithms for adjustment of insulin dosage by patients who monitor blood glucose. Diabetes Care 4:311, 1981.

Symposia on Blood Glucose Self-Monitoring. Diabetes Care 4:392, 1981.

Tamborlane WV, Sherwin RS: Diabetes control and complications: New strategies and insights. J Pediatr 102:805, 1983.

Travis LB: The child with diabetes. *In* Schnatz D (ed): Problems in Management. Menlo, NY: Addison-Wesley Publishing, 1982, pp. 205–221.

Travis LB, Brouhard BH, Johnson T, et al.: Management of the child with diabetes. Texas Med 79:181, 1983.

White NH, Waltman SR, Krupin T: Reversal of abnormalities in ocular fluorophotometry in insulin-dependent diabetes after five to nine months of improved diabetic control. Diabetes 31:80, 1982.

Yue DK, Morris K, McLennan S, Turtle JR: Glycosylation of plasma protein and its relation to glycosylated hemoglobin in diabetes. Diabetes 29:296, 1980.

D. Special Problem Areas

Alberti KGMM, Thomas DJB: The management of diabetes during surgery. Br J Anaesthesia 51:693, 1979.

Androgue HJ, Wilson H, Boyd AE: Plasma acid-base patterns in diabetic ketoacidosis. N Engl J Med 307:1603, 1982.

Baker L, Barcai A, Kaye R, et al.: Beta-adrenergic blockade and juvenile diabetes: Acute studies and long-term therapeutic trial. J Pediatr 75:19, 1969.

Bartosch J: Oral contraceptives: Selection and management. Nurse Pract 8:56, 1983.

Benz M, Kohler E: Baby food exchanges and feeding the diabetic infant. Diabetes Care 3(4):554, 1980.

Bibace R, Walsh ME: Developmental stages in children's conceptions of illness. *In* Stone GC, Cohen F, Adler NE (eds): Health Psychology—A Handbook. San Francisco: Jossey-Bass, 1979.

Boden G, Richard GA, Hoeldtke RD, et al.: Severe insulin-induced hypoglycemia associated with deficiencies in the release of counter-regulatory hormones. N Engl J Med 305:1200, 1981.

Bolli G, Calabiese G, DeFeo P, et al.: Lack of glucogon response in glucose counter-regulation in type I diabetics: Absence of recovery after prolonged optimal insulin therapy. Diabetologia 22:100, 1982.

Cerreto M, Travis LB: Implications of psychological and family factors in the treatment of diabetes. Pediatr Clin North Am 31:689, 1985.

DeFronzo RA, Hendler R, Christensen N: Stimulation of counter-regulatory hormonal response in diabetic man by a fall in glucose concentration. Diabetes 29:125, 1980.

Elkind D: Egocentrism in adolescence. Child Dev 38:1025, 1967.

Entmacher P: Economic aspects, employability, and insurability. *In* Ellenberg M, Rifkin H (eds): Diabetes Mellitus: Theory and Practice. 3rd ed. New York: Medical Examination Publishing Company, 1983.

Fisher JN, Shahshahani MN, Kitabchi AE: Diabetic ketoacidosis: Low-dose insulin therapy by various routes. N Engl J Med 297:239, 1977.

Franz M: Diabetes mellitus: Considerations in the development of guidelines for the occasional use of alcohol. J Am Diet Assoc 83:147, 1983.

Goldstein DE, England JD, Hess R, Rawlings SS, Walker B: A prospective study of symptomatic hypoglycemia in young diabetic patients. Diabetes Care 4:601, 1981.

Gosden C, Ross A, Steel J, Springbett A: Intrauterine contraceptive devices in diabetic women. Lancet 1:530, 1982.

Guisado R and Arieff AI: Neurologic manifestation of diabetic comas: Correlation with biochemical alterations in the brain. Metabolism 24:665, 1975.

Guthrie D: Psychosocial side of diabetes and its complications. Diabetes Educatr 8:24, 1982.

Hauser ST, Pollets D: Psychological aspects of diabetes mellitus: A critical review. Diabetes Care 2:227, 1979.

Hinkle LE: The influence of the patient's behavior and his reaction to his life situation upon the course of diabetes. Diabetes 5:406, 1956.

Hinkle LE, Conger C, Wolf S: Studies on diabetes mellitus: Relation of stressful life situations to the concentration of ketone bodies in the blood of diabetic and nondiabetic humans. J Clin Invest 29:513, 1950.

Hinkle LE, Wolf S: Experimental study of life situations, emotions, and the occurrence of acidosis in a juvenile diabetic. Am J Med Sci 217:130, 1949.

Holyoke A: Family planning for the diabetic. Diabetes Educ 4:6, 1978.

Holyoke A: Drug abuse assessment guide. Diabetes Educ 5(14):24, 1979.

Immerslund O: The prognosis in diabetes with onset before age two. Acta Paediatr 49:243, 1960.

Johnson SB: Psychological factors in juvenile diabetes: A review. J Behavior Med 3:95, 1980.

Madsbad S, McNair P, Christensen M, et al.: Influence of smoking on insulin requirement and metabolic status in diabetes mellitus. Diabetes Care 3:41, 1980.

Meyer EJ, Lorenzi M, Bohannon NV, et al.: Diabetic management by insulin infusion during major surgery. Am J Surg 137:323, 1979.

Partridge JW, Garner AM, Thompson CW, Cherry T: Attitudes of adolescents toward their diabetes. Am J Dis Child 124:226, 1972.

Pedersen O, Beck-Nielsen H, Heding L: Increased insulin receptors after exercise in patients with insulin-dependent diabetes mellitus. N Engl J Med 302:886, 1980.

Santiago JV, White NH, Skor DA, Levandoski LA, Bier

DM, Cryer PE: Defective glucose counterregulation limits intensive therapy of diabetes mellitus. Am J Physiol 247:E215, 1984.

Schade DS, Eaton RP: The temporal relationship between endogenously secreted stress hormones and metabolic decompensation in diabetic man. J Clin Endocrinol Metabol 50:131, 1980.

Schafer LC, Glasgow RE, McCaul KD: Increasing the adherence of diabetic adolescents. J Behavior Med 5:353, 1982.

Service FJ, Molnar GD, Rosevean JW, et al.: Mean amplitude of glycemic excursions, a measure of diabetic instability. Diabetes 19:644, 1970.

Shafer LC, Glasgow RE, McCaul KD, Daehan M: Adherence to IDDM regimens: Relationship to psychosocial variables and metabolic control. J Behavior Med 5:353, 1982.

Speerling MA: Diabetic ketoacidosis. Pediatr Clin North Am 31:591, 1984.

Steel JM, Duncan JP: Contraception for the insulin-dependent diabetic woman: The view from one clinic. Diabetes Care 3:557, 1980.

Sullivan BJ: Self-esteem and depression in adolescent diabetic girls. Diabetes Care 1:18, 1978.

Surwit RS, Scovern AW, Feinglos NM: The role of behavior in diabetes care. Diabetes Care 5:337, 1982.

Traisman HS, Beehn J, Newcomb A: Diabetes mellitus at ages one to five: Findings at onset. Diabetes 8:289, 1959.

Travis LB: Acute complications of type I diabetes: Relationship to coping. *In* Ahmed PI, Ahmed N (eds): Coping with Juvenile Diabetes. Springfield, IL: Charles C Thomas, 1985.

Travis LB, Daeschner CW, Dodge WF, Burns J: Natural history of diabetes mellitus in the child. Tex State J Med 58:502, 1962.

Unger RH: Meticulous control of diabetes: Benefits, risks, precautions. Diabetes 31:479, 1982.

Walts LF, Miller J, Davidson MB, Brown J: Perioperative management of diabetes mellitus. Anaesthesia 55:104, 1981.

Widness J, Cowett R, Zeller W, et al.: Permanent neonatal diabetes in an infant of an insulin-dependent mother. J Pediatr 100:926, 1982.

E. Education: The Team Approach

American Hospital Association: A Patient's Bill of Rights. Chicago: the American Hospital Association, 1972.

Blue Cross Association: White Paper: Patient Health Education. Chicago: Blue Cross Association, 1974.

Blumberg BD: Evaluating patient education programs. Oncol Nursing Forum 8:29, 1981.

Boutaugh M, Hull AL, Davis WK: An examination of diabetes educational assessment forms. Diabetes Educatr 7:29, 1982.

Coyne JR, Stolknacke R: Team approach to the problems of the diabetic patient. Hosp Management 103:82, 1967.

Davis WK, Hull AL, Boutaugh ML: Factors affecting the educational diagnosis of diabetic patients. Diabetes Care 4:275, 1981.

Deckert T, Poulsen J, Larsen M: Importance of outpatient supervision in the prognosis of juvenile diabetes mellitus: A cost/benefit analysis. Diabetes Care 1:281, 1978.

Dries L, Dizzia S: Diabetes teaching: A close-up. Diabetes Educatr 6:26, 1980.

Etzwiler D: What the juvenile diabetic knows about his disease. Pediatrics 29(1):135, 1962.

Giordano B, Edwards L: Meeting the needs of parents of children with diabetes—a babysitter's course. Diabetes Educ 6:26, 1980.

Hansen B, Cohn M: Diabetes research and training centers: Science, application, training and translation. Diabetes Care 3:548, 1980.

Johnson JB: Diabetes education: It is not only what we say. Diabetes Care 5:343, 1982.

Johnson SB, Pollak RT, Silverstein JH, et al.: Cognitive and behavioral knowledge about insulin-dependent diabetes among children and parents. Pediatrics 69:708, 1982.

Joslin E, Sheply H: The ideal diabetic unit: Of the hospital but not in it. Mod Hosp, September, 1946.

Kohler E, Hurwitz L, Milan D: A developmentally staged curriculum for teaching self-care to the child with insulin dependent diabetes mellitus. Diabetes Care 5:300, 1982.

Lawrence PA, Cheely J: Deterioration of diabetic patients' knowledge and management skills as determined during outpatient visits. Diabetes Care 3:214, 1980.

McSweeney M: Measuring the effect of patient teaching. Diabetes Educ 7:9, 1981.

McWeeny MC: The patient's right to learn or not to learn. Nurs Admin Q 4(2):83, 1980.

Miller L, Goldstein J: More efficient care of diabetic patients in a country-hospital setting. N Engl J Med 286:1388, 1972.

Palmer BB, Lewis CE: Development of health attitudes and behavior. J Sch Health 46:401, 1976.

Parcel GS: Skills approach to health education: A framework for integrating cognitive and affective learning. J Sch Health 46:403, 1976.

Pohl S, Hodge R, Evans W, et al.: Diabetes care: An integrated subspecialty and primary care approach. South Med J 74:37, 1981.

Rosenstock IM: What research in motivation suggests for public health. Am J Public Health 50:295, 1960.

Sulway M, Tupling H, Webb K, Harris G: New techniques for changing compliance in diabetes. Diabetes Care 3:108, 1980.

Warren-Boulton E, Anderson BJ, Schwartz NL, Drexler AJ: A group approach to the management of diabetes in adolescents and young adults. Diabetes Care 4:62, 1981.

F. Complications and Consequences

Bodansky HJ, Cudworth AG, Drury PL, Kohner EM: Risk factors associated with severe proliferative retinopathy in insulin dependent diabetes mellitus. Diabetes Care 5:97, 1982.

Brochner-Mortensen J: Glomerular filtration rate and extracellular fluid volumes during normoglycemia and moderate hyperglycemia in diabetics. Scand J Clin Lab Invest 32:311, 1973.

Eisenbarth GS, Wilson PW, Ward F, et al.: The polyglandular failure syndrome: Disease inheritance. HLA type, and immune function. Ann Intern Med 91(4):528, 1979.

Evans N, Robinson VP, Lister J: Growth and bone age of juvenile diabetics. Arch Dis Child 47(254):589, 1972.

Goldstein DA, and Massry SG: Diabetic nephropathy. Nephron 20:286, 1978.

Grgic A, Rosenbloom AL, Weber FT, et al.: Joint contracturia common manifestation of childhood diabetes mellitus. J Pediatr 88(4):584, 1976.

Hung W, August GP, Glasgow A: Hyperthyroidism in juvenile diabetes mellitus. Pediatrics 61(4):583, 1978.

Jivani SKM, Rayner PHW: Does control influence the growth of diabetic children? Arch Dis Child 48:109, 1973.

Kroc Collaborative Study Group: Blood glucose control and the evolution of diabetic retinopathy and albuminuria: A preliminary multicenter trial. N Engl J Med 311:365, 1984.

Lauritzen T, Frost-Larsen KHW, Deckert T: Steno study group. Effect of 1 year of near-normal blood glucose levels in retinopathy in insulin-dependent diabetics. Lancet 1:200, 1983.

Lee RG, Bode HH: Stunted growth and hepatomegaly in diabetes mellitus. J Pediatr 91(1):82, 1977.

Lestradet H, Papoz L, DeMenibus CLH, et al.: Long-term study of mortality and vascular complications in juvenile onset (type I) diabetes. Diabetes 30:175, 1981.

Mauriac P: Gros ventia, heptomegalie, troubles de la croirssance cheziles enfants diabetiques, traites depuis plusieurs annecs parl'insuline. Gas Hebd Sci Med Bordeaux 51:402, 1930.

Morgensen DE: Renal function changes in diabetes. Diabetes 25:872, 1976.

Monnier VM, Cerami A: Nonezymatic glycosylation and browning in diabetes and aging. Diabetes 31:57, 1982.

Oakley WG, Pyke DA, Tattersall RB: Long term diabetes. Q J Med 18:145, 1974.

Peterson HHI, Korsgaard B, Deckert T, Nielson E: Growth, body weight and insulin requirement in diabetic children. Acta Paediatr Scand 67:453, 1978.

Tattersall RB, Pyke DA: Growth in diabetic children: Studies in identical twins. Lancet 2:1105, 1973.

West K, Erdreich LJ, Stober JA: A detailed study of risk factors for retinopathy and nephropathy in diabetes. Diabetes 29:501, 1980.

G. Pregnancy

Churchill JA, Berendes HW, Nemore J: Neuropsychological deficits in children of diabetic mothers. Am J Obstet Gynecol 105:257, 1969.

Gillmer MDG, Beard RW, Brooke FW, Oakley NW: Carbohydrate metabolism in pregnancy. I. Diurnal plasma glucose profile in normal and diabetic women. Br Med J 3:399, 1975.

Hare JW, White P: Pregnancy in diabetes complicated by vascular disease. Diabetes 26:953, 1977.

Jovanovic L, Druzin M, Peterson CM: Effect of euglycemia on the outcome of pregnancy in insulin-dependent diabetic women as compared with normal control subjects. Am J Med 71:921, 1981.

Jovanovic L, Peterson CM, Saxena BB, et al.: Feasibility of maintaining normal glucose profiles in insulin-dependent diabetic women. Am J Med 68:105, 1980.

Miller E, Hare JW, Cloherty JP, et al.: Elevated maternal hemoglobin A1C in early pregnancy and major congenital abnormalities in infants of diabetic mothers. N Engl J Med 304:1331, 1981.

Mintz DH, Skyler JS, Chez RA: Diabetes mellitus and pregnancy. Diabetes Care 1:49, 1978.

O'Sullivan JM, Mahan CM: Criteria for the oral glucose tolerance test in pregnancy. Diabetes 13:278, 1964.

Pedersen J, Molested-Pedersen L, Anderson B: Assessors of fetal perinatal mortality in diabetic pregnancy. Diabetes 23:302, 1974.

Stehbens JA, Baker GL, Kitchell M: Outcome at ages 1, 3 and 5 years of children born to diabetic women. Am J Obstet Gynecol 127:408, 1977.

Yssing M: Long-term prognosis of children born to diabetic mothers when pregnant. *In* Camerini-Davalos RA, Cole HS (eds): Early Diabetes in Early Life. New York: Academic Press, 1976, pp. 575–586.

H. Transplants and Artificial Devices

Anderson A, Borg H, Groth CG, et al.: Survival of isolated human islets of Langerhans maintained in tissue culture. J Clin Invest 57:1295, 1976.

Lacey PE: Pancreatic transplantation as a means of insulin delivery. Diabetes Care 5:93, 1982.

Lacey PE, Davie JM, Finke EH: Prolongation of islet xenograft survival without continuous immuno-suppression. Science 209:283, 1980.

Lillehei RJ, Simmons RL, Najarian JS, et al.: Pancreati-coduodenal allotransplantation. Experimental and clinical experience. Ann Surg 172:405, 1970.

Mauer SM, Steffes MW, Sutherland DER, et al.: Studies of the rate of regression of the glomerular lesions in diabetic rats treated with pancreatic islet transplantation. Diabetes 24:280, 1975.

Najarian JS: Islet cell transplantation in treatment of diabetes. Hosp Pract Oct:63, 1977.

Skyler JS, Seigler DE, Reeves ML: Optionizing pumped insulin delivery. Diabetes Care 5:135, 1982.

Sutherland DER: Report of international human pancreas and islet transplantation registry cases through 1981. Diabetes 31(4):112, 1982.

Sutherland DER, Goetz FC, Elick BA, Najarian JS: Experience with 49 segmental pancreas transplants in 45 diabetic patients. Transplantation 34:330, 1982.

Sutherland DER, Matas AJ, Goetz FC, Najarian JS: Transplantation of dispersed pancreatic islet tissue in humans: Autografts and allografts. Diabetes 29(1):31, 1980.

Symposium on Potentially Implantable Glucose Sensors. Diabetes Care 5:147, 1982.

Symposium on Optimal Insulin Delivery. Diabetes Care 5:1, 1982.

Tamborlane WV, Sherwin RS, Genel M, Felig P: Outpatient treatment of juvenile-onset diabetes with a preprogrammed subcutaneous insulin infusion system. Am J Med 68:190, 1980.

Yasunami Y, Takaki R, Fukuma M, et al.: Adult human pancreatic endocrine cells in culture. Insulin and glucagon release and influence of cold storage. J Lab Clin Med 98:173, 1981.

Appendices

APPENDIX A: PATIENT DATA

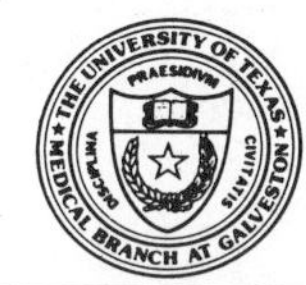

THE UNIVERSITY OF TEXAS MEDICAL BRANCH
GALVESTON, TEXAS 77550

DEPARTMENT OF PEDIATRICS
Divisions of Nephrology and Diabetes
(409) 761-2538
Luther B. Travis, M.D., Director
Ben H. Brouhard, M.D., Associate Director
Alok Kalia, M.D.
Melanie Sweet, M.D.
Vi Quiroga, Administrative Assistant
Barbara Schreiner, RN, MN, Diabetes Nurse Specialist
Shaye Henderson, RN, M.Ed., Diabetes Health Educator
Lisa A. Hollander, RN, MN, Renal Nurse Coordinator
Susan Johnson, RN, Head Nurse, Renal/Diabetes Inpatient Area
Debbie Gonzales, RN, Head Nurse, Pediatric Renal Dialysis
Paula McMahon, RD, Dietitian
Margaret Lovelace, MCSW, Social Worker

Name: _______________

DISCHARGE INSTRUCTIONS

GOOD NEWS! You are ready to go home. Here are some reminders of the things you will need to do for yourself and your diabetes:

INSULIN:

Morning Dose: ____

Evening Dose: ____

Bedtime Dose: ____

MONITORING: Keep Records !!

_______________ Urine tests 3–4 times each day using the 2 drop Clinitest.

_______________ Urine test for ketones if the urine sugar is 2% or higher (Use Acetest or Ketostix)

_______________ Blood test _________________________ using _______________________________
(frequency)

_______________ Urine test for ketones if blood sugar is 240 or higher.

DIET: Constant Carbohydrate with _________________ meals/day and _____________ snacks/day.
Use your Diet Guide for meal planning.

EXERCISE: Plan for exercise every day, either aerobic exercise (like biking, running) or calisthenics (like jumping jacks).

CHANGING INSULIN DOSE:
1) Look for patterns in blood or urine sugars. You should attempt to get your urine sugars to run _________________ OR your blood sugars _________________ most of the time.
2) If sugars are almost always high, raise the insulin responsible by _____________________units.
3) If sugars are almost always low, lower the insulin responsible by _____________________units.
4) Do not change doses more often than every 3–4 days.
5) Call us if you need help with this.
6) other:

HYPOGLYCEMIA:
1) Always carry a quick-acting sugar (like sugar cubes wrapped in foil).
2) Have GLUCAGON at home.
3) Wear an identification tag or bracelet.

KETONES:

1) Call us if you begin to have ketones and need help managing them.
2) Review the information on ketones and sick days.
3) <u>Start</u> treating according to the rules.
    a) Drink plenty of fluids to flush ketones.
    b) Take _______ units Regular insulin every 2–3 hrs if blood sugars are 240 or above <u>AND</u> ketones are moderate to large.
    c) Check blood sugar and ketones every 2–3 hrs.

SCHOOL:

1) Get back to school on the next school day.
2) Have a conference with the school personnel.
3) Give the teacher and school nurse their pamphlets we have given you.

FOLLOW-UP:

__________ Your clinic appointment will be mailed to you.
__________ When you come back to clinic, bring: records, questions, and a snack.
__________ We will call you ____.

THINGS YOU WILL NEED AT HOME:

__________ Insulin (U-100)   Regular and NPH   (have two bottles of each)
__________ Syringes (U-100)   Lo-Dose
__________ Alcohol or alcohol swabs
__________ Clinitest tablets with 2 drop color chart
__________ Acetest tablets (or Ketostix)
__________ Autolet or ____
__________ Monolet Lancets
__________ Blood glucose Monitoring Strips _______________________________
__________ Blood glucose Monitoring Meter _______________________________
__________ Identification bracelet or necklace
__________ Glucagon
__________ Anti-vomiting suppository
__________ Chart or notebook for blood/urine results
__________ Emetrol

HOW TO REACH US: Please call us <u>anytime</u> you need us !

OFFICE: Pediatric Diabetes Office
        Monday–Friday   8:00 am–5:00 pm
        (409) 761–2538

HOME: Physician: _____________   Phone: _____________

        Dietician: _____________   Phone: _____________

        Nurse: _____________   Phone: _____________

        Health Educator: _________   Phone: _____________

If you cannot reach one of us, and there is an emergency:

UTMB Hospital Operator: (409)761–1011, ask her to beep resident on call for Pediatric Nephrology. The doctor on call will talk with you as soon as possible.

CHILDREN'S DIABETES MANAGEMENT CENTER
UTMB, Galveston, Texas

Education Program Evaluation

1. Child's Age: _________________   2. Child's Sex: _______ M   _______ F

3. Is this the first time you have received education in this center?

_______ Yes   _______ No

4. Length of time your child has had diabetes:

_______ 0–1 month   _______ 6–12 months   _______ 2–5 years

_______ 1–6 months   _______ 12–24 months   _______ over 5 years

5. How would you rate the classes in being able to prepare you to manage your diabetes at home?

_______ Very Helpful

_______ Helpful

_______ Somewhat Helpful

_______ Not Helpful

6. What areas of diabetes care do you feel the MOST prepared to handle?
   (Check all that you feel prepared to handle)

_______ What diabetes is

_______ Monitoring (blood and urine tests)

_______ Exercise

_______ Meal Planning/Diet

_______ Insulin use/How it works

_______ How to give shots

_______ Hypoglycemia (insulin reactions)

_______ Hyperglycemia (sick day rules)

_______ Changing insulin doses

7. What areas of diabetes care do you feel the LEAST prepared to handle?
   (Check all that you feel poorly prepared to handle)

_______ What diabetes is

_______ Monitoring (blood and urine tests)

_______ Exercise

_______ Meal planning/Diet

_______ Insulin use/How it works

_______ How to give shots

_______ Hypoglycemia (insulin reactions)

_______ Hyperglycemia (sick day rules)

_______ Changing insulin doses

8. How much of the information in class was new to you?

______   All the information was new

______   Most of the information was new

______   Some of the information was new

______   None of the information was new

9. Please rate the classes. Circle the number closest to how you feel.

Interesting	1	2	3	4	5	Boring
Easy	1	2	3	4	5	Difficult
Too Much	1	2	3	4	5	Not enough
Too fast	1	2	3	4	5	Too slow

Thank you for sharing your thoughts with us.

Person completing form: ______ Child   ______ Parent   Date: ___________

CHILDREN'S DIABETES MANAGEMENT CENTER
The University of Texas Medical Branch
Galveston, Texas
DIABETES CARE

UH# ___________

PRE-CONTACT DATA   Today's date: ___________

INSTRUCTIONS: Please write clearly and answer each item.
Try to be as accurate as possible with dates, but an approximation is better than no answer.

DEMOGRAPHIC DATA

Name _________________________________ Date of birth ___________ Sex _______

Address ____

Home phone_________________________________ Work phone _____________________________

Father's name _________________________________ Address ____________________________

Mother's name_________________________________ Address ____________________________

Referring physician _________________________ Address ____________________________

Other health persons to be notified ____

Child's school and address ____

Contact person _______________________________________ Grade in school _______

DIABETES HEALTH HISTORY

Check the symptoms or signs present *at* or *before* diagnosis:

_______ Increased urination	_______ Fainting episodes
_______ Increased thirst	_______ School problems
_______ Weight loss	_______ Headaches
_______ Leg cramps	_______ Vision changes
_______ Tired feeling (fatigue)	_______ Weakness
_______ Increased appetite	_______ Heavy breathing
_______ Decreased appetite	_______ Breath odor
_______ Personality change	_______ Convulsion (seizure)
_______ Nervousness	_______ Acidosis
_______ Abdominal pain	_______ Coma
_______ Nausea	_______ Behavior changes
_______ Vomiting	_______ Infection
_______ Diarrhea	_______ Immunizations
_______ Dehydration	_______ Emotional trauma/upset
_______ Dizzy spells	

Diagnosis made (date) _______________________ By whom? _________________________ , M.D.

Was child hospitalized? _____ YES (complete next question)   _____ NO (skip next question)

HOSPITALIZATION AFTER DIAGNOSIS:

Where? ____ How long? _______________

Physician's name ____

Were intravenous (IV) fluids given? _____ YES _____ NO _____ Don't know

How sick was your child at time of hospitalization?

_____ Critical   _____ Very sick   _____ Moderately sick   _____ Not very sick

Insulin doses at time of hospital discharge: _____ Don't remember

Morning _____________________   Supper _____________________

Lunch _____________________   Bedtime _____________________

IF YOUR CHILD WAS NOT HOSPITALIZED, what was initial insulin?

Morning _____________________   Supper _____________________

Lunch _____________________   Bedtime _____________________

RANGE OF INSULIN DOSES SINCE DIAGNOSIS:

What was the smallest daily dose ever? _____________________

What was the largest daily dose ever? _____________________

DIABETES EDUCATION RECEIVED AT (place) ____

CHECK ALL TOPICS in which your received instruction:

PHYSIOLOGY
_____ Normal glucose metabolism
_____ What is diabetes?/symptoms
_____ Differences in JODM and AODM
_____ Causes of diabetes
_____ What is good control?

MONITORING
_____ Self-blood glucose
Types: _____________________
_____ Urine testing
Types: _____________________
_____ Record-keeping
_____ Interpreting results
_____ Other _____________________

EXERCISE
_____ Effect of exercise
_____ Planning exercise programs
_____ Precautions

MEAL PLANNING
_____ Food groups
_____ Constant carbohydrate
_____ Special occasions
_____ Reading labels

INSULIN
_____ Insulin action
_____ Types/source of insulin
_____ Care of insulin
_____ Insulin preparation/mixing
_____ Injection technique
_____ Site rotation
_____ Dose adjustment/pattern control
_____ Other _____________________

HYPOGLYCEMIA
_____ Signs and symptoms
_____ Causes
_____ Treatment
_____ Glucagon
_____ Rebound/Overtreatment
_____ Other _____________________

KETONES/SICK DAYS
_____ Signs and symptoms
_____ Causes
_____ Treatment
_____ Managing vomiting
_____ Medicines and diabetes
_____ Other _____________________

LONG-TERM CONSEQUENCES
_____ Statistics and their meaning
_____ General preventive measures
_____ Types
_____ Other _____________________

DAILY LIVING
_____ Goals of therapy
_____ Effects of stress
_____ Stress management
_____ Personal hygiene/foot care
_____ Telling friends, teachers
_____ Resources: ADA, JDF, support groups
_____ Summer camp
_____ General health maintenance
_____ Behavior management
_____ Other _____________________

PRESENT MANAGEMENT

Current insulin doses: Morning ___________________

Lunch   ___________________

Supper   ___________________

Bedtime ___________________

Other   ___________________

Insulin species: _________________________________   Brand _________________________________

Diet: ☐ None   ☐ Keep away from concentrated sugars   ☐ Constant carbohydrate

☐ Other (explain) ____

Total calories _________________   gm Carbodhydrate _________________

gm Protein _________________   gm Fat _________________

Do you: _____ Measure? _____ Weigh? _____ Estimate? _____ Guess?

Write in the number of each exchange your child typically takes during a *weekday*.

	Break-fast	Snack	Lunch	Snack	Supper	Snack
Time of Meal						
Fruit						
Starch						
Milk						
Protein						
Fat						
Free foods						

Circle anything in the chart above that is different during the *weekend*. (For example, if mealtimes are different, circle the time that changes.)

Current exercise program ____
____

Current self-care skills/abilities (X = Child, P = Parent, O = Not done)

_____ Urine checks
    Frequency_________________
    Type _________________
_____ Blood checks
    Frequency_________________
    Type _________________
_____ Test recording
_____ Select meals
_____ Prepares meals
_____ Draws up insulin
    Type of syringe _________________
_____ Gives insulin
_____ Changes insulin dose
_____ Rotates sites
    Sites _________________

_____ Recognizes hypoglycemia
    Symptoms _________________
_____ Treats hypoglycemia
    Treatment _________________
_____ Treats ketosis
    Treatment _________________
_____ Orders supplies
_____ Plans activities

Monitoring: Write the number of times you have had these results in the past 3 months.

	BLOOD TESTS					URINE TESTS				
	Less than 80	80-120	120-180	180-240	Over 240	0	Tri-½	1%	2%	3-5%
Breakfast										
Lunch										
Supper										
Bedtime										

KETONES: Number of days with ketones over past 3 months _______________________________

Cause of ketones____

Treatment of ketones ____

INSULIN REACTIONS (hypoglycemia): ☐ None ☐ Occasional (0-1/mo) ☐ Moderate (2-4/mo)
☐ Frequent (over 1/wk)

Severity of reactions: % Mild _______ % Moderate _______ % Bad_______

Symptoms exhibited ____

Time of day_____________________________

Are reactions recognized by child? _______ Yes _______ No _______ Uncertain

Usual treatment for mild reactions ____

Usual treatment for severe reactions ____

DAILY CARE

Put a check in the box that most closely states how you rate your child's:	GREAT	GOOD	FAIR	POOR	AWFUL
Overall health?					
Control of diabetes?					
Knowledge about diabetes?					
Sticking to diet?					
Getting along with parents?					
Getting along with friends?					
School work?					

Check if the following symptoms are present:

_______ Frequent urination   _______ Nightime urination
_______ Frequent thirst   _______ Bedwetting
_______ Headaches   _______ Feeling poorly
_______ Vision changes   _______ Leg cramps
_______ Mood changes   _______ Stomachaches
_______ Weight changes   _______ Nightmares
_______ Tingling or numbness   _______ Other ___________________________

How many days has your child missed school this year ______________
How many of these were due to diabetes? ______________

How many hospitalizations since diagnosis? ______________
How many of these were due to diabetes? ______________

PAST HEALTH

What other health problems does your child have? ____
____
____

Any allergies? ____

FAMILY HISTORY

a. Father's name ____ Age______________
   Occupation ____________________________________ Health status ____________
b. Mother's name____ Age______________
   Occupation ____________________________________ Health status ____________
c. Sibling #1 ____ Age______________
   Health status ____
d. Sibling #2 ____ Age______________
   Health status ____
e. Sibling #3 ____ Age______________
   Health status ____
f. Sibling #4 ____ Age______________
   Health status ____

HISTORY OF DIABETES IN FAMILY

1. Name/Relation ________________________________ Age on onset ______________
   Current status ____
2. Name/Relation ________________________________ Age at onset ______________
   Current status ____
3. Name/Relation ________________________________ Age at onset ______________
   Current status ____
4. Name/Relation ________________________________ Age at onset ______________
   Current status ____
5. Name/Relation ________________________________ Age at onset ______________
   Current status ____

Family history of chronic illness: check all illness present in your child's family.

_____ Hypertension (high blood pressure)   _____ Cancer   _____ Mental illness
_____ Tuberculosis   _____ Thyroid   _____ Hypoglycemia
_____ Heart disease   _____ Asthma   _____ Other:

Check one box for each statement	Never	Almost Never	Some-times	Almost Always	Always
My child and I agree about diet.					
My child and I agree about his/her appearance.					
My child and I agree about monitoring.					
My child and I agree about his/her friends.					
My child and I agree about school (grades, attendance).					
I let my child manage his/her own diabetes.					
My child remembers to take his/her insulin.					
My child tries to get out of doing chores because of the diabetes.					
My child gets special attention because of the diabetes.					
I have to discipline my child differently because of the diabetes.					
My child takes part in planned exercise every day.					

What DO YOU consider to be the THREE BIGGEST PROBLEM AREAS at this time?

a. ____

____

b. ____

____

c. ____

____

Other than attempting to work with the above problems, are there other things that you would like to discuss at this time?

____

____

____

____

Person completing form _______________________________________

Faculty:________________________ MD

UH# ____________________________

CHILDREN'S DIABETES MANAGEMENT CENTER
The University of Texas Medical Branch
Galveston, Texas
DIABETES CARE

DATA BASE

________ Inpatient (new)
________ Inpatient (re-ed)
________ Outpatient (new)
________ Outpatient (re-ed)

Initial contact date(s) ____________

Name ____ DOB________________ Sex ______

Address ____________________________________ Phone: Home ____________________
____ Work ____________________
____ Other ____________________

Parents' names ________________________________ Sibs ____________________________

Referring physician ____ Phone____________________
    Address ____

Other health-care provider ____ Phone____________________
    Address ____

DIABETES HEALTH HISTORY

Onset symptoms (date) ____________________________ Age ______
Diagnosis made (date) ____________________________ Where ____________________________________
Significant symptoms/signs at onset ____
____
____

Major problems since diagnosis ____
____
____

Previous diabetes education ____
____

Most recent eye exam (date) ____________________________ By____________________________________

Most recent dental exam (date) ____________ Address ____

PRESENT DIABETES MANAGEMENT
(X = Child, P = Parent, O = Not done)

________ Urine checks
    Type ____________________________
________ Blood checks ____________________
    Frequency ____________________________
    Type ____________________________
________ Test recording
________ Selects meals
________ Prepares meals
________ Draws up insulin
    Type of syringe ____________________
________ Gives insulin
________ Changes insulin dose
________ Rotates sites
    Sites ____________________________
________ Recognizes hypoglycemia
    Symptoms ____________________________

________ Treats hypoglycemia
    Treatment ____________________________
________ Wears ID/carries sugar source
________ Treats ketosis
    Treatment ____________________________
________ Orders supplies
________ Plan activities
Current insulin doses:
AM ____________________________
Lunch ____________________________
PM ____________________________
Bedtime ____________________________
Other ____________________________

Insulin:
Species ____________________________
Brand ____________________________

Dietary program ____
____
____

Exercise program ____
____
____

Daily routine:

OTHER HEALTH DATA

Previous health problems ____
____
____

Family health data ____
____
____
____

PRESENT HEALTH

Date ____________   Height _______________ % for age _____________
                     Weight _______________ % for age _____________
                     BP _______________

Abnormalities ____
____
____
____

SOCIAL/FAMILY/EDUCATIONAL DATA

School: Name, city ____
        Contact person ____
        Level in school _________________ Usual performance ____________________
Learning style (how child/parent learns best) _________________________________
____

Family composition/living arrangements/significant others _____________________
____
____

History/Experience with diabetes or other chronic illness ________________________

____

____

____

____

Cultural background ____

____

____

Resources (economic status, ability to seek help) _______________________

____

____

Attitudes (general health benefits, concerns about diabetes)__________________

____

____

Motivation (interest level, willingness to participate, response to education plan) __________

____

____

ASSESSMENT OF STRENGTHS/WEAKNESSES/POTENTIAL BARRIERS

PLAN   _____ Initiate basic education program   _____ newly diagnosed

_____ previously diagnosed

_____ Re-education (patient previously received basic education at CDMC)

focus on ____

____

_____ Pump education   _____ Initial

_____ Re-education

_____ Other ____

Data base initiated by ____________________________________ Date __________

Reviewed by ____

EDUCATION PLAN AND EVALUATION

DATES	TOPIC	METHODS (check all that apply)	ATTENDED BY	EVALUATION
________	**PHYSIOLOGY** Normal glucose metabolism What is diabetes/symptoms Difference in JODM and AODM Causes of diabetes What is good control?	____ Lecture ____ Discussion ____ Demonstration Audiovisuals: ____ My Friend EDI ____ Juvenile Diabetes ____ Managing Diabetes ____ Other ____________ Handouts: ____ An Instruction Aid on JODM ____ Getting Started (B-D) ____ Starter Kit (Monoject) ____ Hypoglycemia vs. Hyperglycemia ____ Other ____________	____________ ____________ ____________ ____________	

________	**MONITORING**
	Self-blood glucose
	    Types: ____________
	Urine testing
	    Types: ____________
	Record-keeping
	Interpreting results
	Other ____________
		____ Lecture
		____ Discussion
		____ Demonstration
		Audiovisuals:
		____ Chemistrip bG slides
		____ Skill slides
		____ Other ____________
		Handouts:
		____ Protocol for SBGM
		____ Supply Houses
		____ Skills graph
		____ Reprints
		____ Other ____________
			____________
			____________
			____________
			
			____________	

________	**EXERCISE** Effect of exercise Planning exercise program Precautions	____ Lecture ____ Discussion ____ Exercise testing Audiovisuals: ____ Other ____________ Handouts: ____ Exercise booklet ____ Reprints ____ Other ____________	____________ ____________ ____________ ____________	
________	**MEAL PLANNING** Food groups Constant carbohydrate Special occasions (see diet ed flow sheet)	____ Lecture ____ Discussion ____ Menu Planning Audiovisuals: ____ The Intakes ____ Living a Health Life Handouts: ____ Picture Diet Guide ____ Liquid Exchange List ____ Reading Labels ____ Reprints ____ Other ____________	____________ ____________ ____________ ____________	

DATES	TOPIC	METHODS (check all that apply)	ATTENDED BY	EVALUATION
______	**INSULIN** Insulin action Types/Source of insulin Care of insulin Insulin preparation/Mixing Injection technique Site rotation Dose adjustment/Pattern control Other ______	______ Lecture ______ Discussion ______ Demonstration Audiovisuals: ______ Mixing Insulin (B-D) ______ Injection Sites (B-D) ______ Insulin I & II (B-D) ______ Skills slides ______ Other ______ Handouts: ______ Two shots/Day ______ Multiple Dose Insulin Therapy ______ Mixing Insulin ______ Diluting Insulin ______ Site Rotation ______ Changing Doses ______ Humulin ______ Reprints ______ Other ______	______ ______ ______	
______	**HYPOGLYCEMIA** Signs and symptoms Causes Treatment Glucagon Rebound/Overtreatment Other ______	______ Lecture ______ Discussion Audiovisuals: ______ Puppet Show ______ DERIN: Hypoglycemia ______ Sugar High, Sugar Low ______ Mixing Glucagon ______ Other ______ Handouts: ______ ID bracelet application ______ Reprints ______ Other ______	______ ______ ______	
______	**KETONES/SICK DAYS** Signs and symptoms Causes Treatment Managing vomiting Medicines and diabetes Other ______	______ Lecture ______ Discussion Audiovisuals: ______ Sugar High, Sugar Low ______ Other ______ Handouts: ______ Ketones and Illness ______ DKA Protocol ______ Reprints ______ Other ______	______ ______ ______	
______	**LONG-TERM CONSEQUENCES** Statistics and their meaning General preventive measures Types Other ______	______ Lecture ______ Discussion Audiovisuals: ______ Posters ______ Other ______ Handouts: ______ Reprints ______	______ ______	

DATES	TOPIC	METHODS (check all that apply)	ATTENDED BY	EVALUATION
_______	**DAILY LIVING** Goals of therapy Effect of stress Stress management Personal hygiene/Foot care Telling friends, teachers Resources: ADA, JDF, support groups Summer camp General health maintenance Behavior management Other _______________	______ Discussion ______ Rap session (group) ______ Counseling ______ Role play ______ Simulation Audiovisuals: ______ Stress tapes ______ Camp slides ______ No Sugar Coating ______ Other _______________ Handouts: ______ Hemoglobin AIC ______ Info for School ______ Info for Parents ______ Info for Babysitter ______ Diabetes in the News ______ Diabetes Forecast ______ Camp Application ______ Other _______________	_______________ _______________ _______________	
___________	**ADOLESCENT ISSUES** Effect of alcohol, drugs, smoking and diabetes Sexuality Peers	______ Lecture ______ Discussion ______ Rap Group ______ Counseling ______ Other _______________ Audiovisuals: ______ Posters ______ Other _______________ Handouts: ______ Reprints ______ Other _______________	_______________ _______________ _______________	
___________	**PUMP THERAPY** Programming pump Care of pump Sites and site care Troubleshooting	______ Lecture ______ Discussion ______ Demonstration Audiovisuals: ______ Betatron II teaching program ______ Flipchart ______ Other _______________ Handouts: ______ Pump manual ______ Site Care ______ Daily Care ______ Alternate Basal booklet ______ Changing Doses ______ Reprints ______ Other _______________	_______________ _______________	

DIET EDUCATION PLAN AND EVALUATION

DATES **TOPIC** **METHODS** **ATTENDED BY** **EVALUATION**

TOPIC

Basic nutrition
Effect of nutrients on blood glucose
Effect of diet, exercise, & insulin on blood glucose
Diet philosophies
Rationale of constant CHO diet
Using the exchange system
Importance of amount, time, & kind
Filling out hospital menu following meal plan
It is a family affair!
Exercise and diet
Hypoglycemia & diet (prevention & treatment)
Getting use to normal blood sugars
Dietetic foods
Parties and diet
Converting labels into exchanges
Converting recipes into exchanges
Illness & diet
Eating out
Measuring foods
Special occasions
Fat in the diet
Fiber in the diet
✦ Weight with diabetes
Tips on getting your child to eat (if applicable)
School & the meal plan
College/Working & the meal plan

METHODS

_____ Lecture
_____ Discussion
_____ Demonstration
Audiovisuals:
_____ The Intakes
_____ Living a Healthy Life I
_____ Living a Health Life II
_____ Labels
_____ Food Models
_____ Measuring Cups & Spoons
_____ Hospital Menu
_____ School Lunch Menu
Handouts:
_____ Picture Diet Guide
_____ Liquid Exchange Diet
_____ Eating Out
_____ Fiber & Exchanges
_____ Labels into Exchanges
_____ Difference between Type I & II diets
_____ Reprints
_____ Other:

OBJECTIVE DATA: Social/Family assessment
Family's eating habits/weights/significant others:

History/experience with diabetic diets or other types of diets:

Economic status

Attitudes (general nutrition beliefs, concerns about diet):

Motivation
(interest level, willingness to participate, willingness to follow meal plan, response to education plan):
Child:

Parent:

ASSESSMENT (Strengths, weaknesses, potential barriers):

PLAN: ____ Basic survival info.
 ____ Initial basic education program:
 with focus on:

 ____ Re-education with focus on:

See diet education session form.

EVALUATION: Summary of Response to Diet Education (skills, knowledge, attitude motivation):
Child:

Parent:

DISCHARGE & FOLLOW-UP PLANS:
Discharge:
 ____ 2 tapes & booklets on diet returned
 ____ 2-day menu written & checked by R.D.
Follow-up:
 ____ Letter to school concerning meal plan (if needed)
 ____ To call: _______________________________________
Future diet educational needs/goals:

Diet education provider(s):

____

EVALUATION Summary of reponses to education (skills, knowledge, attitudes)

Child:

Parent:

DISCHARGE & FOLLOW-UP PLANS (See discharge instruction sheet.)

Discharge checklist: Date ________________

____ Hemoglobin A1C = ________________ %	
____ Autolet/Monojector/Hemalet Returned	
____ Meter returned	
____ Rx for: Insulin	Glucagon
Syringes	Antiemetic supp.
Lancets	Pump:________________
Lancet device: ________________	Pump supplies: ________________
Strips: ________________	________________
Meter: ________________	________________
Ketostix/Acetest	Other: ________________

____ Insurance letter
____ Received written discharge instructions
____ Child/parent completed program evaluation
____ Problem list initiated
____ Continuing ed checklist initiated

Follow-up:
____ Letter to home physician
____ Letter to school
____ Clinic visit
____ To call ____
____ Referral to support agency ____

Future educational needs/goals:

Educator ____

Dietitian ____

Psychologist ____

Social worker ____

Other ____

Faculty ____

Team:_________________ M.D.

_________________ R.N.

CHILDREN'S DIABETES MANAGEMENT CENTER
The University of Texas Medical Branch
Galveston, Texas
DIET EDUCATION

Assessment, Plan, and Evaluation

______ Inpatient (new)
______ Inpatient (re-ed)
______ Outpatient (new)
______ Outpatient (re-ed)

Date(s): _________________

Name ____ Age ______

Parents' names _____________________________ Sibs _______________________

City _____________________________ Phone: Home ____________________

Work ____________________

Best time ____________________

Height __________ cm   Weight __________ kg   Other ____________________

OBJECTIVE DATA: Past Diet History

Date of onset _______________ Symptoms at onset ______ ↓ weight ______ ↑ thirst

Weight before onset ______ ideal ______ above ______ below

Food allergies ____

Previous diet education ____

____

____

Current Self-Care Skills/Abilities
(X = Child; P = Parent; O = Not done; B = Both)

______ Selects snacks
______ Prepares snacks
______ Selects meals
______ Prepares meals
______ Reads labels
______ Follows Liquid Exchange List when ill
______ Always carries fast-acting sugar
        Type _______________________
        Amount ____________________
______ Uses dietetic products
        Type _______________________
        ____

______ Vegetarian
______ Uses vit./min. supplements
______ Knows own (child's) meal plan
______ Pictured diet chart is placed on refrigerator & is used
        when:
______ Eating out
______ Attending social eating parties
______ Special occasions
______ Cooking special recipes

CURRENT MEAL PLAN/FAMILY ROUTINE __________ gm CHO, __________ calories

Time:	Breakfast	Snack	Lunch	Snack	Dinner	Snack
	______	______	______	______	______	______
Fruit ▲						
Starch ◆						
Milk ★						
Protein ■						
Fats ●						
Free ✔						

Satisfaction with meal plan:

______ Yes ______ No

If not, why not?____________________

____

____

____

____

____

____

APPENDIX B: LESSON PLANS

PATHOPHYSIOLOGY AND FOOD METABOLISM

Learner Objectives	Content	Methods	Evaluation

The learner should be able to
1. Describe normal utilization of food
*2. State normal blood glucose levels
3. State role of insulin
4. Identify causes of diabetes
5. Contrast juvenile-onset with adult-onset diabetes
6. Identify symptoms of juvenile-onset diabetes
	1. All food converted to glucose
	2. Normal blood glucose is maintained by insulin
	3. Source of insulin
	4. Insulin moves glucose to cells for energy
	5. Symptoms of lack of insulin
	6. Causes of IDDM
	  a. Hereditary
	  b. Viral
	  c. Autoimmunity
	7. Adult-onset versus juvenile-onset
		Discussion
		Felt board
		Films:
		  Juvenile Diabetes
		  My Friend EDI
		  Managing Diabetes
		Reading assignment
		Poster—Anatomy
		        Physiology
		Charts
			Questions to ask include
			*What is normal blood glucose?
			How does food provide energy?
			Describe diabetes.
			*How long does a person have diabetes?
			How does a person know he or she has diabetes?
			How does a person get diabetes?

*Survival information

MONITORING

Learner Objectives	Content	Methods	Evaluation

The learner should be able to
1. State reasons for monitoring diabetes control
2. State reasons for recording results
*3. Demonstrate urine testing and blood testing
4. Demonstrate appropriate storage and care of testing materials
5. Relate how Hb A_{1C} values correspond to control
	1. Purposes of monitoring
	2. How to monitor
	  a. Urine sugar
	  b. Urine ketones
	  c. Fingerstick blood glucose
	3. Meaning of results
	  a. Relationship of urine glucose to blood glucose
	4. Other lab measures of control
	  a. Hb A_{1C}
		Discussion
		Slide/Tape:
		  Chemstrip bG
		Demonstration
		Skills
		Practice session
		Reading assignment
			Skills assessment
			Questions to ask include
			How do you know your testing materials are okay?
			How often should you check your glucose?
			What method will you use to monitor at home?
			Where will you get supplies?
			Can you afford them?
			What would you do if your Hb A_{1C} was 12?
			What would you do if you ran out of test materials?
			What would you do if you had not kept records and you were due to see your doctor?

*Survival information

DIET

Learner Objectives	Content	Methods	Evaluation

The learner should be able to
1. Name the 3 types of carbohydrates that raise blood glucose
2. Describe the effects of food types on blood glucose
*3. Name 4 foods with fast-acting sugars
*4. Select meals based on meal plan and exchange lists
5. Measure and weigh food accurately
*6. Identify foods to avoid or that need careful planning into diet
7. Discuss way of planning for parties and special occasions
8. Plan ways to keep meals and times of meals constant
	1. Food categories: carbohydrates, protein, fats
	2. Different effects of fruit, starch, and milk on blood glucose
	3. Serving size and use of exchange lists
	4. Special occasions
	5. Reading labels
	6. Sweeteners
	7. Restaurant dining
	8. Role of fiber
	9. Role of dietitian
	10. Special issues
	   a. Dieting
	   b. Changing needs
	   c. Alcohol
	   d. Vegetarian and ethnic diets
		Discussion
		Films
		Slide/Tape: *The Intakes*
		Menu planning
		Food models
		Label reading
			Menu selection and meal planning
			Questions to ask include
			  *What are your exchanges at each meal and snacks?
			  *Name 3 sources of fast acting carbohydrates.
			  What would you do about birthday parties?
			  How can you still go out with your friends?
			  What would you do if your meal was delayed?
			  *Who can you talk with about your diet?
			  How will you know when your child should eat more or less? (to parents)
			  How can you diet or lose weight safely? (to adolescent)

*Survival information

INSULIN

Learner Objectives	Content	Methods	Evaluation

The learner should be able to
*1. State that insulin is necessary for life
*2. Identify own type of insulin
3. Describe characteristics of insulin (appearance, action, storage)
*4. Demonstrate acceptable, safe technique in insulin preparation and injection
5. Prepare a plan for site rotation
6. Adjust insulin dose based on monitoring information
	1. Insulin characteristics
	  a. Source—animal or human
	  b. Appearance of regular and intermediate insulins
	  c. Action: onset, peak, duration
	    (1.) Insulin action in regard to site
	  d. Storage and care of insulin
	2. Injection technique
	  a. Preparing syringe
	  b. Mixing insulins
	  c. Site rotation
	3. Dose adjustment and pattern control
	  a. Goals of therapy
	  b. Deciding which insulin to change
		Discussion
		Films
		Slide/Tape
		Poster
		Pamphlets
		Skills, practice simulation
		Worksheet: "Changing Dose"
			Skills assessment
			Site rotation plan/chart
			Questions to ask include
			  *Why is insulin important?
			  *Which insulin do you take?
			  Describe how Regular/NPH insulin works.
			  *Where do you get insulin and syringes?
			  What if while mixing insulins you put too much in the syringe?
			  What would you do if your insulin got frozen?
			  What would you do if your Regular insulin looked yellow?

*Survival information

EXERCISE

Learner Objectives	Content	Methods	Evaluation
The learner should be able to *1. State the effect of exercise on blood glucose 2. State a plan for daily exercise *3. State that exercise may lead to hypoglycemia *4. Select foods that can be carried for snacks during exercise	1. Benefits of exercise 2. Planning an exercise program 3. Diet adjustments and exercise 4. Prevention of hypoglycemia	Discussion Filmstrip: *Fit to be You* Exercise testing (physical therapist)	Child participates in exercise while hospitalized Questions to ask include What does exercise do for diabetic control? What would you do if it rained all week so you couldn't exercise outside? What would you do if you had an insulin reaction while playing? *What food do you plan to have with you while exercising? How will you decide whether or not to eat an extra snack?

*Survival information

HYPOGLYCEMIA

Learner Objectives	Content	Methods	Evaluation

The learner should be able to
*1. List signs and symptoms of low blood glucose
2. List causes of hypoglycemia
*3. Identify steps in treating an insulin reaction
4. State consequences of not treating hypoglycemia
5. Demonstrate/describe preparation of glucagon (to parent)
6. Describe rebound hyperglycemia in terms of signs, causes, and prevention
	1. Basics of hypoglycemia
	  a. Causes
	  b. Signs and symptoms
	  c. Treatment of mild insulin reactions
	2. Severe reactions
	  a. Causes
	  b. Treatment, including glucagon
	3. Prevention of hypoglycemia
	4. Rebound hyperglycemia
	5. What to tell friends
		Discussion
		Filmstrip: *Low Blood Sugar Emergencies*
		Slides/Tapes: *Derin Talks about Hypoglycemia Sugar High, Sugar Low*
		Realia: Glucagon
		Role play
			Skills assessment
			Questions to ask include
			*What does a reaction feel like? (to child)
			*How will you know if your child is having hypoglycemia? (to parent)
			What causes hypoglycemia?
			What would you do if you began to have a reaction in class?
			*What would you do if your child passed out? (to parent)
			How would you feel about having a reaction with friends around?
			What should your friends know about diabetes and insulin reactions?
			What happens in rebound?

*Survival information

KETONES AND "SICK DAYS"

Learner Objectives	Content	Methods	Evaluation

The learner should be able to
1. Describe how ketones are formed
*2. State times when high blood sugar and ketones may develop
*3. List signs and symptoms of hyperglycemia
*4. List steps in treating "sick days"
5. State when to call for help
	1. Ketones
	  a. Source
	  b. Cause of ketone formation
	2. Hyperglycemia
	  a. Causes
	  b. Signs and symptoms
	3. Sick day management
	  a. Monitoring
	  b. Diet
	  c. Insulin
	4. Managing vomiting
	  a. Dangers
	  b. Treatment
	  c. Who to call for help
		Discussion
		Felt board
		Slide/Tape: *Sugar High, Sugar Low*
		Film strip: *My Friend EDI*
		Worksheet: "Sick Days"
			Questions to ask include
			*When should you check for ketones?
			*Who would you contact for help?
			What insulin should you give to handle sick days?
			What would you do if your parents weren't home and you felt sick and had ketones?
			What would you do if your child started vomiting during an illness (to parent)

*Survival information

DAILY LIVING

Learner Objectives	Content	Methods	Evaluation

Learner should be able to
1. Discuss management goals
2. Relate the impact of emotional stress on control
3. Share behavior management plans
4. Demonstrate skin/foot care
5. Discuss effects of puberty, pregnancy, and alcohol use on diabetic control
6. State plans for returning to school
7. State plans for diabetes follow-up and for follow-up with other health professionals
8. Identify sources of further information
	1. Goals of diabetes management
	  a. Physical well-being
	  b. Normal metabolic tests
	  c. Normal growth and development
	2. Stress reduction
	  a. Effect of stress
	  b. Relaxation techniques
	3. Children's behavior and diabetes
	4. Personal hygiene
	5. Puberty, sexuality, adolescent issues
	6. School, friends
	7. Follow-up plans
	8. Sources of information
	  a. American Diabetes Association (ADA)
	  b. Juvenile Diabetes Foundation (JDF)
	  c. Literature
	9. The future
	  a. Research
	  b. Complications
		Discussion
		"Rap" sessions
		Group discussion
		Referral to local JDF or ADA groups
		Reading in behavior management
		Simulation
		Role play
		Filmstrip: *No Sugar Coating*
			Group participation
			Child's/Parent's ease in sharing feelings
			Questions to ask include
			How do you want to control your diabetes?
			What would you like your sugar levels to be?
			Who will help you?
			How would you tell a friend/date/relative that you have diabetes?
			What would you do if you couldn't decide if your child's misbehavior was his diabetes or him? (to parent)

LONG-TERM COMPLICATIONS

Learner Objectives	Content	Methods	Evaluation

The learner should be able to
1. Identify types of complications for which the person with diabetes is at risk
2. List changes that can occur in the eyes, nerves, kidneys, and large blood vessels
3. Identify preventive health practices related to complications
4. Discuss ways of coping with the possibility of complications in a positive manner
	1. Overview of complications
	  a. Statistics and their meaning
	  b. Types
	  c. Causes
	  d. General preventative measures
	    (1.) Blood glucose control
	    (2.) Exercise
	    (3.) Not smoking
	    (4.) Routine follow-up
	2. Retinopathy
	  a. Structure of eye
	  b. Changes that occur
	    (1.) Background retinopathy
	    (2.) Proliferative retinopathy
	  c. Statistics
	  d. Treatments
	  e. Symptoms unrelated to retinopathy ("don't panic" symptoms)
	3. Neuropathy
	  a. What happens
	  b. Symptoms
	  c. Treatment
	4. Nephropathy
	  a. What happens
	  b. Treatment
	5. Other
	  a. Hypertension
	  b. Atherosclerosis
	6. Putting complications into perspective
	  a. Keeping up to date on new research
	  b. Maintaining good control—one day at a time
	  c. Routine follow-up and reassurance
	  d. Dealing with the possibility of complications
		Discussion
		Posters
		Diabetes Forecast reprints
			Questions to ask include
			What are the complications of diabetes?
			What have you heard about the problems people can later have with diabetes?
			Do you know anyone with complications?
			Are there things about your future health that worry you (that you think about)?
			How would you know if you had complications from your diabetes?
			What can you do to maintain control of your future health?

ADOLESCENT ISSUES

Learner Objectives	Content	Methods	Evaluation
Learner should be able to 1. State the impact of puberty on diabetes control 2. Discuss the effects of alcohol, drugs, and tobacco on diabetes control 3. State that pregnancy in the person with diabetes should be planned in advance 4. Share feelings about telling friends about diabetes	1. Diabetes and puberty a. Changing insulin needs b. Menses and diabetes control 2. Substance use and diabetes a. Effect of alcohol b. Control and drug use c. Effect of tobacco 3. Role of diabetes in family planning a. Pregnancy and diabetes b. Contraception 4. Telling friends, dates a. Pros and cons b. Ways to tell	Discussion Rap sessions Group discussions Simulation Role play Handout: Teen sexuality reprints	Group participation Questions to ask include Why does the need for insulin change during puberty ? How would you know if you needed to change your insulin? What could you do at a party where alcohol is served, if you choose to drink? If you choose not to drink? How would you obtain contraceptive materials? Why should pregnancy be planned in the person with diabetes? Do you tell everyone about your diabetes? Why? Why not?

CONTINUOUS SUBCUTANEOUS INSULIN INFUSION PUMP

Learner Objectives	Content	Methods	Evaluation

Learner should be able to
1. State what the pump may accomplish
2. Demonstrate safety and accuracy in pump self-care skills:
 Programming
 Site care
 Daily pump care
 Changing doses
 Troubleshooting
3. Discuss aspects of living with a pump
4. Cite measures to prevent or manage consequences of pump therapy
	1. Benefits of pump therapy
	 a. Closed-loop vs open-loop systems
	 b. Improved metabolic control
	2. Pump skills
	 a. Programming
	 b. Site selection, care and needle insertion
	 c. Daily pump routine, record keeping
	 d. Changing doses
	 e. Troubleshooting
	  (1.) Alarms
	  (2.) Who to call
	  (3.) Switchback therapy
	3. Life with a pump
	 a. Wearing the pump
	 b. Explaining to friends
	 c. Problem solving
	  (1.) Exercise
	  (2.) Parties, flexible meals
	  (3.) Intimacy
	4. Managing diabetes with a pump
	 a. Hypoglycemia
	 b. Sick days
	 c. Diabetic ketoacidosis
	 d. Site infections
	 e. Body image changes
		Lecture
		Discussion
		Demonstration
		Audiovisual aids:
		 Flipcharts
		 Slide-tape program specific for pump
		Handouts:
		 Flow sheets
		 Reprints
		 Pump care pamphlet
		 Pump manual
		Quizzes
			Skills assessment
			Knowledge quiz
			Verbalized feelings about wearing/caring for pump
			Questions to ask include:
			 Why do you with to use pump therapy?
			 What would you do if your batteries went low at school?
			 How will you manage with your pump during exercise?
			 How will you wear your pump?
			 Where will you have your pump during sleep?
			 What would you do during illness?
			 What would you do if you needed or wanted to stop pump therapy?
			 Who will teach you about your pump?
			 Who will you call about problems and when?

APPENDIX C: SKILLS CHECKLISTS

INSULIN PREPARATION

Actions	Yes	No	Comments
Washes hands	☐	☐	
Knows own dose of insulin	☐	☐	
Rotates cloudy insulin to mix	☐	☐	
Does not shake insulin bottle	☐	☐	
Cleans top of bottle with alcohol	☐	☐	
Fills syringe with air equal to dose	☐	☐	
Inserts needle through top of bottle	☐	☐	
Pushes air into bottle	☐	☐	
Leaves needle in bottle	☐	☐	
Inverts bottle without bending needle	☐	☐	
Pulls plunger back to desired dose	☐	☐	
Checks for air bubbles	☐	☐	
Uses variety of methods to remove air bubbles (flicking, push in– pull back, and so forth)	☐	☐	
Holds bottle and syringe securely while removing air bubbles	☐	☐	
Removes needle from bottle, checks dose	☐	☐	
Replaces needle cover	☐	☐	
Performs above steps with aseptic technique	☐	☐	
States needle may be used a second time, demonstrates care (wipe with alcohol, replace cover)	☐	☐	
Demonstrates disposal technique for syringe and needle	☐	☐	

MIXING INSULINS

Actions	Yes	No	Comments
Washes hands	☐	☐	
Knows own dose of insulin	☐	☐	
Rotates cloudy insulin to mix	☐	☐	
Does not shake insulin bottle	☐	☐	
Cleans tops of bottles with alcohol	☐	☐	
Draws appropriate amount of air into syringe (amount = dose of cloudy insulin)	☐	☐	
Injects air into bottle of cloudy insulin	☐	☐	
Keeps bottle upright	☐	☐	
Does not touch needle to cloudy insulin	☐	☐	
Withdraws needle	☐	☐	
Measures appropriate amount of air into syringe (amount = dose of clear insulin)	☐	☐	
Injects air into bottle of clear insulin	☐	☐	
Leaves needle in bottle	☐	☐	
Inverts bottle to withdraw clear insulin	☐	☐	
Uses safe, aseptic technique in eliminating bubbles	☐	☐	
Holds syringe securely during "flicking" actions	☐	☐	
Withdraws needle	☐	☐	
Does not touch plunger of syringe	☐	☐	
Inserts needle into bottle of cloudy insulin	☐	☐	
Inverting bottle, withdraws insulin slowly to accurate total dose	☐	☐	
Does not push any insulin back into bottle	☐	☐	
If dose is incorrect, discards dose and repeats previous steps	☐	☐	
Places cap on needle after withdrawing from bottle	☐	☐	

INSULIN INJECTION

Actions	Yes	No	Comments
Washes hands	☐	☐	
Chooses acceptable injection site	☐	☐	
Palpates site to assess appropriateness	☐	☐	
Does not inject into area of lipodystrophy	☐	☐	
Cleans site with alcohol	☐	☐	
Allows alcohol to dry on skin	☐	☐	
Does not contaminate site before injection	☐	☐	
Removes needle cap with care	☐	☐	
Pinches up skin with nondominant hand	☐	☐	
Holds syringe appropriately (like dart or pencil)	☐	☐	
Does not contaminate needle before injection	☐	☐	
Releases skin fold	☐	☐	
Holds syringe steadily	☐	☐	
Aspirates to check for blood (optional)	☐	☐	
Pushes plunger down to hub of needle	☐	☐	
Withdraws needle in one quick motion	☐	☐	
Pats site with alcohol	☐	☐	
Does not massage injection site	☐	☐	
Records site on chart or records	☐	☐	
Verbalizes usual site rotation schedule	☐	☐	

TWO-DROP CLINITEST

Actions	Yes	No	Comments
Washes hands	☐	☐	
Places 2 drops urine in test tube	☐	☐	
Places 10 drops of water in test tube	☐	☐	
Holds dropper vertically above test tube	☐	☐	
Drops liquids into middle of tube, not along sides	☐	☐	
Shakes one Clinitest tablet into bottle cap	☐	☐	
Does not touch tablet with fingers	☐	☐	
Drops tablet into test tube from cap	☐	☐	
Immediately replaces cap to bottle	☐	☐	
Observes boiling in test tube	☐	☐	
Does not touch tube while boiling nor for 15 seconds after boiling has stopped	☐	☐	
Uses watch to time reaction	☐	☐	
Holds tube at top	☐	☐	
Swirls tube to mix colors	☐	☐	
Uses adequate light source to read chart	☐	☐	
Holds test tube next to color chart	☐	☐	
Reads color chart accurately	☐	☐	
Records results	☐	☐	
Cleans equipment:			
test tube	☐	☐	
dropper	☐	☐	
work area	☐	☐	
Washes hands	☐	☐	
States appropriate storage for Clinitest tablets:			
Keep in dark bottle	☐	☐	
Keep dry	☐	☐	
Keep away from children	☐	☐	
Identifies "bad" tablets from samples	☐	☐	

URINE TESTING—ACETEST

Actions	Yes	No	Comments
Washes hands	☐	☐	
Prepares clean, dry surface for tablet	☐	☐	
Drops tablet from cap to surface	☐	☐	
Does not touch tablet with fingers	☐	☐	
Immediately replaces cap on bottle	☐	☐	
Place 1 drop of urine directly on top of tablet	☐	☐	
Uses watch to time reaction	☐	☐	
Reads results at 30 seconds	☐	☐	
Uses adequate light source to read chart	☐	☐	
Reads color chart accurately	☐	☐	
Records results	☐	☐	
Cleans work space	☐	☐	
Washes hands	☐	☐	

OBTAINING BLOOD SAMPLE

Actions	Yes	No	Comments
Washes hands	☐	☐	
Identifies two possible areas for blood tests (fingers, toes, ear-lobes)	☐	☐	
Selects fingertip, area no lower than nailbed, not pad of finger	☐	☐	
Identifies 5 ways to increase blood flow	☐	☐	
Demonstrates "milking"	☐	☐	
Cleans site with alcohol	☐	☐	
Allows alcohol to dry	☐	☐	
Does not touch site once cleansed	☐	☐	
Sticks skin smoothly (manually)	☐	☐	
Using Autolet:			
Loads lancet onto Autolet so it is firmly in place	☐	☐	
Places platform firmly against skin	☐	☐	
Pushes button	☐	☐	
"Milks" finger to obtain large drop	☐	☐	
Applies to test strip (see appropriate checklist)	☐	☐	
Wipes site clean	☐	☐	
Clean materials and discards	☐	☐	
Demonstrates care of lancet for reuse (clean with alcohol, replace plastic disc)	☐	☐	

USING CHEMSTRIP bG

Actions	Yes	No	Comments
States that Chemstrip bG may be cut in half lengthwise	☐	☐	
Checks expiration date on bottle	☐	☐	
Removes strip from bottle without touching testing area	☐	☐	
Replaces cap immediately to bottle	☐	☐	
Places strip on clean, dry surface, test side up	☐	☐	
When dropping blood onto strip:			
Covers both zones	☐	☐	
Does not rub blood onto strip	☐	☐	
Does not let skin touch strip	☐	☐	
Does not add blood after first drop	☐	☐	
Times test for one full minute using watch/clock	☐	☐	
Keeps strip on flat surface	☐	☐	
After 1 minute, wipes strip clean with clean cotton or tissue	☐	☐	
Times with watch, 1 full minute (may time longer)	☐	☐	
Compares color results	☐	☐	
Reads color accurately	☐	☐	
Has adequate light to read results	☐	☐	
Holds strip near color chart	☐	☐	
Times an additional minute for blood glucose over 240	☐	☐	
States that if glucose is 240 or more, then ketones should be checked	☐	☐	
Records results	☐	☐	
Cleans work area	☐	☐	
States acceptable storage for Chemstrip bG	☐	☐	

USING DEXTROSTIX

Actions	Yes	No	Comments
States that Dextrostix may not be cut in half	☐	☐	
Checks expiration date on bottle	☐	☐	
Removes strip from bottle without touching testing area	☐	☐	
Replaces bottle cap immediately	☐	☐	
Compares strip with "0" block on color chart	☐	☐	
Places strip on clean, dry surface, test side up	☐	☐	
When dropping blood onto strip:			
Covers test area	☐	☐	
Does not rub blood onto strip	☐	☐	
Does not let skin touch strip	☐	☐	
Does not add blood after first drop	☐	☐	
Times test for 1 full minute using watch/clock	☐	☐	
Keeps strip on flat surface	☐	☐	
After 1 minute, washes strip with wash bottle and steady stream	☐	☐	
Takes no more than 1–2 sec to wash	☐	☐	
Holds strip vertically over waste container	☐	☐	
Blots strip dry	☐	☐	
Note: *If using machine, go to appropriate Skills Checklist.*			
Compares color results	☐	☐	
Reads color accurately	☐	☐	
Has adequate light to read results	☐	☐	
Holds strip near color chart	☐	☐	
Determines results in 1–2 sec	☐	☐	
States that if sugar is 240 or more, then ketones should be checked	☐	☐	
Records results	☐	☐	
Cleans work area	☐	☐	

USING THE GLUCOMETER

Actions	Yes	No	Comments
Places Glucometer on flat surface	☐	☐	
Turns machine on	☐	☐	
Obtains blood sample	☐	☐	
Pushes "Time" button before dropping blood to strip	☐	☐	
When beep sounds, applies blood to strip	☐	☐	
Keeps strip on flat surface during timing	☐	☐	
When buzzer sounds, washes strip with wash bottle	☐	☐	
Blots strip dry	☐	☐	
Places strip color side down in strip guide	☐	☐	
Does not force lid closed	☐	☐	
Presses "Read" button	☐	☐	
Records results	☐	☐	
States the urine ketones must be checked if blood glucose is 240 or higher	☐	☐	
Cleans work area	☐	☐	
Handles Glucometer carefully	☐	☐	
Turns machine off	☐	☐	

CALIBRATING GLUCOMETER (WET AND DRY METHODS)

Actions	Yes	No	Comments
Turns machine on	☐	☐	
Dry Method:			
Presses "cal" button	☐	☐	
Presses time button	☐	☐	
Places low cal chip into strip guide properly	☐	☐	
Does not force lid closed	☐	☐	
Presses "Read"	☐	☐	
Removes chip	☐	☐	
Presses "Time"	☐	☐	
After 60 seconds, places high cal chip in the strip guide	☐	☐	
Presses "Read"	☐	☐	
Knows that "mg/dl" means the machine is in calibration	☐	☐	
Wet Method:			
Presses "cal" button	☐	☐	
Uses Dextro-Chek Calibrator 50 mg/dl first	☐	☐	
Uses Dextrostix properly (may use skills checklist for Dextrostix)	☐	☐	
Uses Dextro-Chek Calibrator 300 mg/dl next	☐	☐	
Keeps test chamber lid closed during calibrating	☐	☐	
Dextro-Chek Control:			
After calibrating machine, drops 1 drop Control on Dextrostix	☐	☐	
Uses Glucometer properly to obtain reading	☐	☐	
States that reading obtained is either in range or not (97–119 for wet, 86–141 for dry)	☐	☐	
States appropriate actions to take if reading is outside range (i.e., recheck calibration)	☐	☐	
States that machine must be calibrated when:			
New batteries are used	☐	☐	
New bottle Dextrostix used	☐	☐	
Different operator	☐	☐	
Machine not used for 1 week or longer	☐	☐	
Control test is out of range	☐	☐	
Temperature has changed more than 10°	☐	☐	
Cleans work area	☐	☐	
Cleans cap and tip of Calibrator and Control bottles	☐	☐	

GLUCAGON

Actions	Yes	No	Comments
Washes hands	☐	☐	
Prepares supplies: Glucagon, 1 ml syringe, alcohol	☐	☐	
Checks expiration date of glucagon	☐	☐	
Swabs tops of both vials	☐	☐	
Injects 1 ml air into vial no. 1	☐	☐	
Withdraws fluid	☐	☐	
Injects diluent into vial no. 2	☐	☐	
Mixes glucagon well	☐	☐	
Withdraws all of glucagon from bottle	☐	☐	
Selects site for injection	☐	☐	
States that ALL of glucagon (1 ml) is to be given SQ or IM	☐	☐	
States that glucagon may be repeated in 15–20 min if there is no response	☐	☐	
States that vomiting may occur after a dose of glucagon	☐	☐	

APPENDIX D: SAMPLE PATIENT EDUCATION HANDOUTS

WHAT DIABETES IS

All parts of your body are made of cells. These cells need sugar to help you do things like walk, talk, ride a bike, think. Your body needs sugar for energy.

Where Does the Sugar Come From?

Sugar comes from the foods you eat. After you eat, most of the food is broken down to very small sugars called *glucose*. When this glucose is taken into your bloodstream, your blood sugar level goes up.

Sugar cannot go into the cells by itself. It needs a special key to help. This key is *insulin*.

Where Does the Insulin Come From?

Insulin is made in the pancreas by special cells called *beta cells*. When the blood sugar level goes up, insulin leaves the pancreas and goes into the bloodstream to meet the sugar.

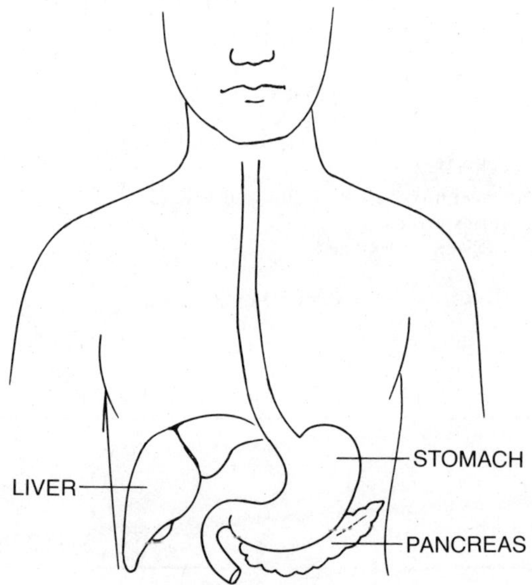

What Does Insulin Do?

Insulin does three things:
1. Insulin unlocks the cell and lets sugar go into the cells. The sugar will make energy for the cells to work.

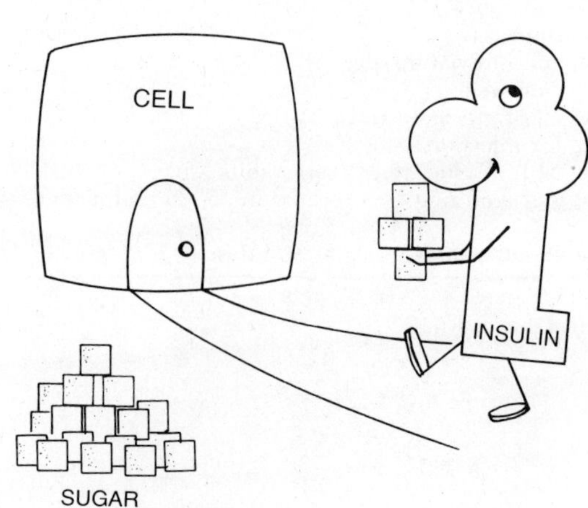

2. Insulin lets the liver store some sugar to use when the body needs it.

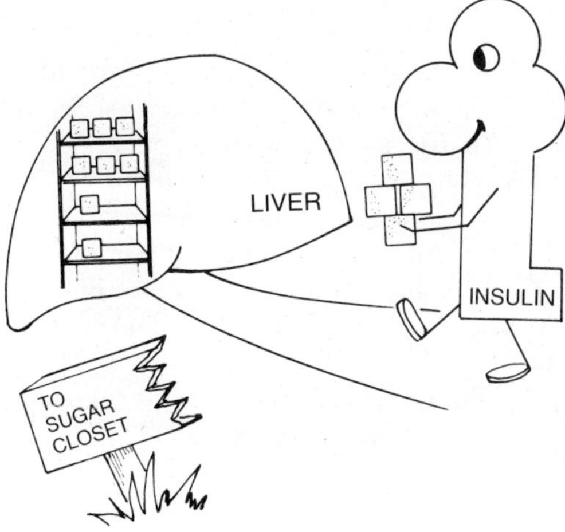

3. Insulin stops your body from breaking down body fat.

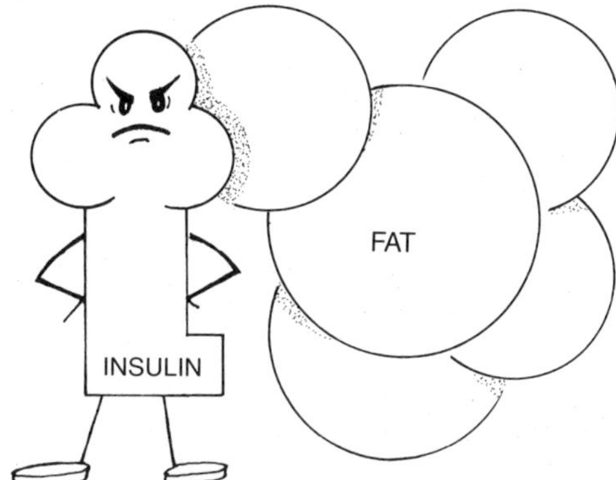

What Happens When There Is Not Enough Insulin (as in Diabetes)?

1. The *blood level sugar level goes up* because the sugar cannot get out of the bloodstream and into the cells.
2. Sugar begins to spill over into the urine. As sugar spills into the urine, you have to urinate (go to the bathroom) more.
3. You become *very thirsty*. This is your body's way of trying to replace all the fluid you are losing by urinating so much.
4. You *lose weight* because fats are being used by your body for energy. If there is not enough insulin, the body cannot stop the fat from breaking down. Also, the cells cannot use sugar so they must use fat for energy.

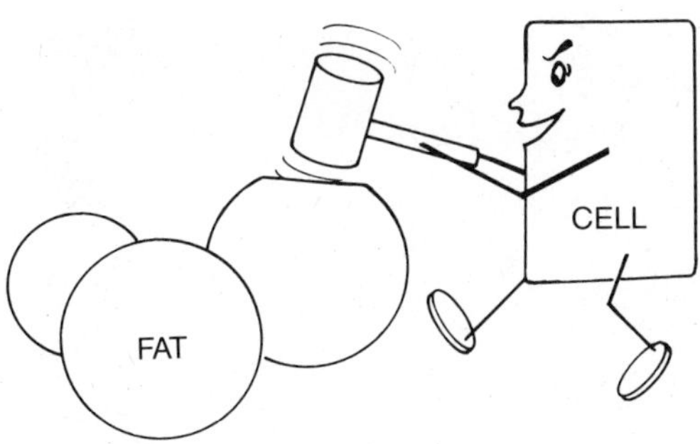

Two Types of Diabetes

In the person with Type I, or juvenile-onset diabetes mellitus, the beta cells in the pancreas do not make insulin. The person must take insulin by shot.

In the person with Type II, or adult-onset diabetes mellitus, some of the beta cells still produce insulin; but usually the person must help his or her pancreas to make more insulin by taking a pill. The pill is not insulin; it just helps insulin to work better. Sometimes, the person must take shots of insulin.

You have Type I, or juvenile-onset diabetes. Your beta cells do not make insulin. That is the only difference between your body and that of someone without diabetes.

Things you need to do to take care of your diabetes:
1. Test your blood sugar at least two times a day.
2. Take your insulin every day at the correct time.
3. Follow your meal plan.
4. Get some kind of exercise every other day.
5. Relax! You will do just fine. You can have control of your diabetes!

INFORMATION PREPARED BY:

The Children's Diabetes Management Center
Division of Nephrology and Diabetes
Department of Pediatrics
University of Texas Medical Branch
Galveston, Texas 77550

SELF BLOOD GLUCOSE MONITORING

What Is It?

Self blood glucose monitoring is a way of checking blood sugar directly with a simple fingerstick and special test strips.

Why Blood Sugar Tests?

Controlling diabetes means controlling *blood sugars*. Until recently, urine testing was the only easy way to monitor diabetes. But urine tests are only an *estimate* of blood sugars. Many things can interfere with the accuracy of urine tests:
1. The kidney's spilling point, or threshold
2. Diluted urine (or concentrated urine)
3. Certain medications and vitamins
4. Inconvenience of testing

Blood sugar testing gives a direct measurement. Using the information from blood sugar tests, the person can achieve much tighter control of diabetes.

Who Should Do Blood Sugar Monitoring?

Anyone. Many children (particularly teens) prefer self blood glucose monitoring as their only monitoring technique.

Some people stay with urine testing but use blood glucose tests during illness or at other times when urine tests may be questionable.

How Do I Do Self Blood Glucose Monitoring?

Basically, you obtain a drop of blood (from finger or toe), place the drop on a special test strip, time the test (usually 60 seconds), remove the blood (by washing or wiping), and read the test result (either visually or with a meter).

How Often Should We Do Blood Sugar Tests?

At least twice a day, before meals, based on which insulin you wish to check on. Blood sugars should be checked more often during illness and during times of difficult diabetes control.

What Supplies Do I Need?

To obtain blood droplet:	Monolet lancets (to puncture skin)
	Spring-loaded devices (Autolet, Hemalet, Autoclix, Monojector)
Blood testing strips:	Chemstrip bG (easiest to use visually)
	Visidex (must read quickly; color unstable)
	Dextrostix (must use meter for accuracy)
Meters (optional):	Glucometer (our current recommendation)
	Accuchek, Glucoscan, and so on are new meters that are only recently being evaluated

Where Do I Get Supplies?

Many local pharmacies are beginning to carry blood testing supplies. In addition, there are a number of supply houses that have mail order services. Be a consumer! Shop around. If you are purchasing a meter, be sure that the seller will train you in its use and will help if there are problems with the machine.

What Does Self Blood Glucose Monitoring Cost?

Generally, more than urine testing. Prices vary, but a current price list may look something like this:

Lancets	$ 8–10/box of 200
Autolet	$20–30 each
Hemalet	$10–12 each
Chemstrip bG Dextrostix	$ 0.50 each strip

Some insurance companies now cover some of these costs.

Where Do I Get More Information?

Check with your physician or diabetes educator. The following are excellent references:

Jovanic, L and Peterson, C: *Is home blood glucose monitoring for you?* Diabetes Forecast, Mar–Apr, 26–30, 1980.

Orzeck, E: *Home blood testing today.* Diabetes Forecast, Nov–Dec, 35–38, 1982.

Self Blood Glucose Monitoring. Juvenile Diabetes Foundation pamphlet.

INFORMATION PREPARED BY:

The Children's Diabetes Management Center
Division of Nephrology and Diabetes
Department of Pediatrics
University of Texas Medical Branch
Galveston, Texas 77550

TWO SHOTS A DAY

The Benefits

Controlling diabetes means controlling blood sugar levels. Nature controls blood sugar in a very perfect way—by the pancreas. Children with diabetes control blood sugar in another way—by insulin injections. Unfortunately, this method is not as perfect as nature's way.

But we are learning better ways to approach or copy how the pancreas usually works.

In nondiabetics, when blood sugar starts to rise, insulin levels also rise to bring the blood sugar to a normal level (80–120 mg/dl).

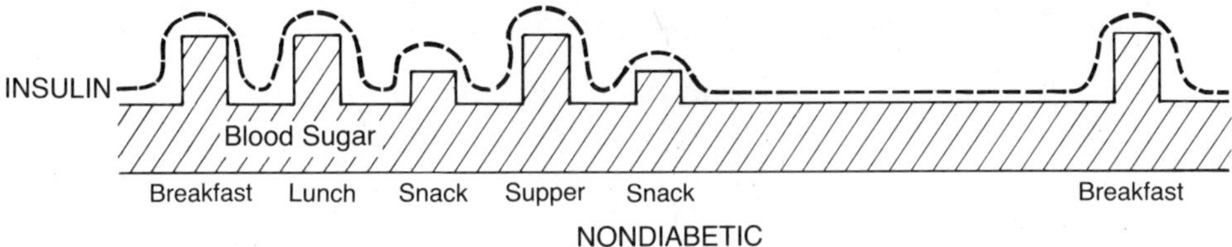

If a person with diabetes takes one shot per day, there may be times when insulin is *not* available or working (such as after breakfast) *or* times when too much insulin is working (such as at afternoon snack or before breakfast).

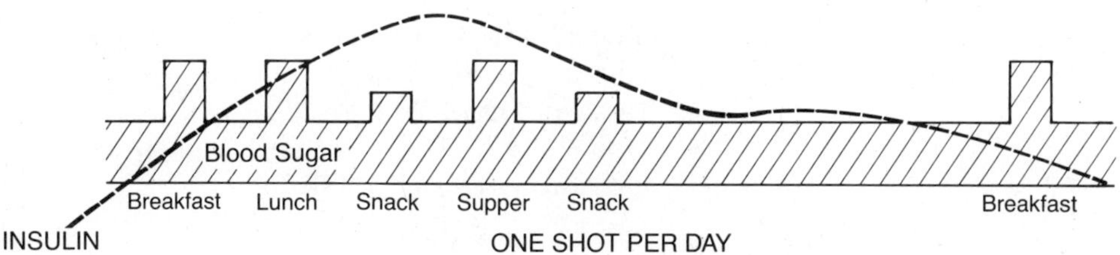

For many children, one shot a day just doesn't copy nature closely enough. You will know that one shot per day is not controlling blood sugars well enough when:

1. There are ups and downs in sugars throughout the day, like a roller coaster; *or*
2. Changing the insulin dose is not helping to control the ups and downs.

This does *not* mean that diabetes has become worse. It simply means that you may need to find a different way to control it. Often, that different way is with two shots per day—given before breakfast and before supper.

Let's see how taking two shots per day looks:

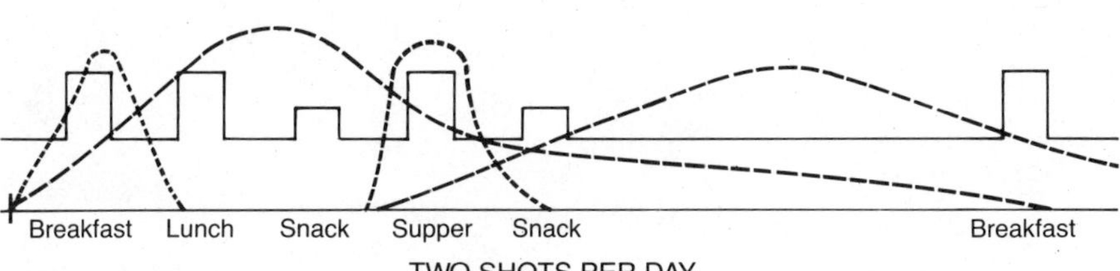

The advantages of two shots per day are:

1. More flexible schedule: The rise in blood sugar from supper is covered by the insulin given before the meal. Supper can therefore be a little later without the danger of low blood sugar.
2. Two shots a day more closely resembles the *peaks* of insulin that the pancreas used to make.
3. Ups and downs in blood sugars are straightened out.
4. The child *feels* better—and diabetes is in better control.

How to switch to two shots a day:

1. Talk this over with your physician. He or she will be able to determine, with you, whether two shots per day will achieve better control.
2. At the Children's Diabetes Management Center, we use the following guidelines to split insulin doses:

> Morning dose = $\frac{2}{3}$–$\frac{3}{4}$ of total daily dose
> ($\frac{2}{3}$–$\frac{3}{4}$ of AM dose is intermediate-acting insulin like NPH)
> ($\frac{1}{3}$–$\frac{1}{4}$ of AM dose is Regular)
> Evening dose = $\frac{1}{3}$–$\frac{1}{4}$ of total daily dose
> ($\frac{1}{2}$ of PM dose is NPH; $\frac{1}{2}$ of PM dose is Regular)

These are *only* used as a starting point. Individual dose changes must be made for each child.

INFORMATION PREPARED BY:

The Children's Diabetes Management Center
Division of Nephrology and Diabetes
Department of Pediatrics
University of Texas Medical Branch
Galveston, Texas 77550

CHANGING INSULIN DOSAGES

Controlling diabetes is a balancing act. Good control comes from a careful balance of diet, exercise, and insulin. Adjusting insulin, therefore, is only *one* of the ways to control diabetes.

To change doses in a safe, effective manner, the child *must*
1. Monitor blood or urine sugars often enough to see patterns
2. Write test results down
3. Know when insulins are working
4. Use insulin adjustments *along with* diet and exercise to control diabetes
5. Follow basic rules for safe dose adjustment

Pattern Control

Looking for patterns in daily sugar levels is one method for controlling diabetes. Let's see what patterns this record of blood sugars shows.

	Breakfast	Lunch	Supper	Bedtime
Mon	80	40	240	80
Tues	80–120	440	180	240
Wed	80	20–40	240	100
Thurs	120	40–80	240	40

Looking down the columns we see that

Before breakfast shows a *normal* pattern

Before lunch shows a pattern of *low* sugars

Before supper shows a pattern of *high* sugars

Before bedtime shows *no* pattern

What would you do with a pattern that shows

Normal sugars?
Low sugars?
High sugars?
No pattern?

When looking at patterns, we are looking at ways to *prevent* frequent times of high sugars or low sugars.

Which Insulin?

Recall how insulins work:

	Starts Working	Peaks	Gone
Regular	½ hr	2 hrs	4–6 hrs
NPH (or Lente)	2 hrs	8–12 hrs	16–24 hrs

If you are taking two shots a day, your insulin peaks look like this:

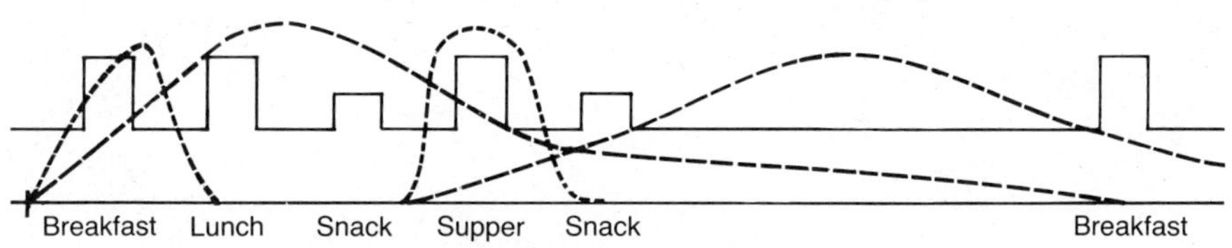

You can check how well the insulins work by checking urine or blood sugar at convenient times (such as mealtimes):

Insulin	Works Best During:	So, Check Before:
AM Regular	Morning	Lunch
AM NPH	Afternoon	Supper
PM Regular	Evening	Bedtime snack
PM NPH	Night	Breakfast

How Much and How Often?

After you have checked the pattern and have decided which insulin to adjust, then use these rules to make the changes:

1. Change only *one* insulin at a time.
2. Change the dose by *only 10 percent* (or, for most people, 1 or 2 units).
3. Wait three to four days for a *new pattern* to develop.
4. Be patient!

A Final Note

Adjusting insulin dosages puts control of your diabetes in your hands. That means some extra responsibilities:

1. Frequent monitoring
2. Careful adjustments following the rules
3. Balancing *all* major areas of diabetes care
4. Asking your doctor or nurse for help *whenever* you are having questions or problems

INFORMATION PREPARED BY:

The Children's Diabetes Management Center
Division of Nephrology and Diabetes
Department of Pediatrics
University of Texas Medical Branch
Galveston, Texas 77550

KETONES AND "SICK DAYS"

Illnesses can be especially difficult times for the child with diabetes. During illness or stress, the diabetic child may have ketones. Ketones may show up during:

1. Illness
2. Emotional stress
3. When there is not enough insulin

By the way, ketones *cannot* happen from "cheating" on the meal plan. Your child's body will not make ketones from overeating.

Ketones are the "ashes" left when the body burns fat for energy. If the cells of the body are not getting enough food or cannot use sugar, then they will look for energy from another place—fat.

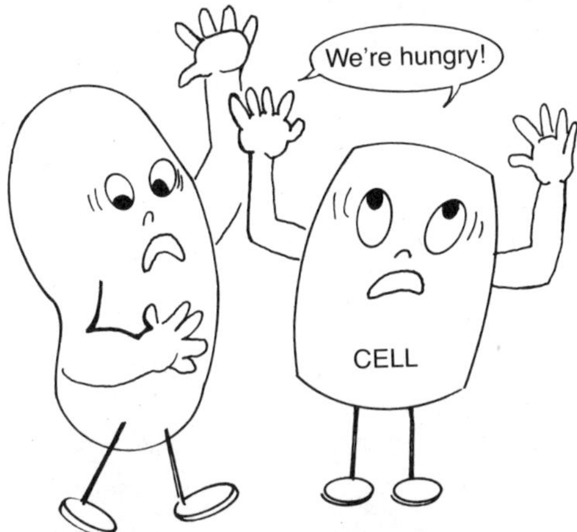

This works okay for awhile. The cells are fed. But ketones build up in the body. Ketones can make the child feel bad. Ketones are acids; these acids can make the body get *very sick, very fast.* Unless ketones are stopped, they can lead to dehydration (being very dry) and diabetic ketoacidosis (DKA).

There are ways to prevent these big problems. The safest way to handle ketones and high sugars at home is to:

1. Follow some rules
2. Start treating immediately
3. Know when to call for help

Here are the Rules for "Sick Days" (days with ketones and high sugars—even if the child doesn't *feel* sick):

1. **Check what is happening.** This is a time to switch to blood sugar testing if you are not already checking blood sugars. Blood sugar checks and urine ketone checks should be done every two to three hours as long as sugar and ketones are high.
2. **Give lots of fluids.** One of the only ways to wash ketones away is with cups and cups of drinks, usually sugar free.
3. **Take the usual dose of insulin.** During "sick days," the body needs insulin to stop ketones and to continue using sugar.

4. **Take extra insulin.** Again, the way to stop ketones is to take extra insulin.
   Which kind? Regular insulin must be used, because it works quickly and may be taken as much as every two to three hours.
   How much extra insulin? The amount of extra insulin is figured on the amount of insulin taken in the morning dose. We suggest 20 percent of the morning NPH or Lente. For example, if you take NPH 20 and Regular 5 in the morning, during "sick days" you would take extra shots of Regular, using 4 units for each dose (that's 20 percent of the morning NPH).)
   When do I take extra Regular insulin? Whenever blood sugars are 240 or more (urine sugars 3 percent or more) *and* ketones are moderate or large. The *"and"* is important. To take extra insulin safely, only take it when *both* sugar *and* ketones are high. Extra Regular insulin may be taken as often as every two to three hours.

5. **Know when to call for help.** Call your physician when/if:

   a. You cannot get blood sugars or ketones down after four to six extra shots
   b. Your child is vomiting and you can't get lots of fluids into him or her
   c. Your child looks sick, is very sleepy, is *not* urinating, is breathing deeply; has a dry mouth and sunken eyes.

What Would You Do for Each Problem?

1. Blood sugar: 180
   Ketones: Moderate   ___________________________
2. Blood sugar: 240–400
   Ketones: Small   ___________________________
3. Blood sugar: 400
   Ketones: Large   ___________________________
4. Blood sugar: 120
   Ketones: Trace   ___________________________
5. Blood sugar: 240–400
   Ketones: Moderate, and it's time
                  for the usual dose of
                  NPH 10/Regular 4   ___________________________

Answers

1. Push liquids; *do not* take extra insulin.
2. Push liquids; *do not* take extra insulin.
3. Push liquids; take extra regular insulin.
4. *Do not* take extra insulin.
5. Push liquids; take usual dose, but do *not* add extra Regular insulin to it. Check in two hours to see how the usual dose is working.

INFORMATION PREPARED BY:

The Children's Diabetes Management Center
Division of Nephrology & Diabetes
Department of Pediatrics
University of Texas Medical Branch
Galveston, Texas 77550

MDIT—ULTRALENTE AND REGULAR

Insulins Used

Regular Crystalline Insulin (any type)
Ultralente (same type)

Description and Rationale

Ultralente is a long-acting insulin that does not reach very much of a peak. In this program, this is given as a *basal insulin,* so there will be a small amount present throughout the day and night. What peak there is will be obtained about 16 to 20 hours after injection, but at the dosage we give this is not a problem in most people. It is usually best given with the Regular insulin before breakfast and before supper.

Regular or Crystalline is pure insulin and works rapidly. It is designed to be given *before each regular meal.* It must be given 30 to 60 minutes before the meal, and the amount given before each meal will obviously vary depending on what is to be eaten at that meal. Usually, the dose before breakfast is greater than that before other meals. The specific dosage for each person will vary and can only be judged by its effect on blood sugar.

How To Do It

1. The starting dose of Ultralente is ______________ units before breakfast and ______________ units before supper each day.
   A. This may be given in the same syringe as the Regular insulin.
   B. You should change this dosage only after consulting with a member of our team.
2. The starting dosages of Regular insulin is:
   ______________ units before breakfast
   ______________ units before lunch
   ______________ units before supper
   ____
   ____

How To Change Doses of Regular

1. *Before Breakfast Dose*
   A. This dose will work best between breakfast and lunch.
   B. Check blood sugars before breakfast *and* either two hours later or before lunch to monitor.
   C. You want blood sugars to be between 80 and 120 mg/dl before the meal, to no more than double (160–240) at the two-hour sample, and to return to between 80 and 150 before lunch.
   D. If blood sugar two hours later or before lunch for three to five days in a row is above these values, *raise* the dose of Regular insulin by 1 or 2 units. Continue to check and change the dose every three to five days until it's where you want it.
   E. If blood sugar before lunch for three to five days in a row is below 80, reduce the dose of Regular insulin by 1 or 2 units.

2. *Before Lunch Dose*
   A. This dose will work best between lunch and supper.
   B. Check blood sugars before breakfast *and* either two hours later or before lunch to monitor.
   C. You want blood sugars to be between 80 and 120 mg/dl before the meal, to no more than double (160–240) at the two-hour sample, and to return to between 80 and 150 before lunch.
   D. Use same rules as in #1.
   E. Use same rules as in #1.
3. *Before Supper Dose*
   A. This dose will work best between supper and bedtime.
   B. Check blood sugars before breakfast *and* either two hours later or before lunch to monitor.
   C. You want blood sugars to be between 80 and 120 mg/dl before the meal, to no more than double (160–240) at the two-hour sample, and to return to between 80 and 150 before lunch.
   D. Use same rules as in #1.
   E. Use same rules as in #1.

Lente Insulin

Occasionally, the super dosage of Ultralente and Regular insulin is not sufficient to keep the blood sugar normal during the night. In such instances, Lente insulin may be added to the night dosage.

Thus, your dosage starting tomorrow should be:
1. Before breakfast: ____

2. Before lunch: ____

3. Before supper: ____

You should continue to check blood sugar before breakfast in the mornings. If blood sugars are out of the 80 to 150 range, then consult with us for some recommendations.

APPENDIX E: OUTPATIENT ASSESSMENT

PEDIATRIC DIABETES - FOLLOW-UP VISIT
DIVISION OF PEDIATRICS

THE UNIVERSITY OF TEXAS MEDICAL BRANCH HOSPITALS
GALVESTON, TEXAS

PLEASE USE BLACK PEN

Patient's Name _______________________ U.H. No. _______________ Date __________

Age _______ (years) _______ (months)   Date of Birth ___________________ Hgt. ________

Date of Onset Diabetes _______________ Current Duration Diabetes __________ Wt. ________

Last Visit _______________

CURRENT INSULIN DOSAGE:
Morning _______________________________________ (type and dose)
Lunch _______________________________________ (type and dose)
Supper _______________________________________ (type and dose)
Bedtime _______________________________________ (type and dose)

How Diabetes control is monitored at home: ☐ Urine Tests ☐ Blood Glucose ☐ Both ☐ Neither

URINE MONITORING	BLOOD GLUCOSE MONITORING

1. What method _______________________
2. Number of times per day _______________
3. Times usually checked _______________
4. When are ketones measured _______________
5. Who records results of sugar and ketones _______________
6. Were records brought to this visit? ☐ Yes ☐ No
7. Ketonuria since last visit? ☐ None
   Number of separate days of ketonuria _______________

1. What method _______________
2. Number of times per day: ☐ One ☐ Two
   ☐ Three or Four ☐ Less than one per day
3. When are these checked _______________
   ____
   ____

Approximate results of Urine Sugars for past 3 to 4 months

Daily Urines	% "0"	% Tr-½%	% 1%	% 2%	% 5%
Breakfast					
Lunch					
Dinner					
Bed					

Approximate results of Blood Glucose for past 3 to 4 months

Time	% less than 80	% between 80-150	% 150-240	% over 240

Insulin Reactions (Hypoglycemia) since last visit: ☐ None ☐ Occasional (0-1/mo) ☐ Moderate (2-4/mo) ☐ Frequent (over 1/wk)

(a) Severity of reactions: % Mild _______ ; % Moderate _______ ; % Bad _______

(b) Symptoms exhibited _______________________________________

(c) Are reactions recognized by child? ☐ Yes ☐ No ☐ Uncertain

(d) Usual treatment _______________________________________

Significant Infections since last visit _______________________________________

Hospitalization since last visit _______________________________________

Current Diabetic symptoms (✔ = Yes, 0 = No)   Explain any current Diabetic symptoms:

(a) Polyuria _______ (e) Enuresis _______ (i) Nocturia _______ _______________
(b) Polydipsia _______ (f) Feel Poorly _______ (j) Nightmares _______ _______________
(c) Headaches _______ (g) Leg Cramps _______ (k) Symptoms of Neuropathy _______ _______________
(d) Visual Problems _______ (h) Abdom. Symptoms _______ (i) Other (what) _______ _______________

Days of school or work missed since last visit _______________________________________

DIET PROGRAM:

(a) ☐ None ☐ Keep away from concentrated sugars ☐ Constant Carbohydrate ☐ Other (explain) _______

(b) Compliance with planned program? _______________________________________

CURRENT EXERCISE PROGRAM _______________________________________

EMOTIONAL OR PSYCHOSOCIAL PROBLEMS _______________________________________

HOME CARE (X=Child Does, P=Parent Does, B=Both Do, O=Not Done)

_____ Order New Insulin   _____ Treats Ketosis   _____ Test Recording   _____ Draws Up Insulin

_____ Urine Checks   _____ Changes Diet   _____ Gives Insulin   _____ Changes Insulin Dose

_____ Plans Activities   _____ Orders New Supplies   _____ Treats Hypoglycemia   _____ Plans Diet

_____ Rotates Shots   _____ Blood Checks   _____ Selects Meals   _____ Is Mostly "In Charge" of Diabetes

NON-DIABETIC PROBLEMS ____

____

____

____

PHYSICAL EXAMINATION: Height __________ cm(% for age _______) Weight __________ cm (% for age _______) BP _______

General ____

____

____

Eyes ____

Nerves ____

Sexual Maturation ____

Injection Sites ____

Other Abnormalities ____

____

____

LABORATORY ASSESSMENT:

Urine Protein ________________ Urine Glucose __________ Ketones __________

Other Urine ____

Urine Culture __________ Other ____

Blood Glucose __________ mg/dl at __________ (timed obtained)

Glycosylated Hemoglobin (A_1C) ____

ASSESSMENT ____

____

____

____

____

PLAN:

1. General ____

____

____

2. Insulin ____

____

____

3. Diet ____

____

____

____

4. Exercise ____

____

5. Education Today On ____

____

____

____

6. Call On __________   Student/Resident ____

7. Return On __________   Fellow ____

Faculty Member ____

FORM 7018 · 11/81

APPENDIX F: EDUCATION RESOURCES FOR CHILDREN WITH DIABETES

DRUG AND SUPPLY COMPANIES

Ames Company
(Blood and urine testing products, patient education materials)

Division of Miles Laboratories, Inc
PO Box 70
Elkhart, IN 46515
(219) 264-8636

Becton-Dickinson
(Syringes, patient education materials, audiovisual materials)

365 West Passaic St
Rochelle Park, NJ 07662
(201) 368-7337

Bio-Dynamics
(Blood and urine testing products, patient education materials, audiovisual materials)

9115 Hague Road
PO Box 50100
Indianapolis, IN 46250
(800) 858-8072

Derata Corporation
(Automatic injector device)

7380 32nd Ave N
Minneapolis, MN 55427

Eli Lilly Company
(Insulin, glucagon, patient education materials)

307 E McCarty
PO Box 618
Indianapolis, IN 46206

Larken Industries, Ltd.
(Blood testing products)

8347 Melrose
Lenexa, KS 66214
(800) 452-7536 (nationwide)
(913) 541-0800 (in Kansas)

Lifescan
(Blood testing products, patient education materials, audiovisual materials)

1025 Terra Bella Ave
Mountain View, CA 94043
(800) 227-8862 (nationwide)
(800) 982-6132 (in California)

Nordisk, USA
(Insulin, patient education materials)

6500 Rock Spring Dr
Bethesda, MD 20817
(301) 897-9220

Sherwood Medical Consumer Products
(Syringes, lancets, patient education materials, audiovisual materials)

1831 Olive St
St Louis, MO 63103
(314) 621-7788

Squibb-Novo, Inc.
(Insulin, patient education materials)

120 Alexander St
Princeton, NJ 08540
(609) 921-8989

Teledyne Avionics
(Hypoglycemia detection device)

PO Box 6098
Charlottesville, VA 22906

SUPPORTIVE AND INFORMATION SERVICES

American Association of Diabetes Educators
(Professional materials for diabetes educators)

N Woodbury Rd
Box 56
Pitman, NJ 08071
(609) 589-4831

American Diabetes Association
(Patient education materials, community information, audiovisual materials, reference list of summer camps nationwide)

2 Park Ave
New York, NY 10016
(212) 683-7444

American Heart Association
(Pamphlets, coloring books, games on exercise)

National Office
44 E 23rd St
New York, NY 10010

Diabetes Education
Metropolitan Medical Center
(Patient education materials, audiovisual materials)

900 S 8th St
Minneapolis, MN 55404

International Diabetes Center
(Patient education materials, audiovisual materials)

4939 Excelsior Blvd
Minneapolis, MN 55416

Juvenile Diabetes Foundation, International
(Patient education materials, community information, audiovisual materials)

23 E 26th St
New York, NY 10010
(800) 223-1138 (nationwide)
(212) 889-7575 (in New York)

Medic Alert
(Diabetes identification)

PO Box 1009
Turlock, CA 95381-1009
(800) 344-3226 (nationwide)
(209) 668-3333 (in California)

National Clearinghouse for Family Planning Information
(Catalogs, free pamphlets concerning teen issues)

PO Box 2225
Rockville, MD 20852

National Diabetes Information Clearinghouse
(Reference lists available on sports and exercise, Spanish materials, teaching guides, educational materials for/about young people, educational materials for patients with low literacy, materials and aids for visually impaired diabetics)

Box NDIC
Bethesda, MD 20205
(301) 496-7433
(202) 842-7630

National Dairy Council
(Food models, nutrition information)

111 N Canal St
Chicago, IL 60606

Patient Education Office, North Carolina Memorial Hospital
(Patient education materials)

Box 515
Chapel Hill, NC 27514

Patient Information Library
(Patient education materials)

PAS Publishing
345-G Serramonte Plaza
Daly City, CA 94015
(415) 994-1150

FILM AND AUDIOVISUAL DISTRIBUTORS

Medfact, Inc.

PO Box 418
Massillon, OH 44648

Milner-Fenwick, Inc.

2125 Greenspring Dr
Timomium, MD 21093

Oracle Film and Video

230½ Hampton Dr
Venice, CA 90291
(213) 399-1497

Professional Research, Inc.

930 Pitner St
Evanston, IL 60202
(800) 421-2362

Sugar Babe, Inc.
  (Injection practice Doll)

PO Box 3133
Princeton, NJ 08540

Vision Multimedia Communications,
  Inc.

PO Box 8527
638 W Winter Park St
Orlando, FL 32804
(305) 422-1912

Walt Disney Educational Media
Company
  (Exercise, fitness, nutrition, well-
  ness audiovisual materials)

Customer Service
500 S Buena Vista St
Burbank, CA 91521

CATALOGS OF PRINTED MATERIALS

Catalog of Evaluated Materials in
Diabetes Education, June, 1982

South Carolina Diabetes Control
Project
South Carolina Department of
Health and Environmental Control
2600 Bull St
Columbia, SC 29201

National Community Resource
Guidelines for Diabetes Educators

American Association of Diabetes
Educators
N Woodbury Rd
Box 56
Pitman, NJ 08071
(609) 589-4831

Recommended Print Materials for
Diabetes Patient Education

Michigan Diabetes Research and
Training Center
University of Michigan Medical
School
Ann Arbor, MI 48109
(313) 763-0200

State and Federal Assistance
Resource Directory for People
with Diabetes

National Diabetes Information
Clearinghouse
Box NDIC
Bethesda, MD 20205
(301) 496-7433
(202) 842-7630

Summer Camps for Children with
Diabetes in the United States and
Canada

American Diabetes Association
2 Park Ave
New York, NY 10016
(212) 683-7444

CATALOGS OF FILMS AND AUDIOVISUALS

Recommended Audiovisual
Resources for Diabetes
Education, 1984
  and
Audiovisual Resources for Diabetes
Education, 4th ed.

Michigan Diabetes Research and
Training Center
University of Michigan Medical
School
Ann Arbor, MI 48109
(313) 763-0200

INSULIN INFUSION PUMP INFORMATION AND MANUFACTURERS

Cardiac Pacemakers, Inc.

PO Box 43079
St Paul, MN 55164
(800) 328-9588

Mill-Hill Infuser

Harvard Apparatus
Natick, ME 01760
(617) 655-7000

Markwell Medical Institute

PO Box 5173
Racine, WI 53405
(414) 632-3841

Orange Medical Instruments

3183-F Airway Ave
Costa Mesa, CA 92626
(714) 641-0674

Pacesetter Systems, Inc.

12884 Bradley Ave
Sylmar, CA 91342
(800) 423-5611

Parker Hannifin Corporation

Biomedical Products Division
17352 Von Karman Ave
Irvine, CA 92714
(714) 851-3664

Pancretec, Inc.

1660 Hotel Circle N
Suite 630
San Diego, CA 92108
(619) 291-3811

PERIODICALS—LAY

Diabetes Forecast

American Diabetes Association
2 Park Ave
New York, NY 10016

Diabetes in the News

Ames Marketing Services
PO Box 70
Elkhart, IN 46515

Diabetes Newsletter

Greater Boston Diabetes Society,
Inc.
1330 Beacon St
Brookline, MA 02146

Good Control

Box 2112
Scottsdale, AZ 85752

Joslin Diabetes Center Newsletter

Joslin Diabetes Center, Inc.
1 Joslin Place
Boston, MA 02215
(617) 732-2400

Pumpers

PO Box 680
Deerfield, IL 60015

PERIODICALS—PROFESSIONAL

Clinical Diabetes
Diabetes
Diabetes Care

American Diabetes Association
2 Park Ave
New York, NY 10016
(212) 683-7444

The Diabetes Educator

American Association of Diabetes
Educators
N Woodbury Rd
Box 56
Pitman, NJ 08071
(609) 589-4831

Diabetologia

European Association for the Study
of Diabetes
Springer-Verlag
175 Fifth Ave
New York, NY 10010
(212) 460-1500

APPENDIX G: HELPFUL BOOKS FOR PARENTS AND CHILDREN

Diabetes—Children

Branfield, John: *Why ME?* Harper & Row, New York, 1973.
  A story of a young girl accepting her diabetes and getting along better with her sister.

Dacquino, VT: *Kiss the Candy Days Goodbye.* Dell Publications, New York, 1983.

Kipnis, Lynne, and Adler, Susan: *You Can't Catch Diabetes from a Friend.* Triad Scientific, Gainesville, FL. 1979.
  Stories of four children dealing with different aspects of diabetes.

Travis, Luther B: *An Instructional Aid of Insulin Dependent Diabetes Mellitus,* ed. 7. UTMB, Galveston, TX, 1985.
  For children and parents, a comprehensive guide to diabetes and its management.

Diabetes—Parents

Biermann, June, and Toohey, Barbara: *The Diabetic's Total Health Book.* Pocket Books, New York, 1980.
  An easy-to-read book covering topics from diet to stress management.

Biermann, June, and Toohey, Barbara: *The Peripatetic Diabetic.* Jeremy Tarcher, Los Angeles, 1984.
  Very helpful information on traveling with diabetes.

Ducat, Lee, and Cohen, Sherry Suib. *Diabetes.* Harper & Row, New York, 1983.
  Written specifically for those with insulin dependent diabetes, the authors present practical tips for children of all ages.

Sims, Dorothea: *Diabetes: Reach for Health and Freedom.* CV Mosby, St Louis, 1980.
  A down-to-earth book that deals with day-to-day management as well as feelings.

General Coping—Children

Marks, Jane: *Help! My Parents are Driving Me Crazy.* Ace Books, New York, 1982.
  Offers suggestions to teenagers for improving relationships with parents.

Schlein, Miriam: *I Hate IT.* Albert Whitman & Co, Chicago, 1978.
  For preschool and young school-age; a reminder that there are many more things to like than to hate.

Simon, Norma: *How Do I Feel?* Albert Whitman & Co, Chicago.
  A beginning book about feelings.

Viorst, Judith: *Alexander and the Terrible, Horrible, No Good, Very Bad Day.* Atheneum, Hartford, CT, 1972.
  For young children, a book on how it feels when nothing seems to go right.

Watson, Jane W, Switzer, Robert, and Hirschberg, J: *Sometimes I'm Afraid,* and *Sometimes I Get Angry,* Golden Press, New York, 1971.
  Both books, written for young children and their parents, are good "trigger" books to help begin discussions about fear and anger.

General Coping—Parents

Johnson, Joy, and Johnson, Mary: *Why Mine?* Centering Corp, Council Bluffs, IA: 1981.
 For parents learning to live with feelings of having a child with a serious illness.

Patterson, Gerald R: *Living with Children,* and *Families.* Research Press, Chicago, 1971.
 Both books describe behavior management techniques.

Stroebel, Charles. *QR: The Quieting Reflex.* Berkley Books, New York, 1982.
 An excellent book that teaches one of many stress reduction techniques.

Index

Page numbers in *italics* refer to illustrations; page numbers followed by t refer to tables.